Acne

Causes and practical management

Acne

Causes and practical management

F. William Danby

Adjunct Assistant Professor of Surgery
Section of Dermatology
Geisel School of Medicine at Dartmouth
Hanover, New Hampshire,
USA

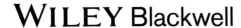

This edition first published 2015; © 2015 by John Wiley & Sons, Ltd.

Registered Office
John Wiley & Sons, Ltd, The Atrium, Southern Gate, Chichester, West Sussex, PO19 8SQ, UK

Editorial Offices
9600 Garsington Road, Oxford, OX4 2DQ, UK
The Atrium, Southern Gate, Chichester, West Sussex, PO19 8SQ, UK
111 River Street, Hoboken, NJ 07030-5774, USA

For details of our global editorial offices, for customer services and for information about how to apply for permission to reuse the copyright material in this book please see our website at www.wiley.com/wiley-blackwell

Library of Congress Cataloging-in-Publication Data
Danby, F. William, author.
    Acne : causes and practical management / F. William Danby.
        p. ; cm.
    Includes bibliographical references and index.
    ISBN 978-1-118-23277-4 (cloth)
I. Title.
    [DNLM: 1. Acne Vulgaris.   2. Hidradenitis Suppurativa.   3. Rosacea.   WR 430]
    RL131
    616.5'3–dc23
                                            2014032057
A catalogue record for this book is available from the British Library.

Wiley also publishes its books in a variety of electronic formats. Some content that appears in print may not be available in electronic books.

Set in 8.5/12pt Meridien by SPi Publisher Services, Pondicherry, India

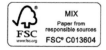

Contents

Preface

This book came to be written for one very simple reason. Somebody suggested that Martin Sugden, my initial contact at Wiley, approach me to write it. While I had considered the possibility of a book—indeed, friends and colleagues had encouraged me to take the leap—the search for a publisher seemed daunting and life's other commitments (plus a serious lifelong expertise in procrastination) ruled.

Martin's invitation arrived at a time when, as the reader will see, there are very significant new thoughts and understandings arriving in the world of the acnes. Indeed, some have not reached the shores of North America, some have not yet been published, and some have just recently popped up as novel considerations. The field is moving fast enough that leaving something out is all but inevitable, and if you find I missed something you consider significant, please do let me know your thoughts. Now seems like a great time to start a file for a second edition.

All of this new material needs to be sifted and evaluated for logical consistency with the whole, and such reflection and consideration takes time. For me such time is usually stolen from the beginning of the day's busy activities, in the shower. Indeed, it would not be too big a stretch to say that this present effort was written, or at least conceived and conceptualized and seriously mulled over, during about 40 years of morning showers.

Ultimately, this book is written for our patients. We commonly use the phrase "suffering from acne," but usually without thinking how deeply the suffering goes.

As a teenager with bad skin, Janis Ian knew about that. She composed and sang "At Seventeen" in the early 1970s. Her poignant lyrics are a lesson in the impact of acne on self-image.

> I learned the truth at seventeen
> That love was meant for beauty queens
> And high school girls with clear skinned smiles
> Who married young and then retired.
> The valentines I never knew,

> The Friday night charades of youth,
> Were spent on one more beautiful.
> At seventeen I learned the truth...

> And those of us with ravaged faces,
> Lacking in the social graces,
> Desperately remained at home
> Inventing lovers on the phone
> Who called to say "come dance with me"
> And murmured vague obscenities.
> It isn't all it seems at seventeen...

> To those of us who knew the pain
> Of valentines that never came
> And those whose names were never called
> When choosing sides for basketball.
> It was long ago and far away,
> the world was younger than today,
> when dreams were all they gave for free
> to ugly duckling girls like me...

These lyrics have haunted me for decades while I've looked for explanations in the hope that the "ugly ducklings" of both sexes can eventually be spared the pains brought on by "the blight of youth."

My initial interest in hormones, the fuel of the acnes, was "by exclusion" rather than by choice. As final-year dermatology residents in Toronto, we were each expected to write a review on a "basic science" topic. The only subject that was of any marginal interest to me and had not been dealt with by my senior residents was "Hormones and the Skin." It has been a long road from 24-hour urine collections for ketogenic steroids, through the early days of dialyzable free testosterone, to the newly revealed mysteries of FoxO1 and mTORC1.

The original stimulus to look into diet as a cause of acne came from the first dermatologist in our family, my father. He had a case of a young dairy farmer whose well water was contaminated by agricultural bromides (see "The Farmer's Boys," Section 2.3.1). That original question got me wondering about diet as a cause of acne, partly because I was curious about the role of chocolate, and that led in due course to this book being written. I set up a semiquantitative patient questionnaire that included just about all common foods and drinks. I suspected the relationship between acne and milk after about two years of patient interviews done over 35 years ago. Osler's admonition to "Listen to your patient, he is telling you the diagnosis" led not to the diagnosis but to a strong suspicion of the etiology of acne.

Already interested in "hormones in the skin," I had been keeping an eye on the literature. I was unaware of the presence of hormones in milk until Janet Darling's early 1970s papers came to my attention. "Chance favored the prepared mind," and I found that a Pasadena dermatologist named Jerome Fisher had been studying acne, milk, and the steroid hormones he suspected in milk for years, since the early 1960s. A reference to his work appeared in *Time* magazine in 1966. I contacted him in 1979 and he sent me the carbon copies of his unpublished 1965 manuscript. Charles Bird at Queen's Endocrinology did our first 'free T' assays. Thus, steroid hormones remained my prime suspects. By 2000 I felt that I was in a position to propose a formal study, so I asked for a meeting with Walter Willett, professor and head of the School of Nutrition at the Harvard School of Public Health.

That study was underway at Harvard in 2002 when Loren Cordain's paper raised the question of the role of a low-glycemic-load (or Paleolithic) diet in preventing acne and other Western diseases. It had not occurred to the multinational team of which Cordain was a member that the absence of acne might have been due to the absence of dairy products. A phone call confirmed that the dairy intake of these tribes was indeed exceptionally low (in the New Guinea group) and absolute zero (in the Paraguay group). In late 2002 Clement Adebamowo, the Harvard group's principal investigator, produced preliminary evidence of the epidemiological link between milk and acne in the Nurses Health Study data. In early 2005, the first of three papers demonstrating the significant association was published.

Meanwhile, another member of the Papua–Paraguay team returned to Australia and was involved in the design and conduct of several clinical studies that linked low-glycemic diets to clinical improvement of acne in a small number of young men. This reinforced the Australian thesis that the prime dietary mover of acne was the high glycemic load of the Western diet. Indeed, the most active collaborator, Robyn Smith, was awarded her PhD on the strength of that high-glycemic-load theory just a few short years after Clement Adebamowo earned his ScD based on the dairy and milk association with acne. Their contributions are reviewed in Appendix B.

Subsequently, Professor Bodo Melnik has presented us with what appear to be the pieces of the jigsaw puzzle that allow us to see almost the complete picture.

Understanding the complex relationships that form the background for these three diseases is essential in order to provide the "deliverable," that is, a book on the acnes that will be, in Martin's succinct description, "practical." Within that word are several messages, including the need to write for a broad audience, from researcher to patient, and from busy dermatologists to patients' parents. The researcher will need to forgive the helping hand of explanation that is occasionally extended to bring readers up to speed, and the beginner in the field will need to put up with (or look up) some unavoidable jargon. If and where I fail, always remember that Wikipedia is your friend, and deserves your support. While much of the book provides the necessary basic science to help with comprehension of the mechanisms discussed, this is not an academic text. Others are better at that than I. Nor will this be a catalog of every paper written on each and every aspect of these disorders, supplemented with my comments. It is instead my personal view, from the practical side, an overarching synthesis supported by selected references.

The first aim of this book is to provide practical guidance to managing the three acnes. There are several other books on acne that aim at being practical, so why is this book different? Simple. Because I believe that the longstanding concepts of the acnes' cause and development, as still held by other authors are, in a word, outdated. That leads to the second aim of the book, to update the concepts upon which therapy must be based. The third and most important aim is to encourage *prevention* of the processes that lead to and perpetuate the acnes, ultimately making active, expensive, drug-based therapy unnecessary.

My intent is to provide the practical options, as I see them, for both patients and prescribers. At the same time I hope it will serve to nudge scholars and researchers in directions that remain both unexplored and promising.

It will also guide you to cost-effective therapy. I am not interested in marketing anything. I have no present financial interest in anything I am discussing, but if you look up the medical literature you will find that I was involved in paid clinical trials in the distant past. That means I may annoy some of my colleagues. My challenge will be to disagree without being disagreeable. Because this work describes three variants of a single disorder, there are shared features and shared pathogenic processes. This leads to unavoidable duplication. The alternative would be to lead the reader on a merry chase through a book filled with links to other chapters and sections. I have kept these internal references to a minimum, providing a cohesive self-contained unit dealing with each of the acnes.

Continuing medical education (CME) standards in the United States require notification of audiences if any drug is used "off label," meaning that it has not been specifically studied to US Food and Drug Administration (FDA) standards for the particular disorder being discussed. Most of the medications used in dermatology are regularly used off label. I will not bore the reader and use valuable space to repeat this caveat throughout the book. Almost this entire book is in my own words but where others' words serve better than I can paraphrase them, I will quote them with attribution. As the sole author, any mistakes are mine and I do appreciate constructive criticism.

Thanks go first to Lynne Margesson. She "came on service" as my junior resident and is my spouse of 39 years, my practice partner, and mother of our two children. She did not hesitate at all in giving me the green light for this project, even though she had a pretty good idea what it would entail. I would love to thank my mentors, if I had any, but I do owe debts of gratitude instead to the several researchers, teachers, writers, and, most importantly, thinkers who have contributed to the field. Howard Donsky nudged his residents to look at the basic sciences in depth. My father, Charles Danby, was a dermatological innovator in his own right. Janet Darling did the initial determinations of the levels of steroid hormones in milk. Sir Kenneth Charles Calman detailed the existence of the first intracrine enzymes in the follicular keratinocytes. The late Jerome Fisher's study of milk and acne and suspicion of hormones helped me down this road. Loren Cordain's studies of aboriginal diets inadvertently set the baseline of "no milk, no acne." Peter Pochi shared a confidence. Walter Willett had the courtesy to listen and then facilitate a fresh look at the Nurses Health Study II and other data. I owe special thanks to Clement Adebamowo for doing all the heavy lifting for that work. Dawn Danby and Paul Waggoner provided the line drawings of the 'FPSU.'

In the acne inversa/hidradenitis suppurativa (AI/HS) area, thanks are due to Michelle Barlow for lighting a fire under us, to Gregor Jemec for support and ongoing collaboration, to Christos Zouboulis for opening doors, to Stuart Maddin for encouraging me to "focus" (always a challenge) and for encouraging me to contact Professor Zouboulis, to Maximilian von Leffert and Prof. Wolfgang Marsch for collaborating on the "follicular support" project, and to Robert Bibb for being the first to try a dairy-free diet in AI/HS. Special thanks go to numerous patients willing to try novel therapies, some out of acquiescence to my requests, some out of curiosity, and many out of the desperation and frustration that often accompany AI/HS.

This book presents an overview of the way I believe the acnes begin and how they progress through their various stages. It also provides personal glimpses into areas not yet fully explored. I will offer new hypotheses, consider areas of controversy, and touch on other hormonally related disorders that need further investigation.

The acnes exist in a four-dimensional spectrum, changing with time. They share a common cause but are unique in their individual three-dimensional presentations. My hope is to persuade you to see the acnes as I see them, and to learn to prevent them. Where others have failed at prevention, I hope to provide you with a few new and original treatment approaches.

Bill Danby
Hopkinton, New Hampshire

Practical acne therapy

There is a common theme in the three acnes. Pores are blocked; they burst, get inflamed, scar down, and heal. Whether the patient (you, perhaps?) experiences acne vulgaris, acne rosacea, or acne inversa/hidradenitis suppurativa (AI/HS) depends upon variables that include lesion location, patient's age, gender, family history, diet, sun exposure, and several others.

So let's start at the beginning.

With a look in the mirror.

How bad is it?

Staging and grading acne are essential in research but of little practical value in individual cases.

If you've got it, you've got it. Measuring it doesn't make it better.

Acne vulgaris that is "the end of my life forever" for one teen can be ignored by another.

Acne rosacea can be embarrassing beyond belief and a huge social handicap, or a minor nuisance.

Acne inversa can be an occasion "boil" every few months, or it can be life-destroying.

Be practical: If you've got it, and you want it gone, take the practical approach.

Genetics

If you inherited the genes for any acne, like 90% of us, that's unfortunate. Nothing fixes genes.

Be practical: You might want to choose a mate someday with *their* genes in mind if you want to look out for your children's risk of acne.

Diet

We know acne is caused by the male hormone dihydrotestosterone (DHT).

DHT works by linking to a male hormone (androgen) receptor.

It is like putting a key in the keyhole to open a door.

The androgen receptor (keyhole) needs to be open to accept the key.

Opening the keyhole requires insulin and/or insulin-like growth factor 1 (IGF-1).

Milk and milk products raise *both* insulin *and* IGF-1, opening the androgen receptor.

Sugar also raises insulin levels, helping even more to open the androgen receptor.

Foods that turn into sugar quickly (high-glycemic-index foods) also raise insulin levels.

Milk and milk products also actually *contain* androgens (the keys to the keyhole).

Milk and milk products also actually contain *other* hormones that turn into androgens.

So *both* dairy and sugary foods can open the androgen receptor.

But dairy also supplies the androgens to turn on acne. Dairy is triple trouble.

Be practical:

Change to a truly natural diet.

Eliminate all dairy.

Go "low glycemic load."

Hormones

Hormones cause acne.

No hormones = no acne.

Eliminating hormones in either sex is not practical.

For males, hormone manipulation is used only rarely. Dutasteride is used in men with acne inversa.

For females, hormones can be modified, replaced, and blocked. It is not natural, but it works.

Birth control pills with *no-* or *low*-androgen progestin are the best.

Look for drospirenone, norgestimate, or norelgestromin. Avoid all other progestins.

Postmenopausal hormone replacement? Progesterone (oral) and estradiol patch only.

Spironolactone blocks androgens and improves almost all acne in almost all women.

Be practical: The acnes are hormonal disorders. Manage your hormones.

Stress

Stress is a contributor to the cause of acne.

Stress also makes preexisting acne worse.

But living a stress-free life is not practical for most of us.

And we have no safe long-term stress-reducing medications.

Reducing stress is worth trying, as long as that effort is not stressful.

Yoga may be worth a try.

Be practical:

Eliminate the stress of looking in your mirror.

How? Follow the other practical rules presented here.

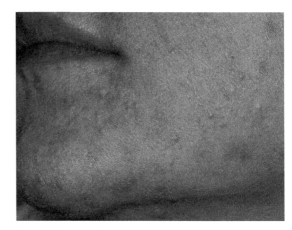

Figure 0.2 Mainly closed comedones with occasional "blackheads."

Comedones (plugs in pores)

In acne vulgaris:

Blackheads are plugged pores with open tops (Figure 0.1).

Whiteheads are plugged pores with closed tops (Figure 0.2).

Both are called *comedones* (open and closed). One (of either) is a single *comedo*.

Both grow until they empty themselves out or explode to the surface.

In acne rosacea, the pores explode superficially before the plug is actually visible (Figure 0.3).

In early acne inversa, the plugged pores are not prominent (Figure 0.4). The plugs tend to be deeper.

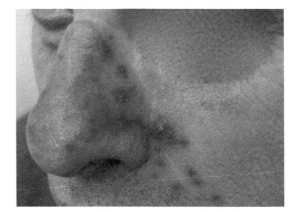

Figure 0.3 Central facial folliculopapules and folliculopustules, with no comedones and minor background erythema.

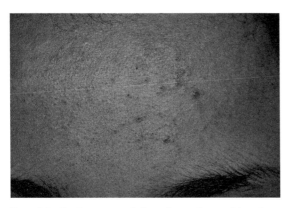

Figure 0.1 Classic open non-inflamed comedones with early inflammation just starting.

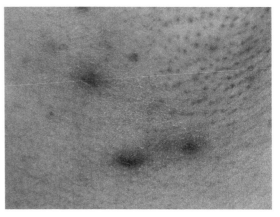

Figure 0.4 These little nodules were the only clue to the disease. Family history was positive.

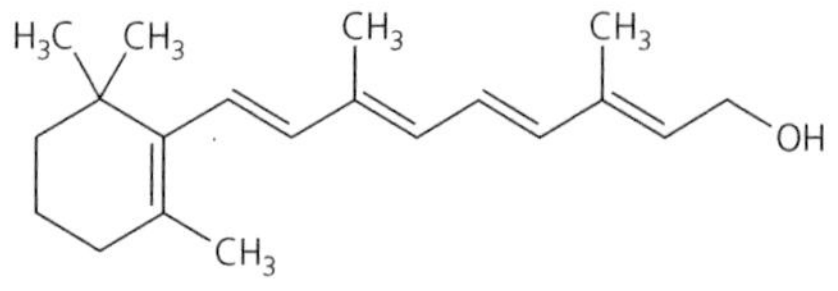

Retinol

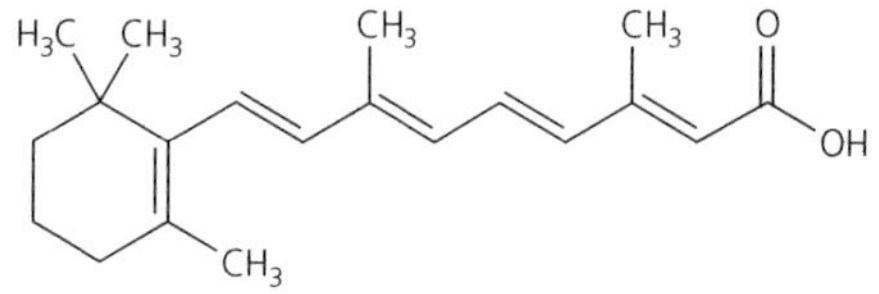

Tretinoin

Figure 0.5 Retinol is the classic vitamin A. Tretinoin, also called *vitamin A acid* and *retinoic acid*, was first marketed as Retin-A®.

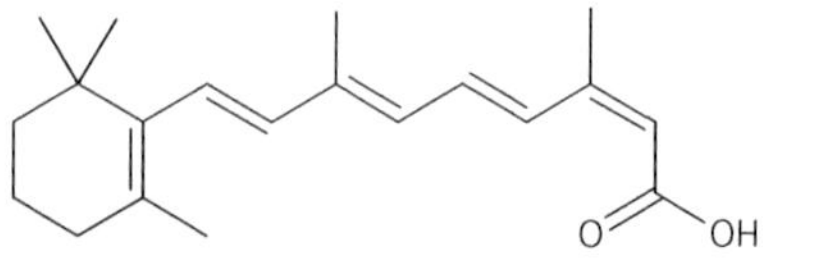

Isotretinoin

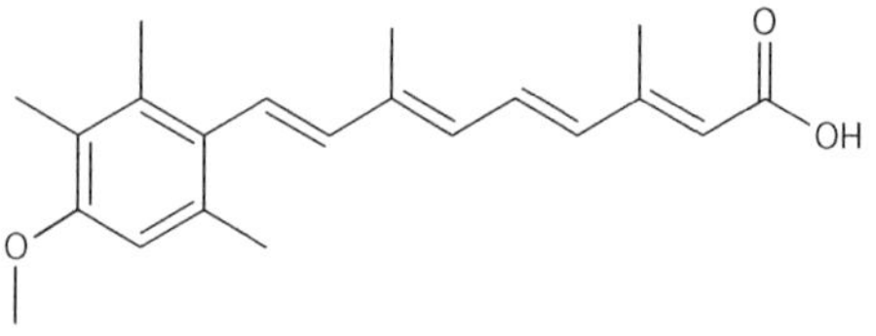

Acitretin

Figure 0.6 Isotretinoin, which is now widely genericized, was originally marketed as Accutane® and Roaccutane®. Acitretin started life as a treatment for psoriasis.

And these deep plugs often explode before the trouble becomes visible.

These plugs are caused by too much androgen (male hormone) activity.

The hormone turns on too many lining cells in the pore and, often with the help of nicotine, they form a traffic jam. The traffic jam leads to the explosion deep in the skin.

The best treatment to empty pores is a class of drugs called *retinoids*. They are cousins of retinol, better known as vitamin A (Figure 0.5).

Oral retinoids (given by mouth) are most effective, but they are usually reserved for worst cases.

Isotretinoin, used in low doses over a period of months, is the gold standard first choice for acne vulgaris (Figure 0.6).

Isotretinoin, used in low doses over months, is also the "last resort" for acne rosacea.

Acitretin, used in low doses over years, is the appropriate choice for acne inversa.

Topical retinoids are used on the skin surface in gels, lotions, and creams. They include tretinoin (the original—also called retinoic acid and vitamin A acid), adapalene, tazarotene, and isotretinoin (not in the United States).

Retinoids do three jobs in acne:
- They empty plugged pores (comedones, both open and closed).
- They prevent open pores from getting plugged.
- They modulate the inflammatory response.

So retinoids must be applied over the entire acne-prone area. Not just on "spots."

Be practical:

No matter what kind of acne you have, you need at least one retinoid.

And absolutely no nicotine.

Blemishes—a brief catalogue

Papules are small elevated bumps; they are usually red and often tender (Figure 0.7).

If there is a collection of pus on top of a papule, it is a *papulopustule* (Figure 0.8).

A collection of pus standing by itself at the opening of a pore is a *pustule* (Figure 0.9).

If a pustule is at the top of a follicle, it is a *folliculopustule*.

Larger papules and larger papulopustules are *nodules* (Figure 0.10).

These are battlegrounds.

The enemy is the "stuff" caught in the pores.

Acne *is* your body trying to get rid of this "stuff."

So what is the stuff down in your pores?

There are bacteria and yeasts and sometimes some little mites plus dead skin cells and hairs and irritating chemicals.

Be practical:

Use oral (isotretinoin) or topical retinoids to empty out the pores.

Eliminate yeast, bacteria, and other organisms.

Empty out the lesion if and when practical.

Cool the inflammation with anti-inflammatory antibiotics.

Use benzoyl peroxide to stop or limit the production of resistant bacteria.

Use other anti-inflammatories like dapsone or steroids as necessary.

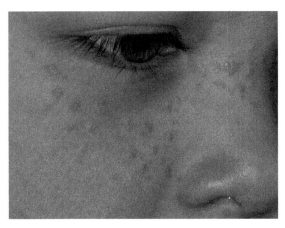

Figure 0.7 Comedones and folliculopapules in juvenile acne. His hormone source was dairy on top of a positive family history.

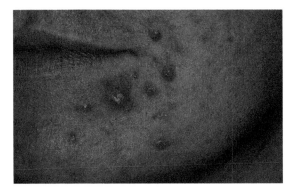

Figure 0.8 Papulopustules with a pustulonodular lesion centrally. She was on an androgenic oral contraceptive and enjoyed her dairy.

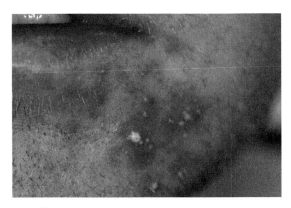

Figure 0.9 Secondary culture-positive staphylococcal pustule superimposed upon folliculopustular acne.

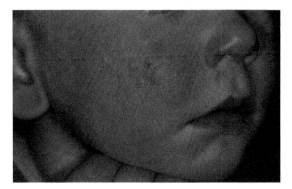

Figure 0.10 Nodular lesions occur even in juvenile acne.

Nodules

Although common in acne inversa (Figure 0.11) and acne vulgaris, these also occur in serious acne rosacea.

These are raised or deep, red or purple bumps, and they are usually tender (Figure 0.12).

They occur anywhere on the body where folliculopilosebaceous units (FPSUs) exist.

They are sometimes crusted, draining, or bleeding (Figure 0.13).

They are filled with inflamed material trying to reach the surface, heal, or scar down (Figure 0.14).

In AI/HS, the ruptured nodules form a gelatinous material. This invasive proliferative gelatinous mass (IPGM) invades and travels deep horizontally under the skin, producing sinus tracts (Figure 0.15).

When the sinus tracts rupture and drain to the surface, they often become secondarily infected (Figure 0.16).

Be practical:

For acne vulgaris and acne rosacea nodules:

Eliminate yeast, bacteria, and other organisms.

Cool the inflammation with anti-inflammatory antibiotics.

Start low-dose isotretinoin as soon as possible, whenever possible.

At the same time, get diet and hormones under immediate full control.

If isotretinoin is impossible, use aggressive anti-inflammatory therapy, including intralesional triamcinolone injections to minimize scarring.

For AI/HS lesions:

Use topical resorcinol cream to dry up small nodules.

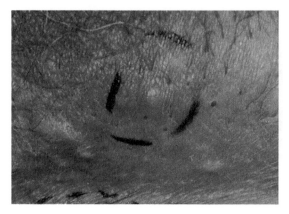

Figure 0.11 Early inflamed nodule on lateral mons pubis, with surrounding scars and tombstone comedones.

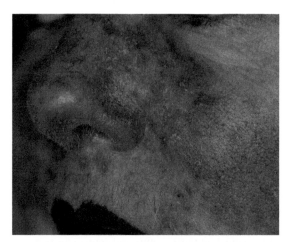

Figure 0.12 Acne rosacea with inflamed facial nodules.

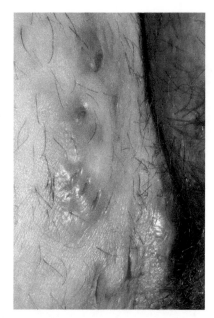

Figure 0.13 Upper inner thigh lateral to inguinal crease showing several interconnected acne inversa nodules, some bleeding to the surface.

Use punch debridement to empty out fresh follicular nodules.

Use unroofing to empty out large nodules and early sinuses.

Use oral zinc and vitamin C, oral antibiotics, and injectable steroids regularly.

Continue all baseline dietary and hormonal care.

Escalate to 'biologics' to cool the lesions before surgical care as needed.

Scars and sinuses

Scars and sinuses are caused by failure to treat acne early and properly.

There is a genetic tendency toward scarring (Figure 0.17).

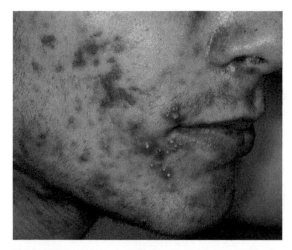

Figure 0.14 Active acne vulgaris showing nodules and pustules ready to drain and areas of subsequent scarring.

Some people scar badly, even in spite of minor lesions and early care.

Others with the same degree of acne do not scar at all.

Most acne scars are hypertrophic—raised above the original acne nodule (Figure 0.18).

True keloid scars, spreading beyond the original nodule, are rare.

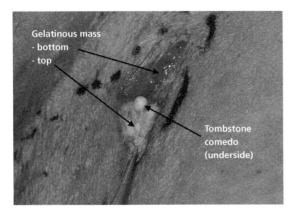

Figure 0.15 Indurated acne inversa/hidradenitis suppurativa lesion being unroofed and showing an ovolinear gelatinous mass in the base of the wound and a dilated epidermoid cystic component of a tombstone comedo with no pilar (hair root) and no sebaceous gland material, attached to the underside of unroofed material.

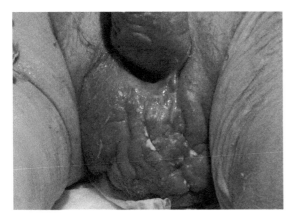

Figure 0.16 Acne inversa/hidradenitis suppurativa of scrotum with purulent secondary infection.

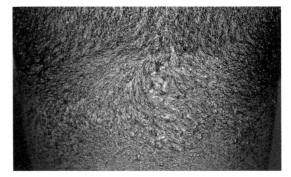

Figure 0.17 Early folliculocentric scarring of individual follicular groups, with coalescence into hypertrophic scarring. These scars are not true keloids (extending beyond the area of injury), but the name is unlikely to be changed to acne hypertrophicus.

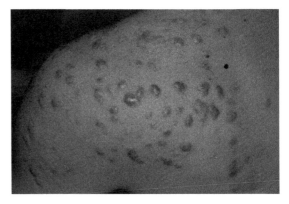

Figure 0.18 Residual hypertrophic and early keloidal shoulder scars following clearance with isotretinoin.

Support

The best support encourages positive, enthusiastic, "full-on" therapy and prevention.

Half-measure support gives half-measure results— and a full measure of frustration.

And a full measure of frustration just gives a full measure of stress.

The best support for continuing therapy is seeing therapy succeed.

You can't succeed if you don't start.

And you can't succeed quickly if you use half measures.

Be practical:

Be part of the solution, not part of the problem.

Get started. Get active. Get finished. Get clear.

Get reading.

Sinuses are likely produced by stem cells. This awaits proof. They must be unroofed as soon as possible.

Be practical:

Treat all acne, especially AI/HS, aggressively and early to prevent scars.

Start with strong medications first, and then reduce to maintenance.

Use intralesional triamcinolone injections early to prevent scars.

Ensure all early AI/HS lesions are punch excised or unroofed as soon as possible.

Introduction

Over one hundred years ago, the von Jacobi–Pringle dermochromes were published [1]. These lovely old books contain colored images of wax models (called *moulages*) of numerous skin diseases, with a summary of what was known about each disorder in 1903 (Figure 0.19).

Regarding acne, the later English version of the text states that the cause "is not yet fully cleared up. Many morbid processes conspire to favour the existence of the disease" [1].

Pringle's translation of Jacobi noted further that "a peculiar seborrhoeic condition is frequently present, which gives rise to the formation of comedones," and "the specific significance attributed to various bacteria found in the pus of acne-pustules is contestable" [1].

Over one hundred years later, the debate continues. The three contenders for the cause of acne have been the plugging of pores, the overproduction of oil, and the results of bacterial colonization of the sebaceous follicle (oil gland). Over the past 40 years, reputations have been built on these three concepts. Strauss [2–6], Pochi [7–12], Kligman [13–17], and Shalita [18–22] built careers on the slippery foundations of seborrhea, plugged pores, and comedolytics, with Leyden [23–28] and others concentrating upon the bacterial microorganisms and their relationships to antibiotics. More recently, Thiboutot [29–34], Zouboulis, and a growing host of other investigators [35–41] have greatly broadened our understanding of the basic science (those "morbid processes") behind the acnes.

Despite all this research, the picture of acne vulgaris did not change much until recently. In a recent monograph, Webster stated honestly and flatly, "The cause of the faulty desquamation that leads to comedo formation is not known" [42]. The situation has been clarified significantly since then. Melnik's molecular-level model of the mechanisms activating acne has changed all that [43–45]. We now have a reasoned and reasonable explanation of the way that the pores are plugged and the acnes develop. This is what physicians call the *pathogenesis of the disease*.

While irrefutable clinical trial–based proof of the cause has eluded us, I believe we now know the best path to follow. Meanwhile, the economic impact of acne has been, and continues to be, immense. The acnes remain the number one reason for visits to dermatologists in the United States.

The acnes generate millions of prescriptions worth hundreds of millions of dollars annually. They form a disease complex whose treatment has spawned an industry in its own right. In turn, it drives other economic

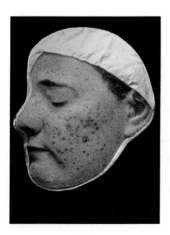
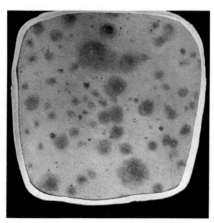

Figure 0.19 Wax models (*moulages*) of acne vulgaris originally in Neisser's Clinic in Breslau, now the Museum of Moulages (Muzeum Mulaży) of the Department of Dermatology in Wrocław (Breslau), Poland. From Jacobi-Pringle. Models in Neisser's Clinic in Breslau.

activities ranging from cosmetic cover-up to surgical repairs and resurfacing. It is now beginning to show up as a driver of several photomediated techniques, from red and blue topical lights to laser-driven photodynamic therapy (PDT).

"The blight of youth" and its fellow travelers, rosacea and acne inversa/hidradenitis suppurativa, are still with us, but we now have many tools to treat them [41].

The next step, in the words of Professor Albert Kligman, is "to actually achieve the ultimate goal in medical practice, namely prevention" [46]. That is also the ultimate goal of this book.

Nomenclature

The three generally recognized types of acne are acne vulgaris, acne rosacea, and acne inversa (usually called hidradenitis suppurativa in the United States). All are caused by a disorder centered on the structure usually called the *pilosebaceous apparatus*, so named because of its two products, hair and sebum.

So that we all understand what I will be talking about, the reader needs to know that I will be using a slightly different but more accurate name for these little appendages. It is essential to understand that there are really *three* parts to this classic little organ, not two. Furthermore, they are responsible for producing *three* products, not two. The three parts (or subunits) are distinctly different, as are their products. The subunit usually ignored in discussions of the cause of acne is the follicular part. Its product, the keratinized lining cells, likewise usually ignored, is often unrecognized but is nevertheless the major factor in the pathogenesis of acne. Fortunately, the appendage lends itself to a very natural subdivision into three distinctly different parts (Figure 0.20):

1 *The follicular canal* is that part of the structure that is represented at its top end by the *pore*. It is basically a tube whose job is to produce lining cells that produce a fibrous protein called *keratin* in cells called *keratinocytes*. These cells are normally shed into the lumen (the central open area of the canal). The size of the lumen varies depending upon a number of local effects, but the most obvious influence is from the size of the hair or hairs that pass through the unit. From almost invisible pores on a baby's face, bearing almost invisible wisps of downy vellus hair, can come thousands of heavy black male beard hairs. Or they may never produce much more than fine "peach fuzz" on a woman's face. The follicle may be up to 4 mm deep and arrow-straight, producing straight hair. It may be curved, producing curly hair, or oval, producing wavy hair. As far as its shape and size are concerned, the follicular canal is the product of the hair-producing (pilar) unit below it. It seems to follow the lead of the hair that it conducts to the surface. Thus, the follicle is a passive bystander or passive guide for the hair coming up from below. For our purposes, it is important to direct attention to the lining cells of the follicular canal. As you will see as we progress, the development of the microcomedo, which is the first stage of the plugging that leads to acne vulgaris, occurs as a result of events in the basal cell layer of the follicle. Although it is possible to make very rough measurements of the size of plugs in the follicular opening, it has never been possible to accurately quantify the output of the lining cells of this highly important unit. That, we shall see elsewhere, may have led generations of investigators down the wrong path.

2 The pilar unit is directly beneath the follicular canal and is a direct extension of the canal. Its job is to produce the hair (the Latin word for hair is *pilus*), and that is its sole reason for existence. The pilar unit's product, each hair, varies tremendously in size and shape under the influence of many factors, from the owner's genes to his or her environment, nutrition, medications, hormonal status, age, general health, and lifestyle. Although it is a challenge, quantification of the pilar units' output of hair can be accurately measured, by shaving a small area at regular intervals and weighing the shaved stubble. That is how the hair growth drug minoxidil was brought to the market [47].

3 The sebaceous gland and its ducts are just as varied as the pilar and follicular structures. They enter the folliculopilar structure from the sides, and this connection area between the hair-producing pilar area below and the keratinocyte-producing follicular area above is called the *isthmus*. Sometimes the sebaceous units stand alone, quietly lubricating large surface areas, but more often they are accompanied by a terminal hair, for example on the scalp. Prior to birth the entire crown, face, neck, shoulders, and upper chest are bathed in a slippery sebum-based material called *vernix caseosa*. Thus, the sebaceous glands produce the lubricant that

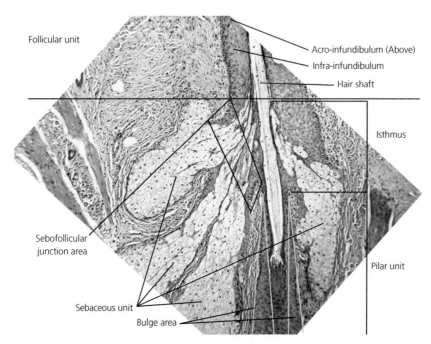

Follicular unit

Acro-infundibulum (Above)

Infra-infundibulum

Hair shaft

Isthmus

Sebofollicular
junction area

Pilar unit

Sebaceous unit

Bulge area

Figure 0.20 The folliculopilosebaceous unit (FPSU) is composed of three distinct structures: the follicular unit, the sebaceous unit, and the pilar unit. The follicular unit (through which the hair shaft and sebum reach the surface) starts at the surface as the acroinfundibulum (the upper portion of the follicle as it penetrates the epidermis) and continues as the infrainfundibulum to the isthmus where the sebaceous glands join the follicular unit and empty sebum into the follicular canal. The necks of the sebaceous glands that form the sebaceous unit attach through the sebofollicular junction area to the isthmus. Deep to (and continuous with) the isthmus is the pilar unit. The hair produced by the pilar unit in acne vulgaris, acne rosacea, and acne inversa/hidradenitis suppurativa may be so small that it is not apparent in biopsies of the FPSU. The bulge area is a thickened area of the upper pilar unit, just below the bottom of the isthmus–sebofollicular junction area. It is the source of the stem cells that repopulate injured epidermis, hair, and sebaceous glands. The FPSU illustrated is likely from the scalp of someone with fair hair.

prevents us getting stuck in the birth canal [48]. At the other end of life, hardly any oil is produced on the skin of the truly aged and dry skin becomes a problem. One of the last areas to lose its oil is the scalp, the area that pushed its way into the world first.

The sebum is measurable with some difficulty, but it takes little in the way of observation to note that patients with acne rosacea have oily skin. This fact is important to the cause of the inflammation in rosacea, to be proposed shortly.

Putting these three terms together produces a bit of a mouthful, the *folliculopilosebaceous unit*. To make things easier, I will use its short form, FPSU, throughout this book. This recognizes the fact that the follicular part that is usually called a *hair follicle* or *sebaceous follicle* is really neither. There is a simple reason why it is neither— because it is *both*. It delivers both the hair and the oil to the surface. It is also highly distinctive in its mission and

in its contribution to the various acnes, so it deserves a place of its own. As you will see later, the junctional area (where these three parts of the FPSU meet) has its own special features (Figure 0.20). Each part contributes to the various diseases of the appendage in its own way. For now, just keep in mind that the three subunits comprising the FPSU behave differently in each of the various kinds of acne.

The three acnes and grading

Acne vulgaris

This is common acne, and it takes many forms. The disorder starts when the follicular portion of the FPSU is plugged, producing two kinds of plugged pores (comedones), open and closed. Open comedones are the classic *blackheads* (Figures 0.21 and 0.22). Closed comedones are called *whiteheads* (Figures 0.23 and 0.24).

Figure 0.21 Folliculopilosebaceous unit with detail and orientation of the sebofollicular junction area. The black oval shows the top and bottom limits of the isthmus section of the pilofollicular tube. The necks of the sebaceous glands that "plug into" the isthmus through 360° form the sebofollicular junction. The bulge area is likewise a 360° wrap around the upper portion of the pilar unit. It is composed of a series of stem cells—the ones closest to the sebofollicular junction are Lgr6 type and may be the source of the invasive proliferative gelatinous mass (IPGM), which is to be further discussed in this book. From http://upload.wikimedia.org/wikipedia/commons/7/7c/Insertion_of_sebaceous_glands_into_hair_shaft_x10.jpg.

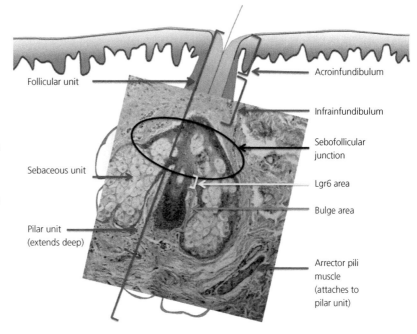

Follicular unit
Acroinfundibulum
Infrainfundibulum
Sebofollicular junction
Sebaceous unit
Lgr6 area
Bulge area
Pilar unit (extends deep)
Arrector pili muscle (attaches to pilar unit)

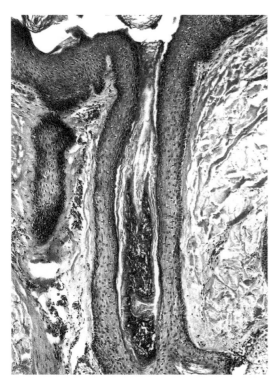

Figure 0.22 Plewig's Follikel-Filament—the earliest form of follicular plugging, with compact pink lamellae of lining keratinocytes, a fine hair that is barely visible, and purple colonies of anerobic *Propionibacterium acnes*. Note that the *stratum corneum equivalent* and the intraductal keratin layer near the hair at the top end are thin and loose, indicating that terminal differentiation and desquamation are occurring normally. From *Acne and rosacea*, 2e, Kligman, Albert M; Plewig, Gerd.

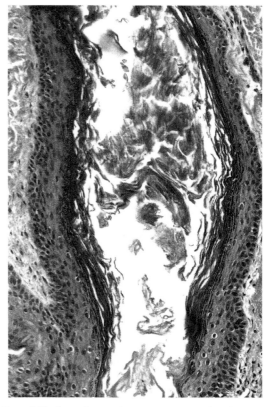

Figure 0.23 The early comedo starting to accumulate deep in the infrainfundibular part of the follicular unit, showing thickening of the stratum corneum underlying multilayered compact keratin as terminal differentiation fails. From *Acne and rosacea*, 2e, Kligman, Albert M; Plewig, Gerd.

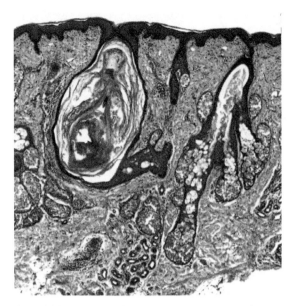

Figure 0.24 Closed comedones do have an opening to the surface, but it is too tight to permit the compacted keratin in the dilated follicular unit to exit. The content may become large enough that the structure is called an *epidermoid cyst*. The term *sebaceous cyst* is a misnomer—the sebaceous glands are normally "squeezed out" to the point that they are rarely detected in these structures. From *Acne and rosacea*, 2e, Kligman, Albert M; Plewig, Gerd.

Acne rosacea

For reasons that are discussed in this book, comedones are not seen in acne rosacea. The diagnosis is made based upon the appearance of folliculopapules (Figure 0.29) and folliculopustules (Figure 0.30) on the convex surfaces of the central face and chin and forehead. The background skin is a rosy pink color that gives the disorder its name (Figure 0.31). It usually onsets after the teen years and may last into the senior years.

There may be accompanying telangiectasia (Figure 0.32). This has led to the definition of a subtype of rosacea called *erythematotelangiectatic rosacea* [49]. More on that later (see Appendix A).

There may also be a peculiar thickening of the involved tissues. The nose is most commonly involved, but cheeks and chin and other facial areas may show swelling, thickening, and eventually a woody firmness (Figure 0.33). This is called *phyma* (nodule or swelling) formation, and the classic involvement of the nose induces *rhinophyma*. Finally there may be, for reasons undetermined, involvement of the soft tissues of the eye, which carries the designation *ocular rosacea* (Figure 0.34).

PRACTICAL TIP BOX 0.1

The "whiteheads" that contain real pus are called *pustules*. Dermatologists use the term *whitehead* to describe pores plugged with keratin (not pus) that show no obvious opening to the surface.

Each comedo can have several possible fates.

An open comedo may simply stop growing, empty out, and disappear. It may get very large and sit quietly for months or even years. It may get inflamed, turn into a folliculopustule (Figure 0.25), empty out its contents onto the surface, and heal up. It may rupture "deep" (Figure 0.26), causing an inflamed acne papule. It may join with other nearby comedones (both open and closed) and nearby papules and pustules to become an acne nodule. If a number of these nodules join together and the inflamed tissues break down between them to form a continuous inflammatory mass, this is called *conglobate acne* (acne conglobata) (Figure 0.27). If this type of acne is

accompanied by a sudden onset of aching joints and fever, it is called *acne fulminans*.

Closed comedones may turn into open comedones and follow the same paths described here, but they may also rupture directly into papules and pustules.

As the inflammation dies down, scarring occurs. It may be so mild that it is unnoticeable, or it may just show as discoloration (post-inflammatory hyperpigmentation, or PIH) that will fade with time.

Destruction of tissue by the inflammation causes total or partial loss of the FPSU plus pits and depressions of various sizes. If the body's attempt to repair the damage has produced tunnels under the skin, these "sinuses" may be permanent (Figure 0.28). And if the body has been overenthusiastic in healing, *hypertrophic scars* are formed, appearing as smooth raised lumps over the active areas. (See Figure 0.18.)

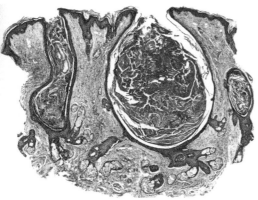

Figure 0.25 Open comedones are not static plugs in the follicle. New keratinocytes are added to their outside layer, and the central keratinocytes are slowly lost through the follicular opening. From *Acne and rosacea*, 2e, Kligman, Albert M; Plewig, Gerd.

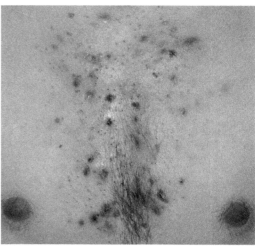

Figure 0.27 Inflammatory papular, pustular, nodular, and scarring acne coexisting with extensive non-inflammatory comedonal acne.

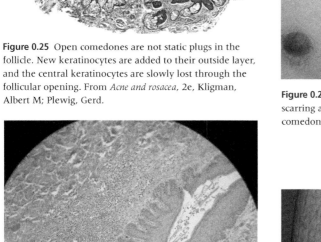

Figure 0.26 The rupture in the wall of this follicular unit has allowed intraductal material to escape, causing the surrounding peri-follicular inflammation and allowing inflammatory cells to enter the duct.

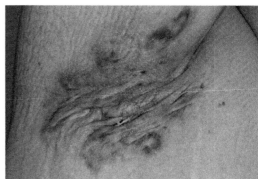

Figure 0.28 The exaggerated webbed scarring that can occur in acne inversa/hidradenitis suppurativa, as in this right armpit/axilla, can be destructive and invasive instead of a healing influence.

PRACTICAL TIP BOX 0.2

The scars that follow acne are called *hypertrophic* because they grow vertically over the injury. Dermatologists use the term *keloid* to describe scars that spread beyond the area of original injury, like burn scars.

Acne inversa (hidradenitis suppurativa)

This variation shows up in areas where the FPSU plugs up and then the follicular wall ruptures deep in the sebofollicular junction area. Most commonly this onsets in the axillae (Figure 0.28), inguinal creases, perineum, genitals (Figure 0.35), and perianal areas, but this

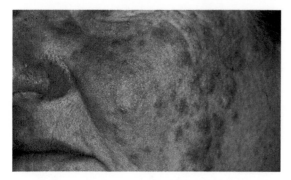

Figure 0.29 Acne rosacea is basically a folliculocentric inflammatory reaction directed at material in the follicular duct. The inflammation varies in depth and degree depending upon the variable content of the pore, the varied immune responses of the patient, and the varied therapies undertaken. This woman failed to respond to topical metronidazole and oral tetracycline group antibiotics but cleared with combined therapy directed at *Demodex* and *Malassezia*.

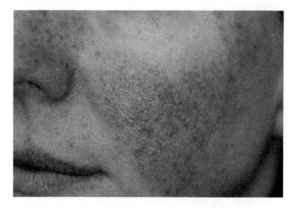

Figure 0.32 The rosy background glow of dilated superficial venules and capillaries gives acne rosacea its name. Most of the dilation of the vessels is due to actinic (from the sun) damage to the support structures of the vessels, allowing them to dilate and contain more red blood cells. This actinic telangiectasia may stand alone or may be left behind, as in this case, when the acne rosacea is cleared.

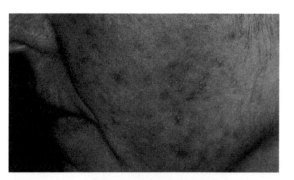

Figure 0.30 These very superficial folliculopustules are the hallmark of *Demodex* involvement in acne rosacea.

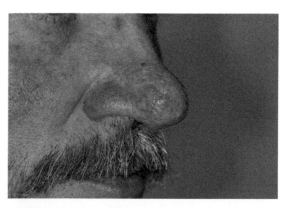

Figure 0.33 This man's rhinophyma involved only the bulb of the nose. It responded to nothing but low-dose oral isotretinoin over several months. The undelying fibrosis has left him with a prominent nasal bulb, but it is much improved from the original bright-red swollen condition.

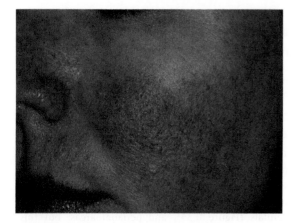

Figure 0.31 This is acne rosacea under treatment with a somewhat irritating, drying, elemental precipitated sulfur and sulfonamide antibiotic topical lotion. Part of the redness is from irritation, some is from the inflammation of the follicles, and some from underlying dilated blood vessels.

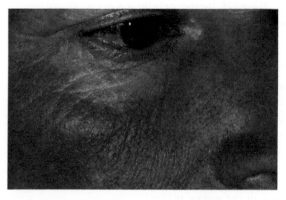

Figure 0.34 This is ocular rosacea. Note the residual conjunctival telangiectasia and cheimosis (edema) despite active treatment.

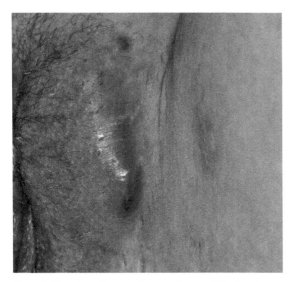

Figure 0.35 A classic location for acne inversa/hidradenitis suppurativa, deep in the left inguinal (groin) crease where friction and pressure combine to rupture the folliculopilosebaceous unit structure at its weak points.

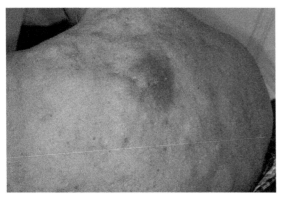

Figure 0.36 In addition to classic acne inversa/hidradenitis suppurativa and acne vulgaris lesions elsewhere, this man suffered from a lifetime of scarring ruptured epidermoid cysts.

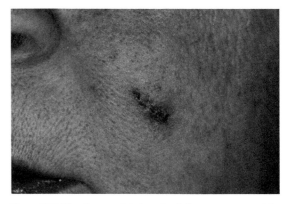

Figure 0.37 The characteristic invasive inflammatory material traveling horizontally just below the skin surface produces this type of indolent invasive linear scarring.

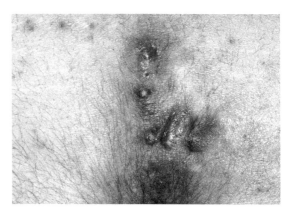

Figure 0.38 In the sacral area, acne inversa/hidradenitis suppurativa is often recurrent due to sitting pressure, and the invasive mass and sinuses are often forced deep by such pressure.

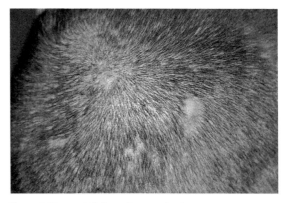

Figure 0.39 Hair follicles, when involved in acne inversa/hidradenitis suppurativa, take the inflammation to new depths. The result can be permanent hair loss if the hair bulb and stem cells are destroyed.

disorder can appear anywhere FPSUs exist, including the trunk (Figure 0.36), the face (Figure 0.37), behind the ears, in the *pilonidal sinus (cyst)* area (Figure 0.38), and the scalp (Figure 0.39); for the latter, it is termed *perifolliculitis capitis abscedens et suffodiens* (dissecting folliculitis of the scalp). There are often no visible comedones early in the disorder, and the first sign of trouble is usually a single deep reddish-purple painful nodule, often thought to be a "boil" caused by infection. It may erupt to the surface of the skin and discharge, or the mass may expand sideways, causing the formation of

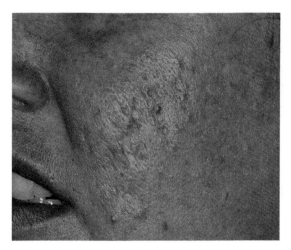

Figure 0.40 Scars like this are heartbreaking to patient and dermatologist alike—so preventable if treated early. Her mother would not permit any oral medication and insisted that consuming lots of healthy dairy foods would help her "grow out of it."

deep and then communicating sinuses lined with squamous epithelium. These may become secondarily infected and drain purulent material for months or years. Secondary scarring can be extensive and complicates therapy (Figure 0.40). Multiheaded comedones, the follicular remnants of the FPSU, serve as the tombstones of burned-out FPSUs.

A special form of this disorder combines AI/HS, pilonidal sinus (cyst) disease, dissecting folliculitis of the scalp, and acne conglobata. These four disorders are referred to as the *follicular occlusion tetrad* [50], but they are all basically the same disorder with variations dictated by local conditions.

Grading the three acnes
Acne vulgaris
Acne researchers have been searching for methods of grading the severity of acne for decades, and the search is still on, but the criteria seem now to be set. A panel of acne experts "concluded that an ideal acne global grading scale would comprise the essential clinical components of primary acne lesions, their quantity, extent, and facial and extrafacial sites of involvement; with features of clinimetric properties, categorization, efficiency, and acceptance" [51].

There are presently three evaluation systems that recognize the need to include extra-facial sites: the Leeds system [52], the Comprehensive Acne Severity Scale (CASS) [53], and the Global Acne Grading System (GAGS) [54]. The Leeds system is complex but has a track record and a separate subcategory for non-inflammatory acne. The CASS is validated but does not discriminate between inflammatory and non-inflammatory lesions. The GAGS is not yet validated. A fourth, the Global Acne Severity Scale (GEA Scale), is designed for France and Europe [55] and could likely be adapted to include extra-facial sites.

Acne rosacea
The classification and grading system proposed by an expert committee in 2004 is still in use. Each feature of the disorder, from flushing to phymatous change, is generally graded as *absent, mild, moderate,* or *severe,* as are the physicians' ratings of the severity of the subtypes proposed and the patients' global assessment [49]. Although the ratings have the disadvantage of being somewhat subjective, they are reasonably accurate, reproducible, and generally manageable in the clinic.

Acne inversa (hidradenitis suppurativa)
Each of the two grading systems used in this disorder follows one of the patterns described for the other two acnes. The original, Hurley's three-"stage" system, is simple enough to use in the clinic [56]. Its three levels of severity serve as useful clinical shorthand for communicating degree of severity among dermatologists and surgeons.

The more refined, more objective, and therefore more complex Sartorius score [57], and its modifications, is of greater use to the researcher than the clinician. As befits a complex disease, the scoring system is complicated at first sight but it does provide the reproducible results essential for tracking of physical improvements over time [58]. Other rating systems are available to quantify quality of life and degree of pain relief, but an overall rating system that would allow global evaluation, including serial follow-up of all aspects of the disorder, has yet to be developed [59].

Overall, in evaluating and grading all the acnes in the clinic, it is hard to beat "So, how are you doing?", "What's your biggest problem right now?", and "May I take a look?" when dealing with patients one on one. As my first supervising surgical resident admonished me, "When all else fails, examine the patient." Those three questions, and their answers, are the best grading system we have and lead naturally and directly to the most important question of all: "How can I help?"

References

1 von Jacobi E. Atlas der Hautkrankheiten. 1st ed. Berlin: Urban & Schwartzenberg; 1903.

2 Strauss JS. Editorial: the sebaceous glands. N Engl J Med 1974 Jul 4;291(1):46–7.

3 Strauss JS, Pochi PE, Downing DT. Skin lipids and acne. Annu Rev Med 1975;26:27–32.

4 Strauss JS, Pochi PE, Downing DT. The role of skin lipids in acne. Cutis 1976 Mar;17(3):485–7.

5 Strauss JS, Stranieri AM. Changes in long-term sebum production from isotretinoin therapy. J Am Acad Dermatol 1982 Apr;6(4 Pt 2 Suppl):751–6.

6 Strauss JS, Stewart ME, Downing DT. The effect of 13-cis-retinoic acid on sebaceous glands. Arch Dermatol 1987 Nov;123(11):1538a–1541.

7 Pochi PE, Strauss JS. Sebum production, casual sebum levels, titratable acidity of sebum, and urinary fractional 17-ketosteroid excretion in males with acne. J Invest Dermatol 1964 Nov;43:383–8.

8 Pochi PE, Strauss JS, Rao GS, Sarda IR, Forchielli E, Dorfman RI. Plasma testosterone and estrogen levels, urine testosterone excretion, and sebum production in males with acne vulgaris. J Clin Endocrinol Metab 1965 Dec;25(12):1660–4.

9 Pochi PE, Strauss JS. Effect of cyclic administration of conjugated equine estrogens on sebum production in women. J Invest Dermatol 1966 Dec;47(6):582–5.

10 Pochi PE, Strauss JS. Sebaceous gland suppression with ethinyl estradiol and diethylstilbestrol. Arch Dermatol 1973 Aug;108(2):210–4.

11 Pochi PE, Strauss JS. Endocrinologic control of the development and activity of the human sebaceous gland. J Invest Dermatol 1974 Mar;62(3):191–201.

12 Pochi PE. Endocrinology of acne. J Invest Dermatol 1983 Jul;81(1):1.

13 Kligman AM, Wheatley VR, Mills OH. Comedogenicity of human sebum. Arch Dermatol 1970 Sep;102(3):267–75.

14 Kligman AM. An overview of acne. J Invest Dermatol 1974 Mar;62(3):268–87.

15 Kligman AM. Pathogenesis of acne vulgaris. Mod Probl Paediatr 1975;17:153–73.

16 Kligman AM. Postadolescent acne in women. Cutis 1991 Jul;48(1):75–7.

17 Kligman AM. How to use topical tretinoin in treating acne. Cutis 1995 Aug;56(2):83–4.

18 Shalita A, Miller B, Menter A, Abramovits W, Loven K, Kakita L. Tazarotene cream versus adapalene cream in the treatment of facial acne vulgaris: a multicenter, double-blind, randomized, parallel-group study. J Drugs Dermatol 2005 Mar;4(2):153–8.

19 Shalita A. The integral role of topical and oral retinoids in the early treatment of acne. J Eur Acad Dermatol Venereol 2001;15 Suppl 3:43–9.

20 Shalita AR. Acne revisited. Arch Dermatol 1994 Mar;130(3):363–4.

21 Shalita AR, Freinkel RK. Acne. J Am Acad Dermatol 1984 Nov;11(5 Pt 2):957–60.

22 Shalita AR. Acne vulgaris: current concepts in pathogenesis and treatment. Int J Dermatol 1976 Apr;15(3):182–7.

23 Leyden JJ, Del Rosso JQ, Webster GF. Clinical considerations in the treatment of acne vulgaris and other inflammatory skin disorders: focus on antibiotic resistance. Cutis 2007 Jun;79(6 Suppl):9–25.

24 Leyden JJ. The evolving role of *Propionibacterium acnes* in acne. Semin Cutan Med Surg 2001 Sep;20(3):139–43.

25 Leyden JJ, McGinley KJ, Cavalieri S, Webster GF, Mills OH, Kligman AM. *Propionibacterium acnes* resistance to antibiotics in acne patients. J Am Acad Dermatol 1983 Jan;8(1):41–5.

26 Leyden JJ. Antibiotic resistant acne. Cutis 1976 Mar;17(3):593–6.

27 Leyden JJ, McGinley KJ, Mills OH, Kligman AM. *Propionibacterium* levels in patients with and without acne vulgaris. J Invest Dermatol 1975 Oct;65(4):382–4.

28 Leyden JJ, Marples RR, Mills OH, Jr., Kligman AM. Gram-negative folliculitis—a complication of antibiotic therapy in acne vulgaris. Br J Dermatol 1973 Jun;88(6):533–8.

29 Thiboutot D. Regulation of human sebaceous glands. J Invest Dermatol 2004 Jul;123(1):1–12.

30 Thiboutot D, Jabara S, McAllister JM, Sivarajah A, Gilliland K, Cong Z, et al. Human skin is a steroidogenic tissue: steroidogenic enzymes and cofactors are expressed in epidermis, normal sebocytes, and an immortalized sebocyte cell line (SEB-1). J Invest Dermatol 2003 Jun;120(6):905–14.

31 Thiboutot DM. Endocrinological evaluation and hormonal therapy for women with difficult acne. J Eur Acad Dermatol Venereol 2001;15 Suppl 3:57–61.

32 Thiboutot D, Gilliland K, Light J, Lookingbill D. Androgen metabolism in sebaceous glands from subjects with and without acne. Arch Dermatol 1999 Sep;135(9):1041–5.

33 Thiboutot D, Martin P, Volikos L, Gilliland K. Oxidative activity of the type 2 isozyme of 17beta-hydroxysteroid dehydrogenase (17beta-HSD) predominates in human sebaceous glands. J Invest Dermatol 1998 Sep;111(3):390–5.

34 Thiboutot DM, Knaggs H, Gilliland K, Hagari S. Activity of type 1 5 alpha-reductase is greater in the follicular infrainfundibulum compared with the epidermis. Br J Dermatol 1997 Feb;136(2):166–71.

35 Ganceviciene R, Bohm M, Fimmel S, Zouboulis CC. The role of neuropeptides in the multifactorial pathogenesis of acne vulgaris. Dermatoendocrinol 2009 May;1(3):170–6.

36 Zouboulis CC, Picardo M, Reichrath J. Letter from the editors: endocrine aspects of acne and related diseases. Dermatoendocrinol 2009 May;1(3):123–4.

37 Kurokawa I, Danby FW, Ju Q, Wang X, Xiang LF, Xia L, *et al.* New developments in our understanding of acne pathogenesis and treatment. Exp Dermatol 2009 Oct;18(10):821–32.

38 Zouboulis CC, Eady A, Philpott M, Goldsmith LA, Orfanos C, Cunliffe WC, *et al.* What is the pathogenesis of acne? Exp Dermatol 2005 Feb;14(2):143–52.

39 Zouboulis CC, Bohm M. Neuroendocrine regulation of sebocytes—a pathogenetic link between stress and acne. Exp Dermatol 2004;13 Suppl 4:31–5.

40 Chen W, Thiboutot D, Zouboulis CC. Cutaneous androgen metabolism: basic research and clinical perspectives. J Invest Dermatol 2002 Nov;119(5):992–1007.

41 Danby FW. New, relevant information and innovative interventions in the management of acne. G Ital Dermatol Venereol 2011 Jun;146(3):197–210.

42 Webster G. Overview of the pathogenesis of acne. In: Webster GF, Rawlings AV, editors. Acne and its therapy. New York: Informa; 2007. p. 1–7.

43 Melnik BC, Schmitz G. Role of insulin, insulin-like growth factor-1, hyperglycaemic food and milk consumption in the pathogenesis of acne vulgaris. Exp Dermatol 2009 Oct;18(10):833–41.

44 Melnik BC. FoxO1—the key for the pathogenesis and therapy of acne? J Dtsch Dermatol Ges 2010 Feb;8(2):105–14.

45 Melnik BC. Evidence for acne-promoting effects of milk and other insulinotropic dairy products. Nestle Nutr Workshop Ser Pediatr Program 2011;67:131–45.

46 Kligman A. Letter of welcome, Second International Conference on the Sebaceous Gland, Acne & Related Disorders. Rome; 2008.

47 Savin RC. Use of topical minoxidil in the treatment of male pattern baldness. J Am Acad Dermatol 1987 Mar;16(3 Pt 2):696–704.

48 Danby FW. Why we have sebaceous glands. J Am Acad Dermatol 2005 Jun;52(6):1071–2.

49 Wilkin J, Dahl M, Detmar M, Drake L, Liang MH, Odom R, *et al.* Standard grading system for rosacea: report of the National Rosacea Society Expert Committee on the classification and staging of rosacea. J Am Acad Dermatol 2004 Jun;50(6):907–12.

50 Plewig G, Steger M. Acne inversa (alias acne triad, acne tetrad or hidradenitis suppurativa). In: Marks R, Plewig G, editors. Acne and related disorders. London: Dunitz; 1989. p. 345–57.

51 Tan J, Wolfe B, Weiss J, Stein-Gold L, Bikowski J, Del RJ, *et al.* Acne severity grading: determining essential clinical components and features using a Delphi consensus. J Am Acad Dermatol 2012 Aug;67(2):187–93.

52 O'Brien SC, Lewis JB, Cunliffe WJ. The Leeds revised acne grading system. J Dermatol Treat 1998;9:215–20.

53 Tan JK, Tang J, Fung K, Gupta AK, Thomas DR, Sapra S, *et al.* Development and validation of a comprehensive acne severity scale. J Cutan Med Surg 2007 Nov;11(6):211–6.

54 Doshi A, Zaheer A, Stiller MJ. A comparison of current acne grading systems and proposal of a novel system. Int J Dermatol 1997 Jun;36(6):416–8.

55 Dreno B, Poli F, Pawin H, Beylot C, Faure M, Chivot M, *et al.* Development and evaluation of a Global Acne Severity Scale (GEA Scale) suitable for France and Europe. J Eur Acad Dermatol Venereol 2011 Jan;25(1):43–8.

56 Hurley HJ. Axillary hyperhidrosis, apocrine bromhidrosis, hidradenitis suppurativa, and familial benign pemphigus: surgical approach. In: Roenigk RK, Roenigk HH, editors. Dermatologic surgery. New York: Dekker; 1989. p. 729–39.

57 Sartorius K, Lapins J, Emtestam L, Jemec GB. Suggestions for uniform outcome variables when reporting treatment effects in hidradenitis suppurativa. Br J Dermatol 2003 Jul;149(1):211–3.

58 Sartorius K, Killasli H, Heilborn J, Jemec GB, Lapins J, Emtestam L. Interobserver variability of clinical scores in hidradenitis suppurativa is low. Br J Dermatol 2010 Jun;162(6):1261–8.

59 Poli F, Jemec GBE, Revuz J. Clinical presentation. In: Jemec GBE, Revuz J, Leyden JJ, editors. Hidradenitis suppurativa. Heidelberg: Springer; 2006. p. 11–24.

CHAPTER 1

The three acnes and their impact

The visibility of the lesions of acne vulgaris and acne rosacea as we present ourselves to the world and interact with others is a source of anguish to many. The hidden lesions of acne inversa (hidradenitis suppurativa) may interfere even with the most basic social interactions. The most profound effect of the acnes is on the psyche, so that aspect will be discussed "up front," but first we need to know what we are talking about.

1.1 Acne vulgaris

Vulgaris is a Latin word, an adjective that means *common*. It is not a pleasant term, but it is descriptive (even a little vulgar). It is also highly accurate because the lifetime risk of acne in developed countries with "Western" diets is 85–90% of the population. Indeed, acne vulgaris is so common that even senior dermatologists (who should know better) have stated, "Children as young as 7 years of age can present with mild, usually comedonal disease, which most often is a normal physiologic occurrence." To avoid embarrassing the author, no reference is provided.

If I agreed with the statement that acne is "normal" (or "physiologic"), there would be no point to this book. My purpose in writing it is to draw together numerous threads of information, from very old to very new. I want to define the problem. Then I want to explain how this disorder (and its relatives) arises. Only then can we sort out how to treat it (and its various types) in as logical a fashion as possible.

So let's get started—at the beginning.

Acne occurs when a plug forms in the follicular portion of the little oil gland and hair follicle organs on the skin called, in the older literature, *pilosebaceous units*. Here they will be called *folliculopilosebaceous units* (FPSUs), for reasons discussed in the Introduction.

There are other small organs that develop from the underside of the skin:

The eccrine sweat glands over most of our skin surfaces produce ordinary sweat.

The apocrine sweat glands in our armpits and groin areas produce a different kind of sweat, plus a peculiar class of chemicals called pheromones.

The mammary glands that form the breasts are derived in the same way, but obviously grow bigger than the others.

These are all referred to as *skin appendages*. They all have their own diseases, and some may be related to acne.

1.1.1 Terminology

The first plugs that lead to acne occur in the structurally quiet, non-inflamed, and non-infected follicular portion of the FPSU. The story starts with a stimulus to the development of a structure named the Follikel-Filament [1], the first tiny accumulation of the lining cells, the keratinocytes, in the follicular duct (Figure 1.1A). These cells produce the tough linear protein called *keratin* that makes up the surface of our skin. When formed into a long thin fiber, keratin makes hair, and when produced in thick flat compact sheets, keratin becomes nail. Thin sheets of keratin, made of individual terminal keratinocytes, form the surface of skin and line the follicular portion of the FPSU. The process of formation of keratin

---

Acne: Causes and Practical Management, First Edition. F. William Danby.
© 2015 John Wiley & Sons, Ltd. Published 2015 by John Wiley & Sons, Ltd.

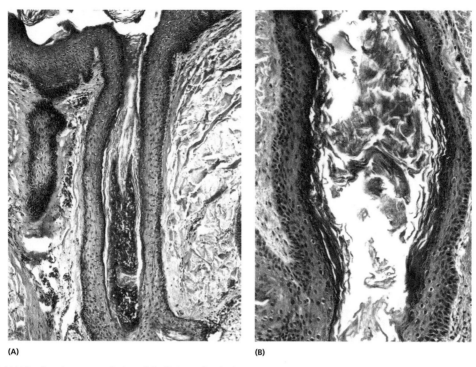

(A)   **(B)**

Figure 1.1 (A) The first tiny accumulation of the lining cells, the keratinocytes, in the follicular duct. (B) Accumulation of these flat cells in the follicle leads to the microcomedo.

by keratinocytes in the follicular canal and on the skin surface is called *keratinization*. Normally, as these cells mature they separate from each other toward the center of the follicular duct, and the loose cells are released into the ductal canal where they are pushed to the top of the duct by the flow of sebum. Accumulation of these flat cells in the follicle leads to the microcomedo (Figure 1.1B). This growth progresses next with larger and larger masses of these lining keratinocytes, leading to the physical plugging of the duct. Next come microbial colonization and overgrowth of preexisting bacterial and yeast colonies. This continues at the same time as the increased plugging. The increase in intrafollicular mass causes expansion, leaking, and then rupture of the follicular unit.

The pilar unit is unaffected in early acne. It just keeps doing its job, which is to make hair, some of which may become trapped in the plugged and dilated follicular unit. That hair normally becomes increasingly coarse during the teen years, especially in boys, and has the effect of keeping the larger FPSUs open and uninvolved in the acne process.

The sebaceous unit is also growing and producing more sebum. At body temperature, that sebum is a liquid. It quietly percolates to the surface, through and around the plugs, and is responsible for von Jacobi–Pringle's "peculiar seborrhoeic condition," the oily skin of acne that we all recognize [2]. It also happens to be the preferred food for the organisms that come to live in the follicular unit, so that encourages their growth. Much more on them later (Section 6.0).

The leaking and rupture of the follicular unit of the FPSU are intimately involved with inflammation. This is a huge and very complex area. Hundreds of papers have been written on the subject. As of this writing, there have been 619 papers since 1952. I don't plan to review them all here, but you need to know that there is serious debate as to what starts the process. Does the plugging of the follicular unit come first, with pressure-induced leakage leading to inflammation [2]? Or does very early inflammation actually stimulate the plugging of the duct to produce excessive numbers of ductal cells [3]? My personal belief is that hormones plug the pore, and that causes the expansion that leads to the leaking, which leads to the inflammation. My reasoning is simple: the organisms said to trigger the inflammation that triggers the keratinization are present in almost everyone, throughout life, and are in no greater number in acne patients than in normal persons [2]. If these organisms were the cause, we would all have acne, all the time. There has to be a factor that comes on at puberty, and generally leaves at the onset of maturity, in order to explain the timeline of acne in our population. More on that later (Section 2.6). There also needs to be a trigger that links the overproduction of the keratinocytes in the follicular duct to the onset of inflammation. That may be a recently described simple product of the pressure and hypoxia that build up in the follicular duct. More on that as well later.

Whether inflammation starts the plugging process or is a response to early leakage of materials from the FPSU, inflammation is seen as a target for therapy. For hundreds of years, physicians have been treating acne by trying to suppress the inflammation. I will try to convince you in this book that treating the inflammation is like chasing the horse after he has left the burning barn. Far more important is preventing the fire in the first place.

The "inflammatory process" doesn't just cause inflammation. It is often forgotten that its main chore is to *repair* the damage caused. Sometimes, the inflammatory process stops with simple healing of the wall of the follicular unit. In the *absence* of repair, the inflammatory reaction just keeps burning. Unfortunately, that leads to much more destruction. The contents of the dilated follicles leak or explode into the tissue under the skin surface. That causes more inflammation and leads to scarring. This prolonged destructive inflammatory activity is the cause of the tender nodules that are so ugly. Untreated, resolution occurs over a long time period, often years. This is referred to as "burning out" of acne. It leads to loss of parts of the FPSU, or the entire FPSU can be destroyed. It also leaves serious scarring behind.

1.1.2 The starting point

The primary target of acne therapy must be the prevention of the environment that produces the Follikel-Filament and so the microcomedo [1]. All the other events are "downstream" and secondary. These downstream events are called *epiphenomena*—things that happen "on top of" (that is what *epi* means) other things. Management of acne has for over a century

concentrated upon suppressing these epiphenomena, while ignoring the real cause of the disease.

It is time to address the cause.

1.2 Acne rosacea

Classic acne rosacea is a variant of the acnes that shows up on the curved surfaces of the face (Figure 1.2). It is made up of blemishes centered on the openings of the follicular units of individual FPSUs. There are little raised bumps (folliculopapules) and very small pustules (folliculopustules). These little bumps and pustules are the "acne," and they appear on a rosy-red background, the "rosacea." The word *rosacea* has been used for a couple of hundred years as an adjective to modify the noun *acne*. So acne rosacea is really just rose-colored acne.

The word *rosacea* is now seen in the public eye and in some dermatological writing. The adjective has become a noun, and rosacea has become a "disease" or "condition" all by itself. See Appendix A for more on the name's change.

It is important to understand that acne rosacea actually has three separate components on the face. The first is the pimply acne, the second is the background redness (Figure 1.3), and the third is a thickening of the skin. There are also eye changes that cause a fourth, separate, but associated condition, but it is not always present.

Just as acne vulgaris always starts with plugs in the follicles that show up as comedones (blackheads) when mature, true acne rosacea always has the folliculopapulopustular lesions instead. Indeed, the presence of

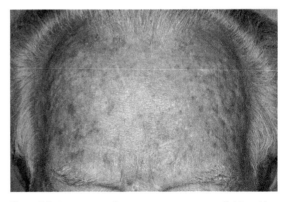

Figure 1.2 Acne rosacea loves convex, sun-exposed skin with a healthy population of well-stimulated FPSUs.

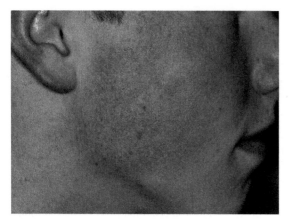

Figure 1.3 Some dermatologists consider this "pre-rosacea." Close inspection reveals a few comedones—almost normal in a 15 year old. He needs lifelong, truly broad-spectrum sun protection to prevent worsening of his actinic telangiectasia; a dairy-free diet; and a gentle topical retinoid.

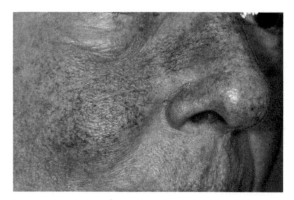

Figure 1.4 Longstanding sun exposure gradually weakens the collagen and other support tissues that wrap around and support the blood vessels, allowing them to dilate. The blood pools in them and turns dark, as on this man's nose.

visible comedones rules out acne rosacea as the prime diagnosis. Just to confuse the issue, there are occasional patients who have *both* acne rosacea and acne vulgaris.

1.2.1 The "pimply" part

The little bumps and pustules are caused by the body's immune systems (both of them) reacting to "stuff" that is caught in the pore. This is an automatic rejection reaction aimed at things like bacteria and yeasts, some tiny beasties called Demodex (see Section 6.4), and little ingrown hairs.

This reaction is the job of the innate immune system. *Innate* means *inborn* or *born with*, and it is the part of the immune system that does not need to "learn" what to do with foreign material. We are able, from birth, to recognize various foreign materials, and this part of the immune system is aimed automatically at anything in the pores or escaping under the skin from the pores that it recognizes as foreign material. It can be triggered by anything from tiny viruses to large ingrown hairs. (See Section 7.1.)

There is also a second part of the reaction caused by the "adaptive" immune system. Its job is to recognize, target, and eliminate foreign material when the innate immune system needs some extra help. It sometimes gets involved as well, but it takes a little while to get going, because it needs time to learn how to "adapt" to a new threat. There is much more on that to come (see Section 7.2).

1.2.2 The "redness" part

The redness (erythema) that causes the rosy color is made up of three separate components:

1 structural erythema,
2 functional erythema, and
3 inflammatory erythema.

The first, structural erythema, is due to dilated blood vessels. These are sometimes called *broken blood vessels*, but they are not really broken. Their structure is actually *dilated*, which just means they are increased in diameter and so are carrying more blood than usual as a result (Figure 1.4). More blood in the blood vessels makes the skin redder than usual. Structural dilation of a blood vessel is due to a gradual weakening of its walls that allows the blood vessel to bulge. Early bulging of very fine facial blood vessels is due to minor injury, most commonly from sun exposure. Even babies (who are usually protected against direct sunlight) will show pink cheeks. This is the earliest sign of *actinic telangiectasia*, the permanent and visible dilated blood vessels just under the skin surface. In a letter to the *British Medical Journal* in 1976, Dr. Ronald Marks stated that

we have pointed out that the upper dermis in rosacea is quite abnormal and shows evidence of both solar elastotic degeneration considerably in advance of what might reasonably be expected for a group of middle-aged Britishers and other dystrophic changes that are not easily categorized. Autoradiographs after injection of tritiated thymidine and enzyme histochemical tests have suggested that small dermal blood vessels are also involved in rosacea (probably secondarily). It is my belief, based on these findings, that the primary disorder is a dermal dystrophy resulting from "weathering" (sun, wind, and cold) and an inherent susceptibility to this process. The dermal attenuation produced in this way causes lack of dermal support for the sub papillary venous plexus, allowing these channels (and the neighboring lymphatics) to dilate enormously. The flushing seen in rosacea is in all probability the result of the vessel dilatation - not its cause. The dilated vessels could become incompetent in addition as a result of the persistent and extreme pooling seen in them and this in turn may lead to diffusion of injurious macromolecules and mediators of the inflammatory process into the dermis. [4]

Dr. Marks labels this as a hypothetical process, with which I agree, but I can conceive of no other reasonable hypothesis that so neatly explains the features we see. Kligman supports this view in his essay on the subject, stating, "I, and others, regard rosacea as fundamentally a vascular disorder" [5].

In researching the literature while writing this chapter, I was delighted to find such valuable support for my working theory of the disorder (which follows shortly), but having read the supportive opinions of the experts, the next question of course must be "What is the vascular abnormality, and what causes it?" The question is neither addressed nor answered by Marks or Kligman. Instead, Kligman pointed out that the "histopathology of rosacea always shows the classic signs of damage to the dermal matrix, namely elastosis, collagenolysis, and increased glycosaminoglycans." He felt the changes were so similar to those seen in the advanced photodamage seen in the fair and often freckled skin of men of Celtic heritage that separating the two "is difficult and may be fruitless because the two may come together," but neither he nor Professor Marks went so far as to suggest that this actinic damage might extend to weakening of the other collagenous supporting tissues in the area. I strongly suspect that damage to the supporting material of the follicular portion of the FPSU occurs simultaneously as a concurrent or parallel process. Furthermore, I would be willing to suggest that both Kligman and Marks would be likely, upon reflection, to admit that as a possibility.

Indeed, the reason that rosacea and actinic damage "may come together," as Kligman wrote, is very simple. *I believe they are one and the same process.* The impact on dermal collagen causes wrinkles; the impact of sun on the collagen that wraps blood vessels causes the *blood vessels* to dilate, producing the condition called *actinic telangiectasia* (discussed in this section); and the impact

on the collagen wrapping the FPSU allows the *follicular part of the FPSU* to dilate when subjected to internal pressure. And when a weakened follicle dilates, it bursts. Where does it burst? Exactly where you would expect— where the damage from the sun is at its worst—at the top of the follicle where the sun has its greatest impact. Older sun-exposed and collagen-damaged follicular units simply have no chance of making comedones, especially if they are the small short follicles in the superficial dermis of a fair-skinned Celt who doesn't have the deep and voluminous FPSUs that harbor deep aggressive acne. The follicular units of these shorter and smaller FPSUs simply leak or rupture first, producing the papules and pustules of classic acne rosacea because they cannot maintain their structural integrity long enough to progress to or support comedo formation.

Actinic means *caused by the sun's rays*, and *telangiectasia* is the condition of having lots of actinic telangiectases (the plural of *telangiectasis*, the word that describes the involvement of a single vessel). If you look closely, even with a magnifying glass, you will see only a pink blush in the early stages. As time passes, however, the little dilated vessels' walls absorb more ultraviolet light from the sun. That causes more sun damage. Extensive telangiectatic sun damage is easily observed on the cheeks of Peruvian children in the mountains near Cuzco, Peru. The combination of high altitude (about 3800 m) and daily exposure worsens and accentuates the damage.

To understand the mechanics of the problem, first take a look at a common garden hose to gain some insight into how blood vessels are constructed. There is an inner lining that forms a very fragile tube to carry the blood. Around that is a layer of supporting tissue that looks like the concentric woven strings you can see in the wall of a garden hose, and then there is the outside support material. Much of this support material in blood vessels is collagen. When collagen is damaged by ultraviolet light, it deteriorates. That is what causes wrinkles. Take a look at stained skin sections under the microscope, noting the pink and highly structured collagen in the dermis of young healthy skin, and then look at the gray-blue mush in sun-damaged skin. The same thing happens, I propose, to the fine supporting strings wrapped around blood vessels. With such loss of the original firm healthy structure, the blood vessels weaken further. That allows them to dilate, and so more blood will be carried. The vessels actually structurally expand in cross-sectional area so they become big enough to be visible just by looking at them up close.

Over the years, these blood vessels can dilate hugely. They become visible at social distances or even from across a room. The tendency to develop this background facial redness is partly genetic, a point not lost on Prof. Marks and emphasized by Prof. Kligman, who estimated "that the prevalence may approach 35% in adult women of Scotch [sic]-Irish-Welsh Celtic ancestry." Further, he states, "I regard rosacea as belonging to the general class of photosensitivity disorders." Certainly, it is generally developed and worsened by sun exposure, so the fair and freckled part of the population is at greatest risk.

This vascular damage is not, by itself, acne rosacea. This is, purely and simply, actinic (or solar, if you prefer) telangiectasia—caused by photodamage that led to dilated blood vessels. It has no hope of clearing with oral antibiotics or topical creams, lotions, gels, foams, or ointments. The best treatment for structural erythema is preemptive and consists of

1 lifelong aggressive preventive sun avoidance,
2 use of true sunblocks such as hats and clothing, and
3 broad-spectrum (UVA and UVB) sunscreen to aggressively minimize the effects of unavoidable exposure.

Second best is active selective photothermolysis with laser or intense pulsed light (IPL) therapy. More on those later (Section 8.8).

The second component of the redness is *functional erythema*, and that relates to the increase in blood flow through the dilated blood vessels. The increased flow reflects temporary wider opening of the vessels. This comes and goes, and these temporary changes are of course reversible. The simple maiden's blush (and the even more embarrassing male counterpart) is a classic temporary high-blood-flow condition. It can come in seconds and vanish in less than a minute. The menopausal "flush" or "hot flash" that can be so embarrassing as a marker of "the change" is a more prominent and longer lasting (but still temporary) episode of high blood flow. Other longer lasting but temporarily dilators of blood vessels that cause functional erythema are sun, cold, wind, hot drinks and soups, caffeinated drinks, some drugs like niacin, and alcohol of all sorts.

And then there is a special third category of redness— that caused by inflammation. This is best called *inflammatory vasodilation*, and is both functional and structural. It is the *only* part of the redness that can actually be treated (even if only partly) with the medications generally used for "rosacea." If it is possible to get rid of the inflammation, the redness will fade to a certain extent. That will help reduce the color. That is where the tetracycline family of anti-inflammatory antibiotics can be very useful.

Note that decreasing or eliminating bacteria or yeast or Demodex-induced inflammation will reduce the associated inflammatory vasodilation but will not touch the redness from structural dilation. Note that the inflammation that causes the functional redness can also damage the walls of the blood vessels, further weakening them and contributing even more to the structural dilation of the blood vessels.

So why is this important? It is absolutely essential that patients understand that only *part* of the redness will respond to medications. I have seen dozens of patients over the years who have been on long-term antibiotics and numerous other medications, either topically or by mouth, who are frustrated by the expense of the medications, their side effects, and the lack of response of the redness to them. Setting reasonable expectations for patients will go a long way toward avoiding therapeutic disappointment. The failure to explain this can lead to misunderstanding, frustration, and friction between patient and physician. Anti-inflammatory medication, whether topical or oral, does absolutely nothing for purely structural erythema or purely functional erythema. Topical brimonidine gel or even topical oxymetazoline nasal drops or spray provide a temporary paling effect.

1.2.3 The third part, the firm fibrosis

The classic "end stage" of acne rosacea is the rhinophyma, or the "drinker's nose." This is relatively rare, fortunately, and is caused by an increase in thickness of the involved tissue that is termed a *phymatous change*, from the Greek word *phyma* meaning *nodule* or *swelling* (Figure 0.33). The nose is most commonly involved, although the cheeks, forehead, and chin may sport the disorder. W.C. Fields is the actor and personality most often associated with rhinophyma, but President William J. Clinton may be a more familiar face. Alcohol intake has been suspected as a co-factor but need not be present. The true cause may (again, hypothetically) be suspected by reference to the progressive fibrosis that occurs in areas of chronic edema of the lower extremities, a component of stasis dermatitis often seen on biopsy. Some individuals may simply be sufficiently susceptible to overproduction of such material either on their lower extremities or as a result of stasis in the dermis of the face, induced secondarily, as Prof. Marks would suggest, by the vascular damage caused by the sun, not only to the venules but to the lymphatics as well. This results in leakage of proteins and induction of a fibrotic reaction that thickens the areas under the skin in the facial area, and occurs on the lower leg due to gravity and senior citizenship. The reason why *all* patients with rosacea do *not* progress to phyma formation remains a mystery. There does seem to be a genetic predisposition, but choosing new parents is not an option in this age group.

1.2.4 Part four—ocular rosacea

If an itchy, scratchy, or gritty feeling in the eyes occurs in association with other signs of acne rosacea, then consider the diagnosis of ocular rosacea. There is dilation of the blood vessels on the surface of the sclerae (the whites of the eyes) and a swelling of the tissues around the eyes, particularly the eyelids and the eyelid margins (see Figure 0.34). This disorder does not seem to appear often as an isolated ophthalmological disease, so it seems to be truly related to cutaneous acne rosacea. The mechanism of its cause, however, is as mysterious as the cause of rhinophyma.

1.2.5 Putting it all together

While there is no denying that acne rosacea is usually associated with background redness, patients with background erythema and telangiectasia may experience redness and flushing alone. Other individuals with actinic telangiectasia may have bumps alone or bumps and pimples together, with or without phyma formation (thickening of the involved skin), and with or without ocular (eye) rosacea. Combinations of all six features are common, but real acne rosacea starts in the little oil- and hair-producing organs, the FPSUs that populate all but a few areas of our body surface.

So what is the common thread that connects the redness with the bumpiness and the little pustules? We need to go back and look at several parts of the whole, and then tie them all together.

First, we need to review what we know about the epidermal appendages that host this disorder. As discussed elsewhere, we need to use a name that is anatomically more accurate, because the follicular component plays an underrecognized role in the pathogenesis of all the acnes. These appendages have three components, so they are better called folliculopilosebaceous units (FPSUs) (see Figure 0.20) to reflect their actual anatomy.

In classic acne rosacea, there are papules and pustules just like those in some forms of acne vulgaris, but in acne rosacea there is something missing. Consider the curious lack of comedones. This is a major clue to what is going on. If you take a close look at the lesions of acne rosacea, and talk to the patients who suffer from this disorder, two facts emerge. First, the folliculo-papules come up fairly quickly, and they turn into folliculopustules fairly quickly, then they burst and heal, also fairly quickly. When they do burst, there is no "core" or "plug" in the material that exits the folliculopustule. There is usually nothing visible except pus. Acne surgery (Section 8.7.1) is not needed to remove retained foreign material. The involved FPSUs do not spend months gradually building up to the point that the wall of the duct is weakened, leaks, and then ruptures as happens with acne vulgaris. Acne rosacea is different from acne vulgaris; it is quicker and shallower. Why should that be? It appears that the same processes that are acting on healthy young FPSUs in acne vulgaris have an entirely different effect on the FPSUs of patients with acne rosacea. For an explanation, we need to look back to the section on actinic telangiectasia (Section 1.2.2, "The 'Redness' Part"). What causes the telangiectases to form? Profs Marks and Kligman agreed that this was caused by damage to the support structure of the thin walls of the capillaries in the upper layers of the dermis. And what causes that damage? Ultraviolet (UV) light, specifically the damaging "superficial" UVB and the "deeper" UVA rays of wavelengths from 280 to 400 nm. This is the same ultraviolet light that damages the collagen supporting the fresh smooth face of youth. For an example, look at another comedonal disease, Favre–Racouchot syndrome. It is not common, but its presentation and location are classic examples of what too much UV light can do on the convex curved surfaces of the face. It is apparent that destruction or weakening of the support tissue, the fibrous root sheath, and its analogs (Section 0.4) allows dilation of the duct and permits development of the classic picture in that disorder. Indeed, the full descriptive name of Favre–Racouchot syndrome is "solar elastosis with comedones" (Figure 1.5).

That picture takes a long time to develop, but the physical location on the convex facial surface of the

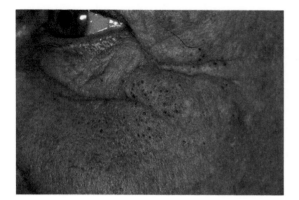

Figure 1.5 Longstanding sun exposure gradually weakens the collagen and other support tissues that wrap around and support the follicular units, allowing them to dilate. The keratin and some sebum pool in them, and some even turn dark, as on this man's cheek.

malar, orbital rim, and zygomatic areas of the face plus the associated actinic damage bear witness to the likelihood that the pathogenesis is mediated by photodamage. There is simply not enough stretch in that thin material, wrapped like a vinyl glove around the FPSU, to push these blackheads out of the weak-walled and dilated follicular canals. If you have ever had the opportunity to (sorry to offend anyone) squeeze the material out of Favre–Racouchot lesions, you will know that the keratinous mass is soft, mushy, and greasy. Its mechanism of formation relies on the weakness of the duct, the duct's expansion, and the failure of the overly compliant follicular wall to contain the mass and generate the pressure required to empty the passively filling follicular unit. This is a compliant variation of the mechanism and sequence of events that produce the hard keratinous plug in acne vulgaris.

So let's apply what we know about sun damage to acne rosacea. Look at the intimate association of the papulopustules of classic acne rosacea with actinic telangiectasia. They are basically located on top of each other. While this has led to a new classification of this disorder, the close relationship of these two features of the disorder has been, I believe, misinterpreted. *This is not just a geographic association of two different processes; it is one single environmental impact that is responsible for the two most prominent features of the disorder.*

I propose that UVA and UVB exposure is sufficiently potent and penetrating to damage the collagenous sheath that supports the wall of the follicular unit. In youth, this support structure is quite strong and forms a natural constrictive resistance. Newly formed keratinocytes and sebum press against it and are forced toward the surface by the resistance provided, so the pressure created empties the duct. That allows no time for the microcomedo to accumulate, and in youth it is unusual to have the sheath (that vinyl glove again) weakened by UV photodamage. But the rupture of the sun-weakened ducts' support does occur on occasion. Acne vulgaris flared by sunlight does occur. But, more importantly, this supports the suggestion that the reason why there are no comedones in acne rosacea and the reason why acne rosacea lesions are short-lived are pretty simple, and they are identical in both cases.

The explanation is simply that the walls of the follicular portion of the FPSU are weakened by the same UV light that caused the actinic telangiectasia. Acne rosacea pores simply lack the ability to resist the early expansion of the follicular canal, and they burst early in the game. Indeed, they burst long before the follicular canal has a chance to make a visible comedo. The break occurs at the top end of the follicle, because that is where the sun damage is the worst. Likewise, these weak follicular canal walls are so thinned that they leak easily, which leads to early activation of the innate and adaptive immune systems, so pustule formation and destruction of the upper end of the FPSU also occur early.

In short, acne rosacea is a distinct variant of the folliculo-occlusive disorders called the acnes. The basic cause of the lesions is identical in all acne types, but acne rosacea is localized to its specific distribution because of solar exposure. That sets the stage for the other players on the field, and that is a whole different story.

1.2.6 The inflammatory epiphenomena in acne rosacea

Each of the three acnes is distinct. The distinctions include location, time of life, the impact of environmental variables, response to therapy, lesion type, and the triggers. The eruptions of acne rosacea occur mainly on the face and in sun-exposed areas, and the general pattern is of follicular plugging, early rupture, inflammatory reaction, and healing. The reasons for the plugging and rupture are explained in this chapter, and ways to prevent, modify, and treat them will be dealt with in this volume. In addition, there are a

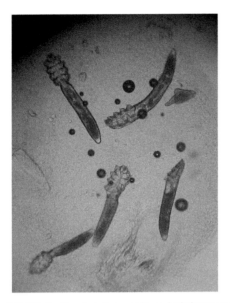

Figure 1.6 This family of adult, juvenile, and a baby Demodex mite had occupied a pustule on the forehead of a rosacea patient. The background shows pus and a keratinous plug (plus some round air bubbles).

number of variables that are important in the development of the inflammatory reaction.

Inflammation in acne rosacea, as in all acnes, is driven by the immune systems responding to materials considered a threat to the organism. As described in Section 7.1, that means that anything that should be "outside" (or above) the basement membrane is considered the enemy (see Figure 2.7). Foreign material on the surface, if it gains access through a scratch or cut, will be attacked. Likewise, anything that is caught under the epidermis (like an ingrown hair) or takes up residence in the pores (there are several organisms to consider) has the potential to stir up trouble. It is time to look at these.

There are five sets of troublemakers that occupy the follicular portion of the FPSU:

1 The classic invader in acne vulgaris is the "acne bacillus" described in Chapter 6.1. It is now known as *Propionibacterium acnes,* or *P. acnes.* It has been the target of dermatologists using antibiotics for over 60 years. For reasons that will be explained in this book, *P. acnes* does not seem to be a major player in acne rosacea.

2 The next most-blamed invader is a mite, a tiny free-living and mobile little beastie called *Demodex folliculorum* (Figure 1.6). It is a cousin of the itch mite that causes scabies. Although usually simply referred to as

Demodex, there are about 65 species. These little fellows and girls live head-down in our open follicular openings. The males actually come out at night on the skin surface, mate, and then return to their pores. One wonders if the females also are night wanderers; otherwise, how would the infestation spread? The mites have been considered by many dermatologists over the years to be simply innocent bystanders, but there are recent clues that they are likely seriously involved in some, although perhaps not all, cases of acne rosacea [6]. One of the clues is from simply sampling the material in the little pustules that show up on patients' faces.

3 There is the interesting and increasingly likely possibility that part of the immune reactivity related to the *Demodex* is due not to the mites themselves but to their colonization by another organism, *Bacillus oleronius.* This bacterium lives in the gut of the *Demodex* and is apparently susceptible to the antibiotics that are useful in cooling acne rosacea [7]. Even more interesting, there is evidence in the serum of patients with acne rosacea of immune reactivity to antigens from *B. oleronius* [8].

4 The fourth of the five troublemakers is not a living organism. It is the contents of the follicle that are actually produced by the FPSU itself. Even in the least hairy areas of the face, tiny little hairs are usually produced by the FPSU. They may be so small that they are essentially invisible, but they show up in microscopic sections prepared from rosacea-bearing skin. In acne vulgaris, they are headed up the follicle to the surface but sometimes they can be seen tightly curled up in the middle of the comedonal plug. Just like ingrown hairs, they seem to be quite capable of causing the acute inflammation that is the hallmark of acne rosacea, and they are sometimes seen in the material prepared for KOH examination from pustule contents (Figure 1.7).

It is assumed that there are also bits of retained adherent keratinocytes in this material, and it is generally understood that loose keratin under the skin is not welcomed by the innate immune system. When an epidermoid cyst ruptures under the skin, exposing released keratin, it is sterile but it causes a massively hot and tender inflammatory reaction that is often mistaken by the unaware for infection. The resolution of such lesions, brought about by simply removing the keratin (and the germinative epithelium surrounding it), is both swift and impressive. Likewise, simply opening these little

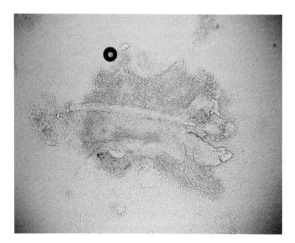

Figure 1.7 The innate immune system reacts to ingrown hairs, likely even the tiny ones like this, caught in a keratinous plug in a folliculopustule in acne rosacea.

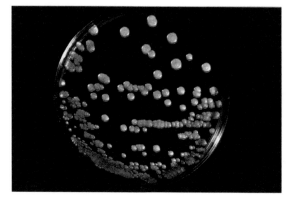

Figure 1.8 Instead of using the olive oil overlay, the nutritional requirement of *Malassezia* is met in Dixon's agar by including glycerol mono-oleate. From http://www.mycology.adelaide. edu.au/gallery/yeast-like_fungi/

rosacea pustules brings about a very quick over-night cooling of the lesions.

5 The last of the troublemakers is not well described at all in the literature on acne, but I have found it to be a factor in most of the referred cases of rosacea I treat. The fact is that the organism is also very important in the pathogenesis of acne vulgaris, a truth ignored for over 30 years, and that story is covered in the section on acne vulgaris (Section 1.1) [9]. The organism in question is the yeast *Malassezia furfur* (Section 6.2). There seems to be only one species involved in the acnes, but it is a challenge to link it with scientific rigor to any particular disorder because of three simple facts:

First, it is everywhere. Cultures of this yeast, using material taken from the scalp, its natural reser-voir, are almost universally positive. It loves to live where its natural food, oil from the sebaceous glands, is present.

Second, it doesn't always cause disease. Indeed, there is a good case to be made that it is the victim, not the aggressor.

Third, it has relatives (there are 14 *Malassezia* species in all), and a close relative, *M. globosa*, appears to be responsible for the seborrheic group of disorders [10]. This trio of facts makes it very difficult to actually prove the relationship between the yeast and several cutaneous disorders. The yeast is accepted as having a causative role in tinea (or pityriasis) versicolor, and the same is generally true of *Malassezia folliculitis* of the upper back, upper chest, and shoulders, but there is ongoing discussion about its role in seborrheic der-matitis, psoriasis, and atopic dermatitis. And when it comes to acne vulgaris and acne rosacea, there is hardly a mention in the modern literature.

In making the case for *Malassezia*'s role in these dis-eases, a conceptual problem arises. Based on early medi-cal school teaching that pus means infection, and pus needs to be cultured, the natural tendency of infectious disease specialists, research dermatologists, and some clinical dermatologists is to culture the pus and see what is growing. If one does that, and the contents of a rosa-cea pustule are sent to a general bacteriological lab, the report comes back as "no growth," "normal skin flora," "no evidence of staphylococci or streptococci," or "light growth of staphylococcus epidermidis." Despite the unconscionable cost of acquiring this essentially useless information, an exercise done in pursuit of satisfaction of the standard-of-care criteria for managing pustular infections, none of these reports is helpful.

The reason for the failure to find the culprit yeast is simple—*Malassezia* is a "picky eater." It must have fatty acids of a chain length of 12–24 carbons, or it cannot grow and thrive. These fatty acids are not present in the usual culture media used for examining putative bacte-rial infections. so the yeast does not grow.

If *Malassezia* doesn't grow, then it cannot be reported and so it is ignored. It is not hard to culture. All one needs to do is put a thin layer of olive oil on the surface of the standard Sabouraud dextrose agar with cyclohexamide culture medium, or mix olive oil into the agar, or use the special Dixon's agar (Figure 1.8), but it is extra work and extra expense, and no commercial lab is generally interested in the yeast so its presence simply is not reported. About 25 years ago, my partner and I interested a local hospital lab in growing *Malassezia* (back when it was called *Pityrosporon*), and after numerous positives we (and the lab) got bored and dropped the practice. The simple fact is that the *Malassezia* yeast is everywhere. Finding it is no surprise, it adds no information, and (unfortunately) it drives nobody to consider therapy.

The other side of the coin is the difficulty in linking it with specific diseases. This is especially difficult when the disease is common (e.g., acne vulgaris, psoriasis, seborrheic dermatitis, atopic dermatitis, and of course acne rosacea). The problem stems from the fact that *Malassezia* itself is normally a simple innocent bystander. It makes no toxins, it does not invade tissue, and it doesn't destroy tissue. Mostly it just sits on the surface of the skin or goes down our follicular orifices looking for more food, the special fatty acids in the oil in the sebum made by the sebaceous part of the FPSU. At least, that is its status until something happens to call attention to its presence, and that is when the fun begins.

So what happens? We humans have an immune system (actually, two of them) always looking for trouble. And if the yeast is present in material that breaks through from the "outside" material in the follicular canal and gets through the leaks in the follicular wall and escapes into the "inside" of the dermis, the trouble starts. The body's "first responders," the innate immune system, recognize the invaders immediately and that starts a "fire drill." A whole cascade of reactions is triggered, and there is redness, swelling, pain, and heat—the classic signs of inflammation. This causes the red bump we know as a folliculopapule, and that is followed in a very short time by a folliculopustule. The reaction continues until the threat is eliminated, which generally means the pustule breaks (or is evacuated by its owner) and healing proceeds.

One problem in proving the relationship of the infection or inflammation to the yeast is the difficulty in satisfying "Koch's postulates." These postulates comprise a set of four rules that were set up in the nineteenth century to "prove" the causal relationship of an infectious organism to the infection it causes:

1 The microorganism must be found in abundance in all organisms suffering from the disease, but should not be found in healthy organisms. The problem here

is obvious; *Malassezia* is everywhere, but not all hosts suffer the disease.

2 The microorganism must be isolated from a diseased organism and grown in pure culture. This is easy to do but is not often done.

3 The cultured microorganism should cause disease when introduced into a healthy organism. The problem here is that the microorganism is already introduced to all of us. Some of us have trouble; most do not.

4 The microorganism must be re-isolated from the inoculated, diseased experimental host and identified as being identical to the original specific causative agent. Again, we all wear the yeast, so this is pointless.

In fairness, Koch's rules have been bent in many directions over the years and are now really of historical interest only, but I still am called to explain this to disbelievers at clinical meetings on a regular basis. It is really best to consider the reaction we see as being more like an allergic contact dermatitis rather than an infection. As an analogy, just about everybody wears jeans at some point, but only a very few of us are allergic to them.

And that is what is happening here—some of us are actually allergic to the yeast. So the problems caused by the inflammation are not caused by the yeast attacking us humans; rather, we humans have immune systems that are attacking the yeasts. We are suffering from "friendly fire." I've seen dozens of women over the years with acne rosacea that is triggered in part by yeast, and there is one story I hear over and over again that tells a tale and reinforces (but does not prove) the theory. Almost invariably, I would say over 90% of the time, if you ask a woman with *Malassezia*-associated acne rosacea if she has ever had problems with vulvovaginal yeast, the response is "Yes, once or twice, many years ago, but not recently." These women, I believe but cannot prove, have a very well-developed adaptive immune response to yeast. That response was triggered years ago as a result of vulvovaginal exposure to *Candida*. That exposure has been sufficiently effective in providing a defense against further episodes of *Candida* that there have been no further problems from the *Candida*, which is *Malassezia*'s cousin. That exposure and response also seem to set up a cross-reactive sensitivity to *Malassezia*. This cross-reaction is strong enough to show up as an itch (likely immunoglobulin E mediated) but is not strong enough to eliminate the *Malassezia* from the skin surface, or from the pores.

It is worth noting that women who have had vulvo-vaginal yeast infections are very quick to recall how itchy the problem was. Consequently, if a woman with rosacea reports that itch is a part of her problem, then *Malassezia* is almost certainly the major troublemaker down in her pores.

One caution is in order here: women with *Malassezia*-mediated acne rosacea have often had the condition for so long that they do not even realize they are itchy. They often will have simply scratched the tops off their little pustules, usually without even realizing it (or admitting it). This often occurs at night, during twilight sleep when they really are not in control of their wish to scratch. But the history of itch or the presentation with excoriated papules, even when itch is denied, is satisfactory evidence of likely *Malassezia*-related inflammation. The differential diagnosis where itchy papules exist is *Demodecosis*, so that presents us with two treatable conditions—more on how to do that treatment later.

The fascinating thing is that these women (and a few men as well) will not be aware of the itch until after successful treatment has been completed. That is why I call *Malassezia*-induced inflammation the Joni Mitchell disease—because of the line "You don't know what you've got 'til it's gone" in her famous song "Big Yellow Taxi." It is a part of rosacea that is actually made worse by the usual antibiotic treatment and generally goes both unrecognized and untreated.

1.2.7 The "acne rosacea" versus "rosacea" controversy

This confusing change in the name occurred when an Expert Committee suggested a change in the criteria for the diagnosis of rosacea. A new classification, erythema-totelangiectatic rosacea, was added [11]. The criteria for making the diagnosis were changed so that anyone with persistent redness of the center of the face (central facial erythema with or without telangiectasia) fits this diagnosis. This is true even though they suffer from nothing more than the sun-induced changes once known simply as "high colour" in the British literature and as rosy cheeks in everyday writing. This tendency of the convex areas of the face, particularly the youthful "apple" of the cheeks, to accumulate sun damage is a very natural aspect of life, a point recognized by artists over the centuries. Surely, all the rosy-cheeked cherubim and

seraphim and the Infant Christ Himself depicted by artists over the past 500 years were not all afflicted with rosacea!

If you would like to explore the nomenclature problem further, you can see the Expert Committee's work at http://www.rosacea.org/class/classysystem.php. My objection to it, and the Committee's response, comprise Appendix A.

In this book, acne rosacea is one of the acnes. And *rosacea* is an adjective, not a disease.

1.2.8 Summary

In summary, where there are numerous dilated blood vessels caused by sun damage, it is proposed that there is also damage done to the supporting structure of the FPSUs in the same area. This weakening of the wall of the follicular duct preempts the development of visible comedones, predisposes to easily ruptured folliculopapules and folliculopustules, and sets the stage for the immune-mediated inflammation that characterizes the rosy clinical picture presented by the combination of actinic telangiectasia and acne rosacea.

1.3 Acne inversa (formerly hidradenitis suppurativa)

The French surgeon Verneuil described a disease in 1864 that he named *hidradenitis suppurativa* (HS), thinking that it was a disorder of the apocrine sweat glands. Subsequently it was realized that the primary area of involvement was, as in acne vulgaris, in the follicular portion of the FPSU. The term *acne inversa* (AI) was first applied in 1991 [12]. That paper set the ground rules for the use of the term at the time.

> Acne inversa is a chronic inflammatory disorder of sebaceous follicles and terminal hair follicles and is one type of (the) acne diseases. The pathogenesis of acne inversa is identical with that of the other types: Hyperkeratosis of the follicular infundibulum leads to a comedo. Bacterial infections result in a rupture of the follicular canal followed by a granulomatous inflammatory reaction with abscesses, panniculitis and draining sinuses.

Although a shift seems to have been gradually occurring recently, particularly in Europe, the newer term AI has not been fully accepted by all workers in the field. This is partly because many of us are traditionalists; partly because some of us are too lazy to think about new names, even when the old name has lost relevance; partly because patients, most physicians, and the medical literature are more familiar with the old term; and partly because AI is a term that suggests that the condition occurs in areas that are upside down (inverted) from the usual location of acne—a concept that doesn't relate well to reality. There is, however, a new and scientifically accurate reason to support this term. That discussion will come a little later.

For now, I am using the term *acne inversa* because it fits with the unitary concept of this book—the concept that all three acne conditions are indeed variants of a single, if somewhat complex, disease process. The differences among the acnes are produced by three factors:

First, they occur in different, but sometime overlapping, geographical areas of the body.

Second, they affect different types of FPSUs.

Third, they actually involve different areas of the FPSUs.

AI has been described, under its synonym *hidradenitis suppurativa*, as an orphan disease. That implies that it has been abandoned by its parents. In day-to-day practice, unfortunately, it is more often than not abandoned by its "foster parents," the physicians and surgeons who should have been caring for it. It is not taught in many medical schools, is poorly taught in most dermatology training programs, sometimes dealt with using the most heavy-handed surgical techniques conceivable, and is regularly ignored or misdiagnosed (or both) by family physicians, emergency room physicians, plastic surgeons, gynecologists, infectious disease physicians, and even our dermatology colleagues. There are dermatology textbooks in which it cannot be found. It is often so completely serially ignored by members of the medical community that the patients themselves, having visited a number of physicians with no results, abandon both hope and care. They hide, lose jobs, lose social contact, lose loved ones, give up on therapy, and fade away from their physicians. They show up in our offices, in urgent care, or in the emergency room, not out of hope for a cure but only out of despair because of the pain, ashamed of their wounds, and embarrassed by the inescapable odor that often accompanies unpredictable discharges.

But there is now some hope. A small group of dedicated researchers and clinicians from around the world has renewed interest in the disease. In 2006, they were cajoled into attending an international meeting by a persuasive Californian suffering from the disorder. Indeed, she helped finance the event. Hosted and chaired by Professor Christos Zouboulis in Dessau, Germany, the group is still in touch, has met once more in San Francisco, and is presently reorganizing as separate but cooperating North American and European Foundations. (See http://www.hs-foundation.org.) Both are working at various aspects of the disorder. At the forefront of the slow but steady push forward is the senior author of the first book in 50 years to deal exclusively with "Hidradenitis Suppurativa," Professor Gregor Jemec of Copenhagen [13].

The disease starts with the same early plugging of the follicular portion of the FPSU that occurs in acne vulgaris. The expanding plug causes gradual dilation and eventually a rupture of the fragile wall of the unit. This in turn leads to an explosion of inflammatory activity but, instead of pushing up to the surface, discharging pus and the keratinous plug, and then healing like most boils and acne vulgaris lesions, the inflammation travels horizontally and over time it creates gel- and pus-filled sinuses under the skin that grow sideways and eventually erupt to the surface. These inflamed and interconnected sinus tracts, initially sterile, may then become secondarily infected, adding to the inflammation and causing swelling, scarring, drainage, pain, odor, and a great deal of patient distress. This is most common in areas that are under pressure from tight underwear, close-fitting clothes, belts, brassieres, bra straps, and the pressure of sitting and other local trauma. It can also occur in areas where regular acne vulgaris is common, on the face and neck and behind the ears, in areas that are not at all "inverse." Patients with this disease who develop facial acne have a deep nodular and scarring variant of resistant acne that is very difficult to treat.

The way this disorder progresses brings us back to the name of this condition. In this variant of acne, the leaks and ruptures that lead to all the trouble occur right next to the *deepest part* of the *follicular* unit of the FSPU. Anatomically, this is where the sebaceous glands originate. They are attached at the lower end of the follicular tube, forming the sebofollicular junction (Figure 1.9). This appears to be the site of the weakness that leads to the leakage and eventual rupture of the wall of the FPSU [2]. That breach in the wall allows the contents to leak, and that starts the inflammatory reaction (Figure 1.10). That reaction can be very intense, causing increasing and self-perpetuating damage to the area and

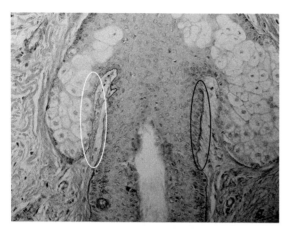

Figure 1.9 Note the variation in the thickness of the PAS+ (periodic acid–Schiff positive) support material, 2–3+ on the outside of the pilar unit (black oval) and 1/2 to 1 1/2+ on the inner aspect of the sebofollicular junction (white oval).

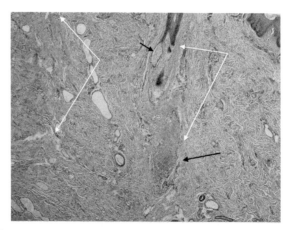

Figure 1.11 Double white arrows show areas of destruction, with smudged scarred collagen. The short black arrow shows a diminished residual sebaceous unit. The long black arrow indicates a pilar papilla under destruction.

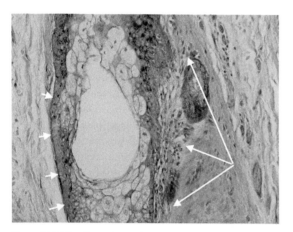

Figure 1.10 The short arrows show periodic acid–Schiff (PAS) 2+ and no inflammation; the long arrows show PAS 0–1+ and active inflammatory infiltrate.

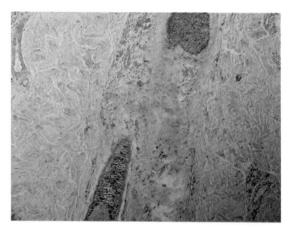

Figure 1.12 The uninflamed healthy collagen on either side of this half-destroyed sebofollicular junction provides evidence of the specificity of the inflammatory attack. No sebaceous gland remains.

destroying the sebaceous glands and the pilar unit in the process (Figures 1.11, 1.12, and 1.13) [14].

This initiating chain of events occurs at the most *inverse* part of the follicular portion of the FPSU. It appears likely that this physical defect and weakness is in this *inverse* location whether the involved duct is present in the classic groin and armpit areas of AI or on the "non-inverse" face and neck. It is for this reason that I have accepted and will use and promote "acne inversa" as a reasoned, and reasonable, name for this variant of acne. Accepting this explanation brings a degree of logic to the name of the disease, correcting a misnomer that

has existed since the inaccurate assignment of responsibility to the "sweat glands" by Verneuil well over a century ago and specifically to the apocrine sweat glands by Brunsting in 1939 [13].

Note that there is no destruction or even inflammation directed at the apocrine glands themselves. They stand unharmed in a sea of inflammation (Figure 1.14). This disease was never a hidradenitis; it has always been a variant of acne. Nor has it ever been a disease that started in the pilar or sebaceous portions of the FPSU, hence the need for the new anatomic and histologic

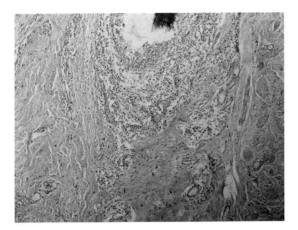

Figure 1.13 The outline of the residual parts of the pilar unit is just barely visible.

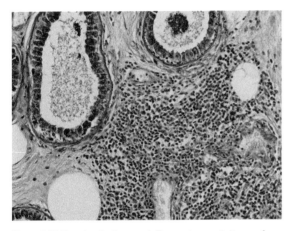

Figure 1.14 Despite the intense inflammatory activity nearby, the apocrine glands show no structural damage.

terminology, recognizing the sebofollicular junction of the FPSU as the site of the problem.

In summary, acne inversa is a disorder of follicular keratinization characterized and caused by plugging of the follicular portion of the FPSU and leading to rupture of the *inverse* end of that structure at the sebofollicular junction.

No matter where it happens to be on the skin surface, acne inversa really *is* acne turned upside down.

1.3.1 Before the rupture, where and why?

If you haven't read the section on the influence of solar damage on the development of acne rosacea, it is time to back up and read it now (Section 1.2). You need to

know what is happening in the top end of the follicle in sun-exposed FPSUs.

So having absorbed that lesson, give some thought to what happens to the follicular support tissue in AI/HS. Think about the effect the sun has on the involved areas. Could it be that the acroinfundibular part (the top end) of the follicles in the intertriginous and genital areas are naturally quite strong, tight, and easily plugged partly because they get NO sun exposure? Suppose we take a giant conceptual leap of faith forward at this point. Could it be that the effectiveness of laser light in managing AI/HS (see Section 8.8.2) is partly dependent upon damaging the support tissue of the upper part of the follicle and allowing it to empty instead of plugging up and rupturing? Of course, there is no proof of this yet, but I think it certainly would be worth a careful scientific look. There are several other links to light (or the lack of it) in this problem—more on that in due course (see Section 8.8.1).

1.3.2 After the rupture, what next?

The events triggered by the rupture of the duct are numerous, interrelated, complex, difficult to treat, destructive, self-perpetuating, and only partially understood. Much of what we see is the result of inflammation caused by the immune system's reaction to material that was in the plugged pores. If you have ever had an ingrown hair, you know that the swelling and tenderness are out of proportion to the size of the hair. Even more important, if the hair is plucked out of the pore or even just flipped free from being trapped (without being plucked), the inflammation goes away almost immediately. No antibiotic is needed.

Why? Because this is an *inflammation*, NOT an *infection*. No bacteria or yeast are required to cause the redness and swelling. This is the kind of inflammatory reaction that is caused by our *innate immune system*, and the reaction may be later augmented by our adaptive immune system. See Sections 7.1 and 7.2.

1.3.3 So what invaders are important in acne inversa?

Just as in acne vulgaris, the contents of the follicular portion of the FPSU make up the foreign materials that set off the inflammatory reaction. Keratin, which is what makes up our hair and nails, the surface of our skin, and the lining of the follicles, was designed to be "on the outside." When keratin is sitting in the pore as a hair or a duct-lining keratinocyte, there is no problem, but if the hair is "ingrown" into the dermis, the innate immune system under the epidermis recognizes it almost immediately and the inflammation starts. But think how amazingly fast the inflammation goes away when the ingrown hair is flicked out of its little tunnel under the epidermis (the top layer of the skin) and onto the surface. No foreign material in the wrong place = no inflammation.

The same thing happens with the keratin of ingrown toenails. It is a bigger procedure, but removing the part of the nail that has become ingrown, or surgically cutting away the overhanging skin tissue, leads to fairly quick relief. This is true even when prolonged use of antibiotics has proven useless. There is a lesson there. No foreign material in the wrong place = no inflammation.

Keratin from the burst follicular portion of the FPSU is instantly spotted by the innate immune system. It causes almost immediate inflammation [15]. We recognize the swelling that shows up around the follicle as an acne vulgaris folliculopapule or as the hot painful early nodule of AI/HS. If the inflammation proceeds to the point that pus is formed, a folliculopustule (pimple) has occurred. The point is that keratin, which is normally our friend, protector, and crowning glory as our skin, nails, and hair, is the enemy when it gets caught where it shouldn't be. If a simple epidermoid cyst on the back bursts, a huge reaction to the keratin occurs, even though the keratin is sterile and may have been sitting quietly protected in the intact cyst sac for decades. All of the antibiotic in the world won't cure that reaction, because the inflammation is NOT caused by infection. Real infected cysts are really rare. But inflamed epidermoid cysts (often misnamed *sebaceous cysts*) are very hot, very sore, and usually very sterile. Total evacuation of the keratin and the entire leaking epithelial sac that surrounds the keratin mass is curative. No foreign material in the wrong place = no inflammation.

If the immune system's recognition of keratin was the only thing causing the inflammation, one could simply empty the keratin and reactive pus and expect healing. But in AI, we have a problem. The problem may be fairly easy to look after if only one fresh new hot spot has occurred, but there may be masses of active spots.

Let's take a look at a solitary inflamed AI/HS nodule first. Remember, the process is upside down in the follicular structure, with the trouble at the bottom or the side of the follicular structure. Just emptying out the keratin and the pus with a stab incision and a squeeze

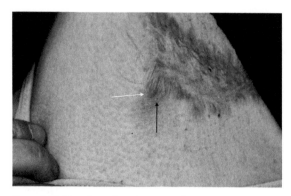

Figure 1.15 Note the red tender area (white arrow) with no comedo and the tombstone comedo (black arrow) next to it.

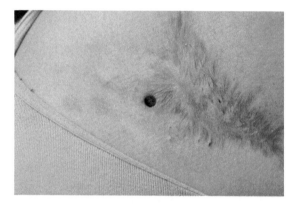

Figure 1.16 Excision site placed to remove both inflamed lesion and tombstone comedo.

will give temporary relief—*but it leaves the damaged follicle behind*. That means the whole process can start all over again. So what is the answer? It is so simple that I wonder why nobody has thought of it before. All that needs to be done is a simple procedure using a biopsy punch, basically a sharp and disposable little instrument that works like a round cookie-cutter. We usually use these in dermatology to do biopsies and they come in various sizes. A 4, 5, 6, or 7 mm biopsy punch can be used to take out the whole plugged and leaking inflamed FPSU. It is really quite simple to do and, because local anesthetic is used, it is then possible to aggressively squeeze out and debride any residual pus and keratin (Figure 1.15). The wound is sealed with a chemical coagulant bleeding-stopper (ferric chloride is preferred) and left open with nothing but a petrolatum dressing, to leave a small scar (Figure 1.16). This works well on fairly small, early, solitary lesions of AI. For painful spots in the areas under breasts, under bra straps, along panty lines, and on buttocks, the pain relief is a joy. (See Section 8.7.2.1 for full operative details.)

A much more involved problem occurs when the lesions are multiple or have been untreated for too long. This happens far too often and is generally caused by delays in diagnosis, misdiagnosis, inadequate treatment, inadequate prevention, and inappropriate incision and drainage (I&D) procedures in doctors' offices, operating rooms, urgent care facilities, and emergency rooms around the world. It is sad but true that AI/HS is so commonly mismanaged that mismanagement is the de facto standard of care. Why does this disease cause so much trouble, and what is the best way to treat it?

One needs to understand that, from a practical point of view, there are three ways to treat AI/HS surgically. The first is described above, punch ablation or debridement and mini-unroofing of a single complete inflamed FPSU. It is appropriate for solitary lesions and works best in new lesions. The second is the unroofing technique, described below, which is useful in managing the older and well-established localized single or multiple nodules and sinuses. These *can* be rendered quiet with aggressive medical care prior to the unroofing, but the medical care is at best a temporary substitute for, or preparation for, the surgical unroofing. At the other end of the line is the need for the third option, full surgical excision of the entire involved area with appropriate margins. This may be the only way to manage the massive, draining, malodorous, scarred, and sinus-ridden involvement of the axillae, groin, perineum, buttocks, or genitals (or, even worse, combinations of these).

The Hurley three-stage classification that is used in HS/AI is based upon the number of lesions, the number of areas, and the extent of the involvement of the entire patient rather than the individual lesion types. While the Hurley stage gives us a classification of the severity of the disease in general, it is only a rough therapeutic guide. Thus, even the worst Hurley Stage III patients may benefit from selective use of all three of these surgical techniques, depending upon the age, type, activity, and location of the lesions. And the preventive medical dietary and behavioral changes must continue in place for years, if not for a lifetime. (See Chapter 8.)

So what does one do for patients who have large nodules and abscesses that involve more than one FPSU but are not bad enough to need the full surgical excision and repair? Basically, one must recognize first that what

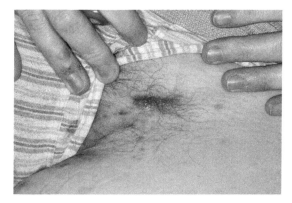

Figure 1.17 This is actually the first of several lesions, some of them communicating, that involve this left inguinal crease.

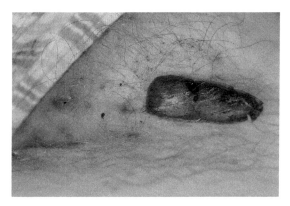

Figure 1.18 A simple oval cut with scissors cleared the area nicely. Further extensive work was needed to the left, inferomedial to this lesion.

we are dealing with is NOT primarily an infection, even though there may be some secondary infection. The inflammatory chaos that the patient presents to the physician is due to a massive innate immune response to retained keratin and other debris. It is in essence an out-of-control "ingrown hair" reaction that has "gone nuclear." It may sound simplistic, but Grandma was right; if you get the core out, then everything settles down. Even the ancient Romans knew that, and gave us the instructions "*Ubi pus, ibi evacua,*" Latin for "Where there is pus, evacuate it." The debris must be removed and the wound provided with the best conditions possible for healing. Removal of debris is called *debridement,* and the only way to fully debride that material from under the skin surface is to remove the entire roof from the nodules, sinuses, and abscesses, and clean them out (Figures 1.17 and 1.18).

Unroofing is remarkably simple compared to the major surgery used for Hurley III. It can usually be done in the doctor's office, the outpatient clinic, or the emergency room. No hospital admission is needed, and there are several other advantages. Time off work is usually minimal. (See Section 8.7.2.2 for full operative details.)

1.3.4 What makes this disease behave so much worse than acne vulgaris?

The major difference, recently demonstrated, is the location of the break in the follicular wall and the sequence of destructive events that follow. There has been a series of papers published recently that tell us more about this area than we ever knew before. The important features are the following:

There is apparently a defect in the support structure of the FPSU, with no support (or very weak support) right at the spot where the sebaceous glands originate from the follicular unit, just above the upper level of the pilar unit [16].

Inflammation appears in areas where the support structure is thin or missing. That pinpoints the area where the breakdown occurs.

The inflammation consists of all the regular series of inflammatory cells one would expect [15].

The sebaceous glands have been shown to almost disappear, blown off by inflammation [14].

In areas where the sebaceous glands are gone, there is visible inflammation and scarring. The destructive inflammatory process leaves behind little stumps where the sebofollicular junction previously existed.

Just below the sebofollicular junction in the pilar unit of the FPSU is a group of cells that produces a visible bulge, so it is called the bulge region. This is a segment of the pilar unit between the attachment site of the arrector pili muscle to the pilofollicular structure below, and the beginning of the sebofollicular junction at the isthmus above (Figure 1.19). The arrector pili muscles make the hair on the back of your arms stand up in a chill. More importantly, that bulge area is where stem cells come from.

The main job of these stem cells is to make sure the hair follicle and hair root are stimulated to grow and replace themselves, to be sure that the FPSU continues to grow hair even if it is damaged, and to repair all portions of the FPSU if and when damaged. Thus,

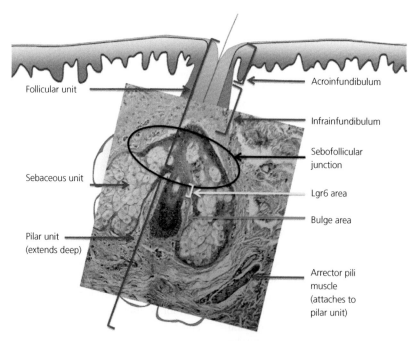

Figure 1.19 The stem cells that form the bulge migrate from the deeper part of the bulge upward toward the sebofollicular junction, and their characteristics and potentials change as they move "north." The stem cells bearing the Lgr6 marker (in yellow) are, at the time of writing, the best candidates for producing the epithelialized sinuses that represent the FPSU's attempt to heal.

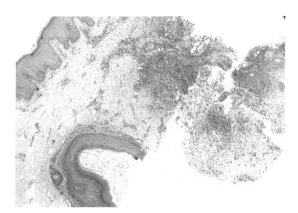

Figure 1.20 This biopsy was taken early in the development of a single lesion, and was done with a 6 mm punch. The material recovered contained a localized area of gelatinous material at the lower right in addition to the fragment of exploded FPSU and the intense inflammatory activity located more superficially.

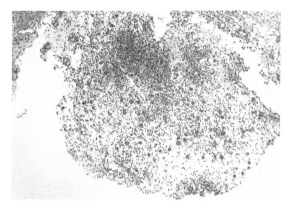

Figure 1.21 Scattered throughout this loose gelatinous matrix are several cell types, including keratinocytes, inflammatory cells, evolving new capillaries, and about 20 little round bundles of cells that are suspected to be "activated keratinocytes," likely of stem cell origin, likely from the Lgr6+ population, and the likely source of the small structures in Figures 1.23 and 1.24.

stem cells can turn into all sorts of cells. When the sebofollicular area ruptures, the break occurs right next to the area occupied by the stem cells, and the closest stem cell variety to the sebofollicular junction is the Lgr6 series. The inflammation appears to allow (or perhaps stimulates) the stem cells to break loose, and they float off into the surrounding mixture of inflammatory cells and fluid. A population of "stem-like cells" has been identified in this inflammatory material by Gniadecki, and it is hypothesized that they are the source of the characteristic material found in AI/HS lesions [17].

These stem-like cells and accompanying inflammatory (and reparative) cells exist in a gelatinous soup. It is rich in nutrients because the body makes sure that the environment for healing is as good as possible. The hormones needed to stimulate the growth of hairs and indeed the entire androgen-driven FPSU are surely present. The stem-like cells appear to be quite capable of living life on their own, and newly created islands of actively growing and dividing cells appear (Figures 1.20 and 1.21) floating in the gelatinous mass. Indeed, the "stem-like" cells are suggested to initiate the growth of these islands by changing themselves into more specialized structures, which is exactly what stem cells are programmed to do. All this needs proof, of course, and the technology is improving every day.

In summary, it is beginning to look like AI/HS is caused by the coincidental physical proximity of a congenital weakness in the follicular wall right next to the congenital strength of the stem cell line. Quite the coincidence!

When these islands come together in the invasive proliferative gelatinous mass (IPGM), genetic programming appears to get to work. Because the source of these activated keratinocytes appears to be from stem cells and stem cells are tasked to perpetuate and repair the folliculopilar structure, they attempt to create a hollow structure whose first product is a protective PAS + (periodic acid–Schiff positive) basement membrane equivalent, most likely fabricated by the basal cells it is protecting on the outside, and lined on the inside, as these structures mature, with squamous epithelium. This presumed genetic stimulus, carried by the stem cells, almost certainly pushes the little round collection of cells to become the little islands (Figure 1.22) that continue to grow and coalesce, making groups of hollow structures that join together (Figure 1.23). This seems likely, barring another explanation, to be the source of the extensive network of interconnecting sinuses that extend under the skin in AI/HS (Figures 1.24, 1.25, and 1.26).

Importantly, there is no histological evidence that these epithelialized sinuses originate as down-growths from the plugged and ruptured follicles, as has been suggested. To the contrary, the residual upper part of the FPSU retires from the field of battle and becomes the receptacle in which the open tombstone comedo occurs.

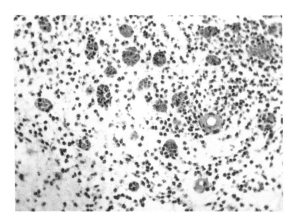

Figure 1.22 The difference in morphology between the newly formed capillary (right central) and the other little round bundles of cells is apparent. Marker studies to accurately identify these structures are under way.

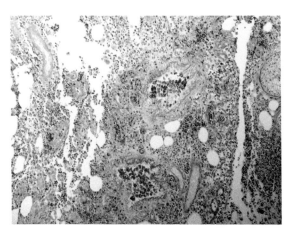

Figure 1.24 The structure appears to be no accident. The remarkably PAS+ (periodic acid–Schiff positive) cells in the center are a feature of the pilofollicular structure. See Figure 1.12 and the bulge area in Figure 1.19.

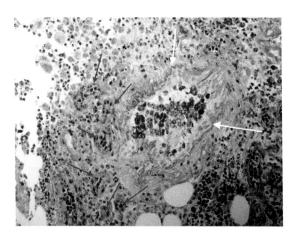

Figure 1.23 The central structure is apparently the precursor of the sinus tracts. Its first chore appears to be the fabrication of a protective barrier of PAS+ (periodic acid–Schiff positive) material. This is obvious centrally (white arrow), but on closer observation one can see several other younger structures (likely evolved from the "little round bundles") showing faint early PAS+ barrier development (red arrows).

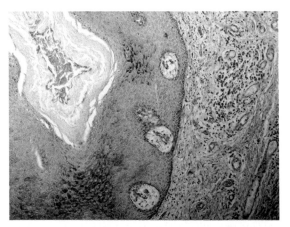

Figure 1.25 The protective PAS+ (periodic acid–Schiff positive) layer has allowed coalescence of several of the primordial sinus structures. Note the outer PAS+ material, the basal cell layer, the acanthotic "epidermoid" sinus lining, and the immature but recognizable laminated keratin, all under development.

The proliferative gelatinous mass in which 'stem-like' cells do their growth magic is a unique material, not well described in the literature. Histologically, one observes areas of acute and chronic cell inflammation nearby, but the gel is relatively sparsely populated. The initial accumulations of epithelioid cells do not seem to attract much in the way of inflammatory activity. They seem to live charmed lives and are apparently avoided by both immune systems. The new structures remain undisturbed during their formation and early growth. This may be due to preferential protection conferred by their status as stem cell products, or due to their PAS+ outer layer. As these structures mature, enlarge, and rupture, they are doubtless recognized eventually as foreign material. They are then responsible for turning on the innate immune system and all its inflammatory mediators, in the same way as ingrown hairs under the skin do. We are, however,

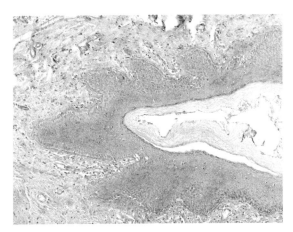

Figure 1.26 The PAS+ (periodic acid–Schiff positive) layer is better developed, now a healthy and protective 3+; the epidermoid lining is better defined; a stratum granulosum has developed; and the keratin is truly laminated.

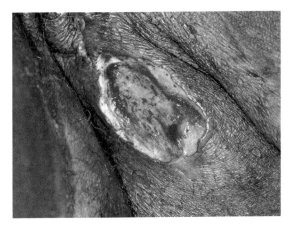

Figure 1.28 Clean healthy base. This tissue wants to heal; it just needs to be given the opportunity. Ferric chloride and petrolatum normally heal such wounds in about 10–14 days.

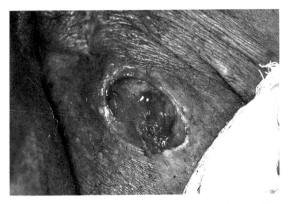

Figure 1.27 This indolent lesion had been present for months. Note the invasive proliferative gelatinous mass (IPGM) at the base.

fortunate that these stem cell islands never seem to organize to produce terminal hairs, a missing complication for which we can be very thankful. Nor do they seem to produce any sebaceous glandular material, restricting themselves to attempting to reconstitute the follicular unit.

Despite the severity of the inflammation, it must be emphasized that the IPGM (Figure 1.27) caught under the dermis and progressing laterally is not infected, although it is certainly inflamed and very uncomfortable. More importantly, when one opens a nodule by unroofing it, pus is released only if there is active inflammation, due to either the foreign body effect of

the trapped material or secondary infection. Instead, the proliferative mass is revealed as amorphous gelatinous tissue that can often be simply curetted or wiped away, leaving clean dermis and subcutaneous fat that heals quickly with topical petrolatum alone, normally needing no antibiotic (Figure 1.28). This is not the pink to bright-red bleeding vascular matter of which granulation tissue is made. Nor is it the "slimy" intraductal material that comprises bacterial biofilm [18]. IPGM is a unique gelatinous substance that populates almost every chronic AI nodule. It is both the cradle and the royal jelly of the sinus tracts. It is another feature of AI that warrants much more investigation.

1.3.5 So what can one possibly do to settle down all this inflammation?

There is to date no known way to dissolve the IPGM by taking oral medication, or by injecting intralesional steroids or other anti-inflammatories. It is actively growing tissue and is very healthy. It appears to be spawned by fresh stem cell activity induced to repair the damaged follicle. It produces, and provides a matrix for the development of, a structure composed of well-defined collagen and glycoprotein-based supporting material. This material supports a brand new and healthy basal cell layer (I suspect this is a cooperative effort between the basal cells and IPGM-resident cells, likely fibroblasts) and gives the sinus tracts protection from the destructive activity of the inflammation.

The inflammatory component can be cooled in several ways, but usually only temporarily.

1 *Steroids*: The classic use of prednisone orally, the regular and repeated use of intralesional triamcinolone acetonide, and the occasional use of intramuscular triamcinolone have all shown variable effectiveness against individual lesions and areas of involvement.

2 *Antibiotics*: Over the years, the most popular anti-inflammatory medications have been the tetracycline family of antibiotics that just happen to be very efficient anti-inflammatories as well. Tetracycline (no longer inexpensively available in the United States), minocycline, doxycycline, and lymecycline have all been used, and other regimens have included clindamycin and rifampicin (alone and in combination). The polyantibiotic approach has recently been escalated to include a troika of very potent antimicrobials—rifampin, moxifloxacin, and metronidazole combined [19]—each of which in its own right has significant anti-inflammatory activity. A novel antibiotic monotherapy using intravenous ertapenem, which is claimed to have no such anti-inflammatory activity, has been shown in a limited early series to have similar results. Long-term follow-up is not yet available.

3 *Nonsteroidal anti-inflammatory drugs (NSAIDs)*: While these have been used, their effect is unpredictable and episodic unless used in doses that otherwise threaten health.

4 *Narcotic analgesics*: These are sometimes necessary postoperatively or for short-term management of painful nodules. We have seen a few enterprising drug seekers who take no interest in any management other than for their pain, which they contend, of course, is unrelenting and unresponsive to anything but the requested narcotic of choice.

5 *Biologics*: The demonstration that tumor necrosis factor alpha (TNFα), interleukin 23 (IL-23), IL-17, and innumerable other cytokines are involved in the inflammatory reaction of AI/HS is no surprise—where there is inflammation, one will find inflammatory mediators. Ever more potent, ever more specific, and ever more expensive, the "biologics" do work in the short term to cool the inflammation. While significant success has been achieved in cooling parts of the inflammatory process, the search for the magic bullet, the one medication that will settle everything down, continues. None has yet produced a lasting cure of AI, but the inflamed tissue can be significantly cooled to the point that surgery is easier on both the patient and the surgeon. Long-term reliance on these drugs for maintenance therapy threatens both the bank account and the health of patients relying on them.

Knowing, as we do now, that all these anti-inflammatory weapons are usually ineffective (there are occasional exceptions) in the long run, what is the option? One needs to remove the substances causing the inflammation and prevent more from forming. And the earlier this is done, the better the result.

As a case in point, consider the bright young woman who presented as I was writing this chapter. Imagine how this painful, draining, and smelly involvement of her vulva interferes with her everyday life as a busy and intelligent college student. Her love life? I did not embarrass her by asking. The point here is that she came to see my partner and me having already been started elsewhere on what many consider the last best hope—a "biologic." She had been using adalimumab (Humira®) for the prior six months. It may have cooled her a bit, but it will never address the underlying problem. It was simply not working, really. She needed immediate unroofing to spare her from ineffective I&D at her college's emergency room, and to spare her from the mutilating plastic surgery (a partial vulvectomy) that was being planned. After gentle peripheral local anesthesia by a well-trained medical assistant (who can take the time needed for proper unhurried anesthesia), all her wounds were unroofed. Several threatening milia, comedones, and small cysts were also detected and unroofed. She had the areas dried up with ferric chloride and coated with petrolatum, and she and her mother got on a plane for the 1000-mile trip home, thence back to school in a distant state (Figures 1.29, 1.30, 1.31, 1.32, 1.33, and 1.34).

In contrast, a patient with labial involvement untreated with the anti-inflammatory biologic discharged copious amounts of purulent material (Figure 1.35). Gently sponging away the draining pus revealed classic IPGM that was then removed (Figures 1.36 and 1.37). Worthy of note is that an I&D procedure (discussed further in Section 1.3.6) would have produced pain relief and a satisfying amount of blameworthy pus, but would have done nothing to eliminate the IPGM.

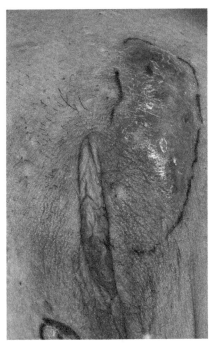

Figure 1.29 The lesion was uncomfortable, was not as painful as it had been, and was not as swollen, but it "just won't go away and keeps getting bigger."

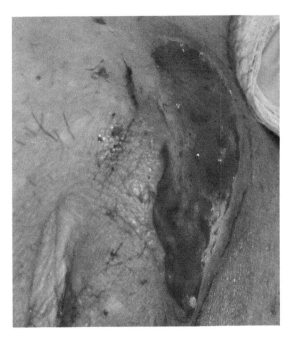

Figure 1.31 Looks pretty clean. Maybe just a little ferric chloride and petrolatum, and that's all that is needed?

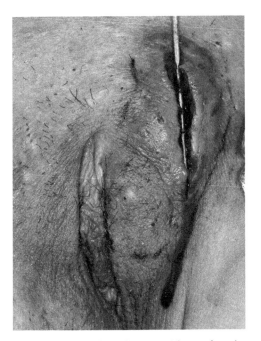

Figure 1.30 Not a drop of purulent material was released, a useful condition most likely attributable to the adalimumab.

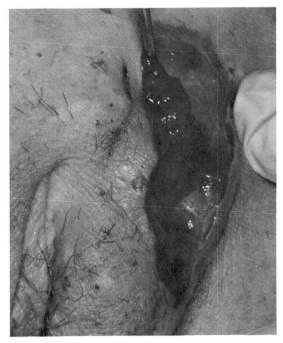

Figure 1.32 Looks like there is something else here besides pus or keratinous debris.

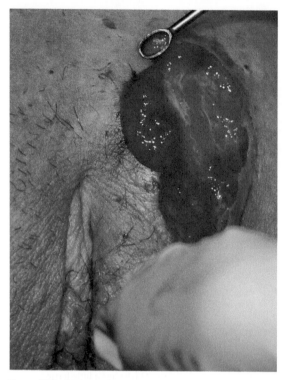

Figure 1.33 This is not keratin, it is not pus, it is not granulation tissue, and it is not fat. This is the invasive proliferative gelatinous mass (IPGM).

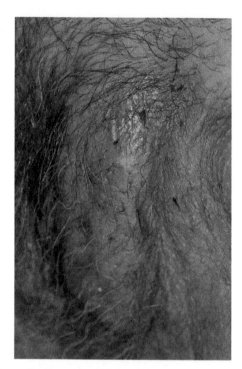

Figure 1.35 This very tender lesion was about 2 cm × 5 cm. It was a much more impressive red before the local anesthetic was placed.

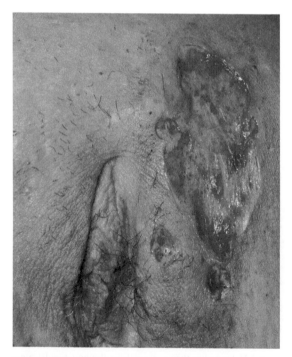

Figure 1.34 Here is the clean base of the lesion: uninfected dermis that will heal beautifully with nothing more than petrolatum.

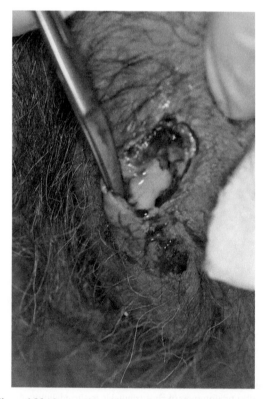

Figure 1.36 The purulent drainage is a reliable indicator of the degree of pain.

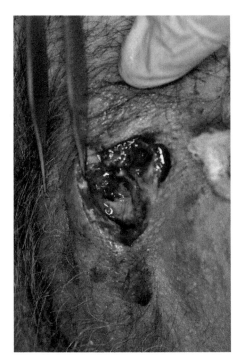

Figure 1.37 Under the purulent material, there is characteristic invasive proliferative gelatinous mass (IPGM).

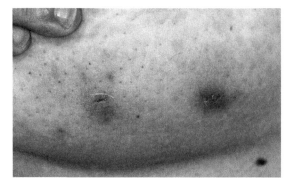

Figure 1.38 These were both incised and drained (I&D'd) about 5 days prior with simple stab wounds. Note the profusion of plugged pores in this inframammary area.

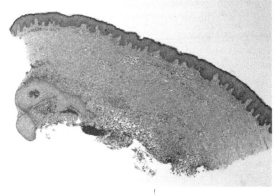

Figure 1.39 This is the top of the specimen removed using a punch biopsy, about a week after the patient had had an I&D in the emergency room. Note the residual mass of actively growing keratinocytes trying and failing to repair the ruptured FPSU. The inflammatory infiltrate that was producing the swelling and pain is obvious; indeed, beneath this there was significant abscess formation and foreign body reaction.

1.3.6 So how do you get rid of all this material?

The first step is, of course, making the correct diagnosis. Sufferers from AI/HS will almost always have had experience with receiving the erroneous diagnosis of "boils" and having the I&D (incision and drainage) procedure done in their physician's office, a clinic, or the emergency room (ER). Hot, fluctuant, secondarily infected lesions are unbearably painful and the I&D gives almost instant relief, even if it is little more than a stab wound administered after a quick blast of ethyl chloride spray. Unfortunately, as succinctly put by Professor Jemec in the *New England Journal of Medicine*, "Lesions treated with incision and drainage routinely recur" [20]. The reason is simple. Failure to remove the IPGM perpetuates the problem.

Figure 1.38 illustrates a case in point, a patient who had two flared AI nodules on the underside of her left breast. She was unable to arrange to attend our office, so instead she visited a local ER where I&Ds were performed and she was placed on antibiotics. The relief was short-lived so she sought further help, and when she arrived I was able to obtain punch biopsies of both I&D sites. The

residual debris contains fragments of the destroyed follicle wall (Figure 1.39). This material not only is the stimulus that triggered her innate immune system's hot response but also is thought to be the source of the stem cells that would, if left behind, lead to development of the sinus tracts that are the hallmark of AI/HS.

So, how does one avoid such local recurrences? See Section 8.7.2.1, "Mini-unroofing."

1.3.7 What does the future offer?

A recent excellent review concluded with the words, "Future investigations should be dual and more focused on the pathogenesis of HS at immunological and bio-molecular level. The focus should be on molecular genetics, biophysical effects on the hair follicles in response to shearing forces, the role of microbiotic flora and aberrant immunological pathways" [21].

Current research aims to identify the prime factors that cause and allow the follicles to burst. The bacteria, their biofilms, and the immune response to these organisms are all secondary—they are epiphenomena. Shearing forces are doubtless triggers, but what is the biomolecular abnormality that differentiates the unfortunate individual, whose sheared follicular unit leads to AI/HS, from the rest of us in whom no such problem ever occurs despite identical trauma?

Recent research demonstrates a defect in the lower part of the follicular unit, at the sebofollicular junction [16]. Present speculation suggests that this defect may have to do with an error in metabolism of collagen or another component of support protein. It is likely hereditary and may perhaps be contributed to in part by low ascorbic acid levels, either on a dietary basis or as a result of smoking. This occurs in a follicular unit that is overexpanded as a result of dietary hormones and growth factors in dairy foods and high-glycemic-load diets, just as happens in acne inversa's little brother, acne vulgaris. The combination of dairy, our modern high-glycemic-load diet, a simple vitamin deficiency, nicotine, and a genetic weakness may eventually be shown to be the kindling and fuel for a lifetime of misery.

1.4 The psychology of acne

If one were to list the stresses of the teenage years, I suspect the top seven would be acne, drugs, family, friends, money, school, and sex. The numerical rating given each would vary from teen to teen but, for many, acne and its psychological impacts overshadow everything they do. Acne vulgaris is bad enough, but AI/HS in a young person can be truly devastating.

1.4.1 Acne as a stress
When I discuss the hormonal causes of acne with patients, I tell them that the hormones that make acne worse come from three sources. The first is their own internal hormones from their ovaries or testes. The second is from various factors in their diet. The third is a small group of hormones related to stress.

The original paper on stress and acne was based on a small study done on students [22], but it doesn't take many days of working with patients to realize the profound and tight interactions between stress and acne. If you practice in a college town, the cyclic impact of midterms and finals is undeniable.

I point out that one of the ways to reduce the impact of stress is to get the acne better as fast as possible so that patients will feel better about themselves. Gaining control as quickly as possible means they will not need to "stress out" about new acne lesions popping up at irregular, unpredictable, and downright "just not fair" times.

This gives me the opportunity to explain to them that acne caused by stress has been considered for years to be a response to hormones from our "stress glands," the two adrenal glands that sit on top of our kidneys. Most have heard of adrenalin, and they can easily associate that with adrenal glands. They need to know that the adrenalin (*epinephrine* is a synonym) reaction to stress is the "first responder," and the adrenal steroid hormones that trigger acne are much slower to respond. They also come from a totally different part of the gland.

Until recently, the accepted chain of events has been as follows. Stress triggers the release from the pituitary gland of a small polypeptide hormone called *adrenal corticotropic hormone* (ACTH). ACTH's job is to turn on the adrenal glands, increasing their production of several hormones. In addition to cortisol (which helps the body deal with stress), the adrenals also produce testosterone and other hormones like dehydroepiandrosterone sulfate (DHEAS) that can turn into testosterone right in the FPSU, causing more acne.

It has been thought and taught for years that stress-induced acne was an exaggerated response to these adrenal androgenic (and so acnegenic) hormones in predisposed individuals. This is termed "functional androgenic hyper-responsiveness to ACTH" [23]. It resembles an exaggeration of adrenarche, the "start-up" of the adrenal glands that is the real first sign of puberty, even before pubarche, which is the start-up of the ovaries and testes.

This slow pathway likely still contributes to the chronic steady hormone load that operates to help trigger acne, but there is a new player that seems to have a quicker and more direct effect. This faster pathway is stimulated by a chemical called corticotropin-releasing hormone (CRH) that is one step before ACTH. It is the first polypeptide hormone in the chain of command

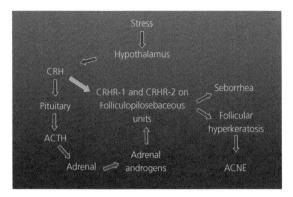

Figure 1.40 The red arrows illustrate the traditional link between stress, the corticotropin-releasing hormone (CRH) it stimulates, and acne. The green arrow illustrates what is now considered the "shortcut." Just to make life interesting, CRH receptors are also present on eccrine sweat glands (that may be linked to the sweaty palms and soles caused by stress), and the FPSU seems to be capable of making its own CRH in its own intracrine system.

from the brain. CRH is activated by stress and is released from deep in the brain, in the hypothalamus. The classical sequence of events was that CRH was viewed as the hormone that released the ACTH, and the ACTH would take the stimulation message to the adrenal glands and they would then multiply the androgenic and acnegenic effects.

We now have evidence that corticotropin-releasing hormone (CRH) may have a life of its own. Recent studies show that the sebocytes in the FPSU have a pair of CRH receptors (CRHR1 and CRHR2), and these appear to be responsive to CRH from the hypothalamus (Figure 1.40) [24, 25].

So, in short, it may be that acne causes stress, stress elevates CRH, CRH triggers ACTH, and ACTH raises levels of acnegenic adrenal steroid hormones that cause acne, but CRH also may directly impact the FPSU, also causing acne. And that, of course, causes more stress, and around we go again.

To break the cycle, we cannot shut down the hypothalamus, or the pituitary, or the adrenal glands, so we need to shut down the acne. The stress will cool as the acne fades, at least as far as the stress is due to the patient's concern about his or her acne. The whole system will slowly but surely decelerate, like a car when you take your foot off the accelerator. This slowing takes months in acne vulgaris and years in AI/HS, but the results are worth the wait.

1.4.2 Acne and self-image

The physical consequences of acne are painful, unsightly, and even messy. The scars are too often permanent. The socioeconomic consequences include interpersonal difficulties, social isolation, altered job prospects, and sometimes chronic unemployment. Then there is the added expense of medications and medical care that leads to a decrease in disposable income. That limits some of life's pleasures.

The psychological consequences include loss of self-esteem, personality change, depression, anxiety, the self-destructive use of alcohol and drugs, and the aspect that concerns us most, the risk of suicide (curiously termed *suicidality*). If all acne patients could gather their strengths around them and turn their energies to overcoming this disorder, they could put the whole thing behind them.

1.4.3 Isotretinoin therapy and the psyche

If you have done any reading about the care of acne, you will have run into the question of isotretinoin and the risk of depression. There is a vast "literature" on the Internet, and a discussion follows in Section 8.4.2.2. But before wading into that very muddy water, it would be fair and wise to provide some scientific balance. Good news seems to travel so much more slowly than bad news, so this time I am going to put the good news up front.

Of recent special and particular interest is the news that isotretinoin, contrary to its Internet profile, seems to directly improve mood. Two fairly recent studies looked at this. The first looked at the psychological profile of patients treated with various topical preparations compared to oral isotretinoin therapy. At the end of the second month, quality of life remained more impaired in the topical treatment group compared to the isotretinoin group. At the end of the fourth month, quality of life and all psychological test scores had improved more in the isotretinoin group [26].

The second paper studied changes in psychiatric parameters and their relationships to oral isotretinoin in acne patients. Two psychiatrists employed four psychiatric assessment tools to evaluate 38 acne patients [27]. The patients were examined before oral isotretinoin and at two and eight weeks after starting the drug, using the Leeds revised acne grading system. Not unexpectedly, the severity of depression (using the Assessment of the Psychological and Social Effects of Acne [APSEA]) and the acne score improved after eight weeks of oral isotretinoin treatment. What was not expected was the finding that the severity of depression decreased after only two weeks of treatment.

Unexpected or not, this observation certainly parallels what we regularly see in patients starting isotretinoin. Those of us in clinical practice have long noted that oral isotretinoin therapy alleviates depressive symptoms. There really is no treatment that brings with it such hope, and delivers such results, as isotretinoin. This second study details improvements in depression directly related to acne-related life quality improvements rather than to improvement in acne lesion grade. These results suggest a direct positive effect on mood, independent of the improvement in mood due to the disappearance of the skin lesions. In my patients, it usually abolishes the negative impact upon mood caused by the Internet as well.

We have known for decades that isotretinoin is the only medication that actively miniaturizes sebaceous glands, reduces sebaceous gland output, and reverses retention hyperkeratosis. It now appears that isotretinoin has been shown to lower Beck's Depression Inventory (BDI) scores as well.

1.4.4 The isotretinoin–depression question

Teenagers are not an easy group to study. This is particularly true when looking at questions of depression and suicide. There have been, for many decades, numerous cases of suicide occurring in individuals with (and without) acne in whom there was no prior sign of distress obvious to friends and family. When this has occurred in someone taking isotretinoin, the drug has been blamed. This leads to the question that we hear whenever we consider prescribing this drug. "What about the risk of depression, doctor? It is all over the Internet." It's a tough and serious question, and it usually is a front for the real and unspoken question, "What about the risk of suicide, doctor?" There is only one safe answer: "If you believe there is a risk and you wish to avoid that risk, you must avoid the drug." Some dermatologists have decided to do exactly that and will not prescribe it. More on this in Section 8.4.3.2.

But let's get back to the population at risk of suicide. Given the subject, which is "touchy" at best and almost a taboo subject, there are barriers to discussing this problem. Interviews with this age group and collection

of sufficient data to be statistically significant are challenging, indeed problematic.

Nevertheless, a baseline of sorts was set out in a study of 9567 New Zealand secondary school students aged 12–18 years [28]. The study centered on "self-reported" acne, depressive symptoms, anxiety, and suicide attempts. The results showed that "problem acne" was associated with increased risk of psychological problems. Note that this refers to acne that is considered a "problem" by the teen reporting in the study. The study showed elevated odds ratios of 2.04 for depressive symptoms, 2.30 for anxiety, and 1.83 for suicide attempts. Basically, the mere presence of problem acne approximately doubled the risks of each of these three conditions. The New Zealand experience may be somewhat more concerning than the North American and European situation, but the reasons for this are not known. It may simply be that the well-contained population of New Zealand is easier to study, and the data more centralized, giving more accurate estimates than are available in the scattered health care "nonsystem" in the United States. Importantly, even after controlling (adjusting the data) for depressive symptoms and anxiety, the odds ratio remained at 1.50 for suicide attempts associated with problem acne. In simple terms, that means that even when there appear to be no signs of depression (visible or admitted) and no signs of anxiety, the risk of suicide is about 50% higher if you have problem acne but are otherwise identical to someone of your age, sex, and so on. This suggests the possibility that a significant number of suicides occur among a small subgroup of patients who concealed their true depressive and anxious feelings. This underlines the authors' conclusions: "Young people presenting with acne are at increased risk of depression, anxiety and suicide attempts. Attention should be paid to their mental health, and the importance of asking directly regarding suicide is emphasized" [28].

The bottom line? Suicide sometimes occurs in teens (and others) who hide their suicidal tendencies, whether they are taking isotretinoin or not. Their final act is a shock to all who thought they knew them well, including parents, teachers, fellow students, coworkers, siblings, and significant others. Reports of these incidents are filled with statements of disbelief, usually to the effect that the victim was happy, well-adjusted, and well-liked, and showed great promise for the future.

As Ms. Ian has sung, "It isn't all it seems ... at seventeen."

So dermatologists must not expect such information to be volunteered. We need to ask; we need to open the door. For those of you concerned about the possibility or risk of planting the seed of "suicidal thoughts" that might be acted upon, the psychiatrists have assured us that this is unlikely. Indeed, it is the unusual teenager who hasn't thought casually about suicide, or experienced it in friends, classmates, or relatives. It may have even been a subject for discussion among teenage friends. A recent US study found that "9 percent of male teenagers and 15 percent of female teenagers experienced some stretch of having persistent suicidal thoughts" [29]. Bottom line? If you are a patient reading this, please be honest with your dermatologist or indeed whoever is doing his or her best to help you. If you are a dermatologist, ask.

A second baseline has been set by Dreno *et al.*, who found that rates of depression among isotretinoin users ranged from 1% to 11% across several studies, with similar rates compared to those taking oral antibiotic [30]. They concluded that "isolated clinical case reports indicate a possible clinical relationship between depressive symptoms and isotretinoin. In these conditions, it appears today that the link between suicides and severe depressions has not yet been clearly demonstrated" [30].

There are indeed numerous other small studies and "isolated clinical case reports" concerned with depression, suicidality, and a possible link to isotretinoin. Several purport to show a link between the use of isotretinoin for treatment of severe acne and self-injury, suicide, and negative thoughts. Evidence to the contrary is now provided by analyses of two large databases. The review by the Guptas of 9.6 million US patient visits "failed to demonstrate an association between isotretinoin use and suicide" and further suggests that "suicidal behavior with isotretinoin represents an uncommon, idiosyncratic phenomenon" [31].

While any life lost to suicide is a tragedy, the blame must not be laid unfairly on any innocent bystander, whether family, friend, colleague, teacher, classmate, prescriber, or isotretinoin itself.

To put this in perspective, and I appreciate that this may be thought to be a somewhat self-serving statement, I have not seen one single illness precipitated by the discontinuation of dairy products by my personal patients over the last 35 years. Nor has anyone committed suicide because I stopped their dairy, although I have heard on several occasions the teen hyperbole "I can't live without my milk."

1.4.5 Isotretinoin in perspective

Isotretinoin is one of the few "wonder drugs" in medicine. Having practiced before it became available, and having seen lives ruined by the inability to control rampant acne, my perspective is broad and deep [32–35]. This drug has changed the lives of hundreds of thousands of patients, and yet the positive impact is not much in evidence on the Internet. The reason is pretty simple—nobody likes to dwell on past problems once they are satisfactorily resolved. Isotretinoin success allows patients to put their acne behind them, usually permanently, and get on with their lives. They really don't want to even remember the problems. They destroy their old photos and ask me to get rid of the "before" photos I've taken for their records.

Enough time has now passed that I see parents previously treated with isotretinoin bringing in their children and specifically asking for isotretinoin. This is the reverse of the situation years ago when the occasional parent would ask, after their offspring was cleared, "Can you please do me now?" Nobody knows the value of isotretinoin better than those whose lives have been turned around.

The positive psychological impact of isotretinoin on hundreds of thousands of patients has been massive, and has been massively underdocumented.

References

1 Plewig G, Wolff HH. Sebaceous filaments [in German; author's trans.]. Arch Dermatol Res 1976 Mar 10;255(1): 9–21.

2 Plewig G. How acne vulgaris develops [in German; author's trans.]. Hautarzt 2010 Feb;61(2):99–104, 106.

3 Zouboulis CC. Is acne vulgaris a genuine inflammatory disease? Dermatology 2001;203(4):277–9.

4 Marks R. Letter: the problem of rosacea. Br Med J 1976 Jan 10;1(6001):94.

5 Kligman AM. A personal critique on the state of knowledge of rosacea. Dermatology 2004;208(3):191–7.

6 Powell FC. Rosacea and the pilosebaceous follicle. Cutis 2004 Sep;74(3 Suppl):9–12, 32–4.

7 Lacey N, Delaney S, Kavanagh K, Powell FC. Mite-related bacterial antigens stimulate inflammatory cells in rosacea. Br J Dermatol 2007 Sep;157(3):474–81.

8 Li J, O'Reilly N, Sheha H, Katz R, Raju VK, Kavanagh K, *et al.* Correlation between ocular *Demodex* infestation and serum immunoreactivity to *Bacillus* proteins in patients with facial rosacea. Ophthalmology 2010 May;117(5):870–7.

9 Leeming JP, Holland KT, Cuncliffe WJ. The microbial colonization of inflamed acne vulgaris lesions. Br J Dermatol 1988 Feb;118(2):203–8.

10 Bikowski J. Facial seborrheic dermatitis: a report on current status and therapeutic horizons. J Drugs Dermatol 2009 Feb;8(2):125–33.

11 Wilkin J, Dahl M, Detmar M, Drake L, Liang MH, Odom R, *et al.* Standard grading system for rosacea: report of the National Rosacea Society Expert Committee on the classification and staging of rosacea. J Am Acad Dermatol 2004 Jun;50(6):907–12.

12 Kuster W, Rodder-Wehrmann O, Plewig G. Acne and genetics [in German; author's trans.]. Hautarzt 1991 Jan;42(1):2–4.

13 Jemec GB, Revuz J, Leyden JJ. Hidradenitis suppurativa. Berlin: Springer; 2006.

14 Kamp S, Fiehn AM, Stenderup K, Rosada C, Pakkenberg B, Kemp K, *et al.* Hidradenitis suppurativa: a disease of the absent sebaceous gland? Sebaceous gland number and volume are significantly reduced in uninvolved hair follicles from patients with hidradenitis suppurativa. Br J Dermatol 2011 May;164(5):1017–22.

15 van der Zee HH, de RL, Boer J, van den Broecke DG, den Hollander JC, Laman JD, *et al.* Alterations in leucocyte subsets and histomorphology in normal-appearing perilesional skin and early and chronic hidradenitis suppurativa lesions. Br J Dermatol 2012 Jan;166(1):98–106.

16 Danby FW, Jemec GB, Marsch WC, von Laffert M. Preliminary findings suggest hidradenitis suppurativa may be due to defective follicular support. Br J Dermatol 2013 May;168(5):1034–9.

17 Gniadecki R, Bang B. Flotillas of lipid rafts in transit amplifying cell-like keratinocytes. J Invest Dermatol 2003 Sep;121(3):522–8.

18 Kathju S, Lasko LA, Stoodley P. Considering hidradenitis suppurativa as a bacterial biofilm disease. FEMS Immunol Med Microbiol 2012 Jul;65(2):385–9.

19 Join-Lambert O, Coignard H, Jais JP, Guet-Revillet H, Poiree S, Fraitag S, *et al.* Efficacy of rifampin-moxifloxacin-metronidazole combination therapy in hidradenitis suppurativa. Dermatology 2011 Feb;222(1):49–58.

20 Jemec GB. Clinical practice. Hidradenitis suppurativa. N Engl J Med 2012 Jan 12;366(2):158–64.

21 Nazary M, van der Zee HH, Prens EP, Folkerts G, Boer J. Pathogenesis and pharmacotherapy of hidradenitis suppurativa. Eur J Pharmacol 2011 Dec 15;672(1-3):1–8.

22 Chiu A, Chon SY, Kimball AB. The response of skin disease to stress: changes in the severity of acne vulgaris as affected by examination stress. Arch Dermatol 2003 Jul;139(7): 897–900.

23 Lucky AW. Quantitative documentation of a premenstrual flare of facial acne in adult women. Arch Dermatol 2004 Apr;140(4):423–4.

24 Ganceviciene R, Graziene V, Fimmel S, Zouboulis CC. Involvement of the corticotropin-releasing hormone system in the pathogenesis of acne vulgaris. Br J Dermatol 2009 Feb;160(2):345–52.

25 Zouboulis CC, Seltmann H, Hiroi N, Chen W, Young M, Oeff M, *et al.* Corticotropin-releasing hormone: an autocrine hormone that promotes lipogenesis in human sebocytes. Proc Natl Acad Sci USA 2002 May 14;99(10):7148–53.

26 Kaymak Y, Taner E, Taner Y. Comparison of depression, anxiety and life quality in acne vulgaris patients who were treated with either isotretinoin or topical agents. Int J Dermatol 2009 Jan;48(1):41–6.

27 Hahm BJ, Min SU, Yoon MY, Shin YW, Kim JS, Jung JY, *et al.* Changes of psychiatric parameters and their relationships by oral isotretinoin in acne patients. J Dermatol 2009 May;36(5):255–61.

28 Purvis D, Robinson E, Merry S, Watson P. Acne, anxiety, depression and suicide in teenagers: a cross-sectional survey of New Zealand secondary school students. J Paediatr Child Health 2006 Dec;42(12):793–6.

29 Nock MK, Green JG, Hwang I, McLaughlin KA, Sampson NA, Zaslavsky AM, *et al.* Prevalence, correlates, and treatment of lifetime suicidal behavior among adolescents: results from the National Comorbidity Survey Replication Adolescent Supplement. JAMA Psychiatry 2013 Jan 9; 1–11.

30 Dreno B, Chosidow O. Isotretinoin and psychiatric side effects: facts and hypothesis. Expert Rev Dermatol 2008; 3(6):711–20.

31 Gupta M, Gupta AK. National Ambulatory Medical Care Survey National Hospital Medical Care Survey 1993–2003 [Internet]. 2008 [cited 2014 Aug 24]. Available from: http://www.icpsr.umich.edu/icpsrweb/ICPSR/studies/29922

32 iPLEDGE. The guide to best practices for the iPLEDGE Program [Internet]. 2012 [cited 2014 Aug 24]. Available from: https://www.ipledgeprogram.com/Documents/Guide%20to%20Best%20Practices%20-%20iPLEDGE%20Program.pdf

33 Layton AM, Dreno B, Gollnick HP, Zouboulis CC. A review of the European Directive for prescribing systemic isotretinoin for acne vulgaris. J Eur Acad Dermatol Venereol 2006 Aug;20(7):773–6.

34 Danby FW. Night blindness, vitamin A deficiency, and isotretinoin psychotoxicity. Dermatol Online J 2003 Dec;9(5):30.

35 Danby FW. Oral isotretinoin, neuropathy and hypovitaminosis A. Clin Exp Dermatol 2009 Oct;34(7):e260.

CHAPTER 2

The folliculopilosebaceous unit—the normal FPSU

The epidermal appendage previously referred to as the *pilosebaceous unit*, and renamed the folliculopilosebaceous unit (FPSU), is an extraordinarily complex organ (Figure 2.1). It has still not given up all its secrets, and this chapter provides a summary of what is known of the normal FPSU, and what influences our numerous FPSUs to swing them from their normal paths, creating the acnes.

2.1 Anatomy

The sebocytes in the sebaceous glands are the sebum-producing units of the FPSU. These glands are found most densely populating the shawl distribution over the convex surfaces from the vertex of the scalp to the horizontal nipple line of the upper trunk, reflecting their role of providing the prime lubricant in the process of parturition (birth and delivery) [1]. Their concentration elsewhere is related to the somewhat variable coverage of the remainder of the trunk and limbs by hair-bearing FPSUs.

The number of sebaceous lobules attached to the base of the follicle at the sebofollicular junction varies from zero to a cluster of perhaps six. The number of FPSUs is likely genetically determined, and the size of the lobules reflects both genetics and the quantity and quality of hormonal stimulation. With age, the sebaceous gland activity fades gradually as hormone levels drop. Significantly, where the prime function of these glands dictates the highest population, over the face

and scalp, oiliness persists into old age, especially in those areas that enjoy a lifelong testosterone stimulus. The hands and feet are spared this oily population, likely on a survival basis. A slightly moist grip and plantar surface is better suited to fight or flight than a greasy one.

A few sebaceous glands may be found around several orifices, ectopically on the labial vermilion of the lips and the genital labia minora, and naturally in the external auditory canal, in the nasal vestibule, and modified as Meibomian glands in the eyelid margins.

2.2 Genetics

2.2.1 Acne vulgaris

The double strands of DNA that carry the genes we inherit from our parents determine whether or not we are likely to suffer from acne, which kind, and probably how bad it can be. If you have acne, the genes had to come from somebody, and even if you figure out who gave you the acne genes, it is too late to change your parents now. You must do the best you can with the genes you were dealt. It is just like playing poker.

On the other hand, if you do not have acne, that does not mean you do not have the genes. The problem is that some genes are fully expressed in all the people who have them (like brown eyes), while other genes (like for freckles) only show up (are "fully expressed") if the conditions are right. For freckles, you need to add sun exposure.

Acne: Causes and Practical Management, First Edition. F. William Danby.
© 2015 John Wiley & Sons, Ltd. Published 2015 by John Wiley & Sons, Ltd.

The FolliculoPiloSebaceous Unit (FPSU)

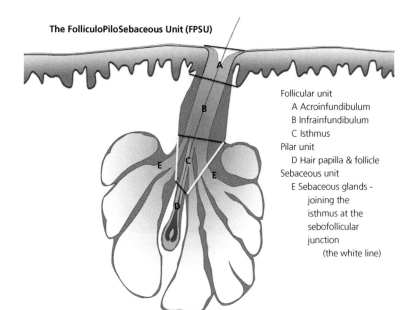

Follicular unit
  A Acroinfundibulum
  B Infrainfundibulum
  C Isthmus
Pilar unit
  D Hair papilla & follicle
Sebaceous unit
  E Sebaceous glands -
    joining the
    isthmus at the
    sebofollicular
    junction
      (the white line)

Figure 2.1 The follicular unit consists of the intraepidermal acroinfundibulum (A), the intradermal infrainfundibulum (B) that extends to the top end of the isthmus (C), and then continues as the pilar unit (D) containing the hair papilla and follicle. The sebaceous unit is composed of all the sebaceous glands that join the isthmus (C) at the sebofollicular junction (E). It is a 360° structure that wraps around the isthmus.

For acne, you need to add hormones. And if you add the hormones without having the genes for acne, you will not get acne. Lucky you! So let's get a little deeper into this.

If neither of your two parents had acne, it does not mean that they are not your parents. The rules of heredity are complicated, and if your mother had just enough acne genes to give you a "half dose," then she could easily have had no acne as a teen. The same may be true with your father, but with two half doses, one from each parent, you could get a single full dose of the genes required to give you acne. You just got unlucky. To use an analogy that you will see again, you were born with a loaded gun. You will need to avoid anything that wants to pull the trigger. A recent study from Italy rates the risk of acne, if one has affected first-degree relatives, at 3.41. So if you have one parent or sibling with acne, the risk of getting acne is almost 3 1/2 times that of the rest of the population who is your age but does not have affected relatives [2].

Just about every patient I see with acne vulgaris has a positive family history. Acne is not always present in other family members, but when the family history is positive, it is both variable and complex. For instance, I am aware of a family with two daughters. One of them has never been troubled by acne. The other one had acne that was so bad at age 11 that she required a course

of isotretinoin. The father and his side of the family have almost no acne, and the mother also had very little. The girls' maternal uncle, on the other hand, suffered terribly with acne on his face and back as a teenager, and still has problems as a senior. Although their mother was not affected, she seems to have carried the gene, whatever it (or they) might be, through to the younger daughter.

There are some very good studies on genetics and acne, the best being those that studied twins. It's not a surprise to me that there is a relationship, but it is worth noting that the expression of some genes rests upon environmental exposures long after the genes are provided by the parents. New babies are born with unfreckled skin but, under the influence of sunlight, one will develop freckles later, and another will not. There are related markers, such as red hair, that can predict which one will likely develop freckles, but there's no guarantee. There are redheads who have flawless "peaches and cream" complexions that never freckle. This is a very rough illustration of the direct influence of our environment on the actual expression of our genes. It is simple and straightforward activation of the genes that were set at the time of conception.

There is another, more complicated influence that needs consideration, a more subtle process that is hidden in the background, and about which we are only now learning. This is the problem of our genes' exposure to various chemical and other influences *after* conception, during gestation (pregnancy), during early life, and during the process of sexual development and maturity. This field of study is called *epigenetics*. More about that in Section 2.3.

Meanwhile, for clarification, the "instruction set" that you are born with, located in the DNA within your genes, is called your *genotype*. What those instructions actually turn out as a product (what you actually look like) is called the *phenotype* (from the Greek word *pheno* meaning "to show, to appear, or to display").

A genotypic freckled redhead (someone who has the genes to make red hair and freckles) who is never exposed to the sun will never be troubled with freckles. His or her genotype will not be expressed as a freckled phenotype unless there is a certain environmental exposure, in this case sunlight, but the red hair will be there whether there is sunlight or not.

I raise this point because some people simply do not seem capable of getting acne. While this makes life a lot easier for them than their pimply brothers and sisters, it does make life difficult for researchers experimenting on the cause of acne. Some study subjects are simply incapable of developing acne. Including such individuals in a study designed to trigger acne would give inaccurate results, because the results of the studies would always be negative in such persons. Only persons who *can* get acne should be included in dietary studies on acne, for instance.

Lucky people with flawless complexions just won't get acne. This is a small percentage of our Western population, but other populations may be different. Over a decade ago, Loren Cordain described two tribes on different sides of the world that did not have acne, both tribes in their aboriginal habitat. One group inhabits the island of Kitava, one of the Trobriand Islands in Papua New Guinea's archipelago. The other, the Aché, live in the jungles of Paraguay. Both groups are hunter-gatherers with predominantly vegetarian diets. The Trobriander people have been thoroughly studied by social anthropologists and human ethnologists, but medical reports have been few. As isolated groups, the tribes' genetics were stable and the environmental influences from person to person within the tribe were likewise pretty much the same, particularly their diet.

Lindeberg *et al.* reported, "The residents of Kitava lived exclusively on root vegetables (yam, sweet potato, taro, tapioca), fruit (banana, papaya, pineapple, mango, guava, water melon, pumpkin), vegetables, fish and coconuts. Less than 0.2% of the caloric intake came from Western food, such as edible fats, dairy products, sugar, cereals, and alcohol" [3]. In eastern Paraguay, the Aché tribal diet contains wild, foraged foods; locally cultivated foods; and 8% Western foods (mainly pasta, flour, sugar, yerba tea, and bread). Cordain's study reported that members of these tribes had no problems with acne whatsoever [4].

The diets, very low in processed food and generally presenting a low glycemic load [5], were given credit for this lack of acne. At the time, the paper was criticized for attributing the lack of acne to the diet because it was thought that these populations might have been genetically incapable of developing acne. It was even suggested that these populations be subjected to a Western diet to see whether or not they would develop acne [6], a reasonable scientific approach in an ethics-free world. Following up this question in discussion with Prof. Cordain, I learned that some of these individuals, when exposed to a so-called Western diet, do indeed develop acne, which certainly suggests that some of them really do harbor the acne genotype. That certainly has been the pattern in other previously isolated groups. Further testing with dietary challenges would be needed to determine the frequency of the gene(s) for acne in that population, work that would challenge ethnologic ethics.

There are other populations that had essentially no acne before the advent of the Western diet. Acne is now endemic among the previously clear-skinned Inuit in the Canadian Arctic [7]. The Japanese and others have been the subjects of several papers [8]. It seems, therefore, that the genetic tendency toward acne is present in most human populations, probably all of them.

The likelihood is that the genetic background is expressed only when the FPSUs are challenged by a specific stimulus, and it is generally accepted that a change in the hormonal environment has that effect. This theme and its mechanism will be fully developed elsewhere. (See Section 2.8.)

It is not only aboriginal populations that develop acne when genes and diets meet. The multicenter study in Italy quoted above [2] has shown acne positively correlated not only with family history, but also with dairy intake and mild obesity. In the population studied, three factors stood out. In addition to an increased risk of 3.41 times triggered by a family history of acne in parents or siblings, being overweight increased the risk of acne by 1.3 to 3.3 times. Third, milk consumption (three 250 mL glasses or more per week) increased risk in the entire population by 1.78 times for any kind of milk and 2.20 times for skim milk [2]. There was no significant correlation to menses and a negative correlation to one serving of fish per week.

It is important to consider that these dietary risks apply to the entire population studied. That includes, at one end of the curve, the subjects who may have no genetic risk of acne at all. They bring down the risk artificially because they have no innate risk of developing acne no matter what diet they consume. At the other end of the curve are those whose acne will be triggered by only small amounts of milk. Remember these results when you get to Section 2.8.

2.2.2 Acne rosacea

The discussion above relates mainly to acne vulgaris, the acne that is common among 85–90% of North American teenagers. With regard to acne rosacea, many of my rosacea patients report that their parents, in their middle and later years, also had acne rosacea. There is little doubt in my mind that this is also genetically influenced, but early work done on this facet of this disease is only beginning to surface.

It is said that "genes rule." While there is little doubt that they load the gun, there are many different influences that can pull the trigger. One study suggests that of the numerous inflammatory mediators that are active in acne, some are heritable as single genes that often control enzymes, neuroendocrine transmitters, and cytokines found in the pathways that lead to acne rosacea's signs and symptoms [9]. A specific genetically determined defect in the skin's ability to handle reactive oxygen species (small, chemically active substances that cause damage) has been correlated with rosacea [10]. On the other hand, in a study of twins, only one of a pair of homozygous (identical) twins developed acne rosacea, suggesting that a nonheritable variable made the difference and was the trigger [11].

It would certainly be no surprise to learn that, ultimately, heredity and environment interact. Just like the freckles and the sun we started with.

2.2.3 Acne inversa/hidradenitis suppurativa (AI/HS)

That this disorder is hereditary to some degree is accepted. A positive family history occurs in 35–40% via autosomal dominant inheritance. That means that each child has a 50:50 chance of inheriting the disorder, and that if you had 100 children then 50 of them would likely inherit the gene (provided only one parent is a carrier). But Mother Nature can be a devious parent at times and it is possible to have four to six involved (or uninvolved) children in a row. Explanations other than random selection and luck are lacking. The family history in AI is often less well defined than in acne vulgaris because family members do not always report the existence of their disease. It is somewhat hidden from view, it is often undiagnosed, and its existence is often denied. Indeed, without the trigger, the genotype would not show up as the phenotype. Nevertheless, I have treated many mother–daughter (and even one granddaughter) groups with this disorder, and a few father–daughter families have shown up over the years. Interestingly, the father–daughter pairs shared a very disfiguring and scarring nodular form of facial acne as well as the acne inversa. And last year a mother showed up with her four-and-a-half-year-old son, who has a history of small "boils" on his buttocks. The mother has mild AI/HS herself. So did her father. And his father. Four generations.

Details of the molecular genetics are emerging. For example, two novel mutations of the nicastrin gene have been associated with the disorder in two Chinese families [12], but it will be a while before we know exactly how they are related to expression of the disorder. Meanwhile it appears that this same problem is not common among AI patients. How the pieces of this giant puzzle fit together remains a mystery.

2.2.4 The Scottish twins

I met Meghan when she was 28. She had had acne since she was 12, and was getting more than a little tired of it. Although there was some variation with her periods, the problem persisted and was active pretty much all the time. She was not sexually active, had never been on any hormonal contraceptives, and was generally content with her life, with minimal stress.

She presented during the early years of my practice when I was collecting dietary data. Meghan had moderately severe nodular acne involving both cheeks, particularly the jawline and under the chin. She had tried numerous treatments; had been on antibiotics, particularly tetracycline, for years; and was pretty fed up. During the "family history," she told me that she was an identical twin, and her sister had never had so much as a single "spot" for as long as she had known her. When I got to asking her about her dietary intake, and in particular her dairy intake, her face lit up. Her eyes widened, and she said to me, "Oh, my goodness, it must be the cream in the milk."

She told me that when she grew up in Scotland, the milk arrived on the doorstep in bottles, and was not homogenized. That meant that the cream had separated, was sitting on top of the milk, and would pour off first when the lid was removed from the milk bottle. She told me that she always wanted to be the first to bring in the milk bottles in the morning, because she loved to use the cream from the top of the bottle. Her sister, quite to the contrary, would drink milk only when forced, and only from the bottom of the bottle.

Meagan agreed to continue with her standard therapy, which at that time consisted of oral tetracycline and topical retinoic acid cream, but to discontinue all dairy products. She started to clear within 2 months, at the end of 6 months she was able to discontinue the tetracycline, but it took a full year before I could convince her to let go of the retinoic acid. I did not ask her to return to her dairy, and I never saw her again as a patient.

She was one of my first successes in dietary management involving twins. Fortunately, it was not necessary to "double blind" the study, because her identical twin sister had already served as a control. Asking a pair of twins to decide which one of them should go off dairy and which should stay on dairy presents problems not only in interpersonal relationships but also in ethics. This is especially true in private practice, where patients present themselves for the best care possible, and are not expecting to be "guinea pigs."

Lesson learned: Twin studies are valuable even with just one set of twins!

2.3 Epigenetics

This is a relatively new field of study. We know that DNA-based genes set the basic rules for reproduction, growth, and function, but there are ways in which the guidance provided by your original genes can be modified. One of the influences on the development of acne may be through epigenetic changes mediated by diet.

The sum total of all our genes (what we now call our *genome*) governs our genotype, basically our genetic typeset. It is represented as a long string of code made up of four letters, typed in on a keyboard that has only four keys—C, A, T, and G. These four letters spell out the DNA code for everything our 23,000 genes can possibly do. Your DNA has instructions for thousands of individual biological reactions. They can be combined in an almost infinite number of ways to direct the many things you do every day, like making oil in your oil glands or growing nails and hair. Others are things you do only once in a while, like heal a cut or have a baby. And there are things your body may never do, like have a bad reaction to a certain drug. The instructions are there in your DNA, waiting.

At conception, your parents load your genome with your special customized mix of Mom DNA and Dad DNA. Your personal unique genotype produces you as a unique person. What is produced (hair and eye color and acne tendency) is your phenotype. The *pheno* part, as mentioned, comes from a Greek word meaning "to show." So your genotype is what is hidden in your genes and your phenotype is what shows.

For DNA to direct a specific task, a mirror copy of a small part of your DNA is made of RNA. This bit of RNA is the messenger that tells your body what protein or other body chemical to make, to do whatever is needed. It is called, logically enough, *messenger RNA* or *mRNA*.

Epigenetics adds to the mix by causing some very small changes in the DNA. One such change is the addition of a methyl group to cytosine (the C) or adenine (the A) in the DNA itself, a chemical change in DNA called *methylation*. Another is the formation of "bookmarks" in the chromatin. These (and several other mechanisms) can lead to certain genes in your DNA being turned on (or off) so they are allowed to make (or are prevented from making) a certain RNA. This changes the DNA's message from doing a certain thing to not doing it, like an on-off switch. In actively reproducing cells, these changes may continue throughout the life of that cell line. There is evidence that, if these tiny changes impact the DNA in sperm and ova, they may be hereditary and can be passed along to offspring.

Think of epigenetic change as a "program update" downloaded from your environment onto part of your genome. The source may be a drug, a toxin, or even a dietary change [13]. Unfortunately, we have no effective protection against such changes, triggered by influences as different as a low intake of folic acid or a high intake of arsenic. Foods, alcohol, drugs, hormones, heavy metals, cigarette smoke, and occupational chemicals—all are suspect. The list is growing, but so far there are no specific studies in acne. As an illustration, however, it has been shown that feeding royal jelly to create queen bees from worker bees (both of whom have the same genome) seems to be mediated by some 550 methylation differences between the queens and the worker bees [14]. These direct the remarkable changes, based on diet alone, that produce a new queen.

It is not difficult to imagine that changes in dietary hormonal intake over a period of time can make significant changes. In one Harvard study, preteen boys who drank milk were about one inch taller than those who did not [15]. There was no other significant difference in their diets, and a recent study confirms this dietary influence on linear growth [16]. This raises the question of the average increase in height that is apparent throughout the entire population in North America, compared to the population in China or other societies consuming less or no dairy. Is this just better nutrition in general, the effect of increased amounts of insulin-like growth hormone 1 from drinking milk, or is this the result of an epigenetic influence?

"You are what you eat" may boil down to "You are what your dietary epigenetic influences tell you to be."

2.3.1 The farmer's boys

My father was a dermatologist, and I joined his practice when I completed my training. He had been caring for a patient from upstate New York, a farmer's son, with terrible acne. At that time, there was a "digestant" on the market in Canada that contained bromide salts and there is a disorder called bromoderma that looks like acne. My father had seen a couple of cases, and he wondered whether there might be a link between bromides and this teenage boy's acne. As it happened, there had been some contamination of the well on the farmer's property, and methyl bromide was at fault. It had been used in the agricultural process of soil fumigation and had gotten into the well. Suspecting that this was the cause of the acne, and being unable to obtain blood levels of bromine at that time, my father attempted to

"wash out" the bromide by the pragmatic prescription of sodium chloride tablets to tolerance. Achieving no significant results after a month of this, he asked me for some assistance with the case.

I had just begun working with milk and other dairy products as a possible cause of acne, and I went through this young man's dietary history for a few minutes. It turns out that the farm was a dairy farm, and the lad consumed roughly two quarts of unpasteurized whole milk daily. He was 17 at the time, and was accompanied to the visit by his 15-year-old brother as well as their parents. The younger brother was likewise involved with acne, over his face, neck, shoulders, and trunk. He was also a very aggressive consumer of his cows' product. At that time, isotretinoin was just becoming available but these young lads were from over the border in New York State, and so I could not prescribe it for them. Instead, I simply asked them to discontinue their entire intake of dairy products, continue on the tetracycline that was the standard at that time, reduce it if possible, and check back in a few months. Winter intervened, but they did show up the following spring, and their active lesions were essentially clear.

A couple of years later, I got a telephone call from the boys' mother. Their 11-year-old brother was now 13, and he was starting to develop acne. What should she do? Could she bring him over to see me? I was surprised to learn that, despite the fairly solid relationship between dairy withdrawal and her older sons' clearance, the youngest son was still drinking lots of raw farm milk. I suggested that this be discontinued, she agreed, and that was the end of the story. Some years later, the mother saw me for an unrelated problem and confirmed that once the youngest brother stopped the dairy, they never needed my services.

Lesson learned: Even the apparently obvious lessons need reinforcement.

2.4 Embryology

The epidermal appendages, true to their Latin roots, "hang down from" the epidermis. They start life in the fetus at an early age, during the fourth month of gestation. They need time to grow because they have work to do in assisting the fetus to eventually leave its watery home and enter the outside world.

The first sign of the FPSU is a small collection of cells budding down into the dermis from the thin fetal epidermis. As the bud grows, it extends deeper into the dermis, during the fourth and fifth months, as a cord or column of undifferentiated epithelial cells. Those destined to become sweat glands head deeper into the fetal dermis. The cord that is the FPSU-to-be develops a collection of cells at its deepest extent that becomes the hair papilla, and this generates the fine fetal lanugo hair, starting at five months.

Outgrowths near the top of the FPSU become differentiated into sebaceous glands; the cords forming eccrine sweat glands elongate and coil in the deeper dermis; and the cords destined to become mammary glands sit quietly in their designated and appropriate locations awaiting adrenarche and pubarche (the two phases of puberty).

The FPSUs get to work almost immediately, producing both the fatty, oily lipid called *sebum* and the keratinocytic part of the slippery, complex, and multifunctional *vernix caseosa* that covers us as newborns.

Among the several postulated functions of *vernix*, the most important, in my opinion, is lubrication. I quote (with a blush) the only published reference relating the hormonal stimulation of the sebaceous glands' prime function to their subsequent role in the problem of acne:

To understand the function of sebum and by extension the reason for our sebaceous glands, one needs to look at the beginning of our lives. We enter the world through a marginally accommodating passage that, under the pressure of the birthing process, is stretched beyond its capacity to provide its own lubrication. Substantial secondary lubrication must be supplied and it needs sufficient substantivity to avoid being squeezed out by the pressures involved. The extra lubrication is supplied by the sebaceous glands that cover the very surfaces that require it, namely those convex surfaces in direct contact with the birth canal. These include the vertex itself and the scalp anteriorly over the forehead and nose to the lower jawline and posteriorly over the shoulders and upper aspect of arms and chest to the extent of what has been called the "shawl distribution."

Evolution has provided fewer sebaceous units inferior to the jawline, in the axillae, on the lateral chest surfaces, and on both the flexural forearm surfaces and the medial aspects of the upper arms — all sites that normally require no such lubrication, having no "trail-breaking" role in a normal vertex presentation and delivery.

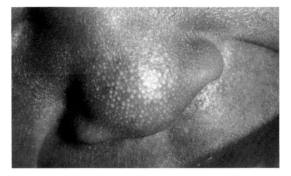

Figure 2.2 We have more natural sebaceous gland activity at birth than at any other time of life. The sebum and water mix called *vernix caseosa* is what lubricates our way into the world.

Evolution has also provided us with apparent proof of this explanation, in the form of an absence rather than the presence of a clinical disorder. Although there does exist a strain of sebaceous gland-deficient (asebia) mice, and although congenital atrichia and anhidrosis are compatible with life in human beings, evolution appears to have selected out as incompatible with efficient reproduction any gene that would lead to what would be termed "asebia totalis congenita," if it existed.

Physical examination of newborns, once one achieves the firm but gentle grip required to evade the lubricating function of the vernix caseosa, often reveals a very prominent population of hyperactive sebaceous glands over the cutaneous convexities (Figure 2.2).

Indeed, although never subjected to measurement, the ratio of sebaceous gland mass to body mass by simple observation is doubtless greater at the time of birth than at any subsequent point in human life. How is it that these little oil glands achieve such prominence just before delivery? It is likely because of the concurrent stimuli of two placental products, the 300 mg/d of progesterone piped directly to the fetus through the umbilical cord and the somatomammotropin known as placental lactogen. Whether the latter should be renamed placental sebolactogen will not be debated here, but this molecule has two targets (fetal sebaceous glands and maternal mammary glands) that share both their embryologic origins and their need for maximal stimulation at this point in the reproductive story.

Later in life, a different somatomammotropin, growth hormone, acts synergistically with progesterone's more potent androgenic relatives to re-stimulate these same sebaceous glands and plague us with acne.

I would like to suggest that the lowly sebaceous glands' crowning achievement is to actually achieve "crowning." This is the penultimate act of the birthing sequence and heralds the arrival of a new life in our beautiful but troubled world. Thanks to our sebaceous glands, the voyage is less traumatic than it would be otherwise. [1]

2.5 Histology

Acne is classically referred to as a disorder of the pilosebaceous apparatus. The problem with that designation is that acne is *not* a disorder of the pilar unit. And acne is *not* a disorder of the sebaceous gland unit, except secondarily. It is actually a disorder of the function of the sebo follicular junction (See Figures 0.21 and 2.1.)

To discuss its intricacies and its disorders, we need a new name for this multifunctional, multitasking, and multipotential cutaneous appendage. For reasons that will be more obvious and relevant in the discussion on acne inversa, I use the term *folliculopilosebaceous unit*, or FPSU. (See the Introduction.)

2.5.1 Onwards and downwards

The follicular part of the FPSU is classically called the infundibulum, and there is no reason to change that. It is basically a tube made up of layers of concentric maturing cells. If you cut it in cross-section, it looks like the layers of an onion or the rings of growth in a tree. The actively growing cells start in the outside basal cell layer and move inwards. With time and as a result of metabolic changes, they turn into thin flattened *ductal keratinocytes*. These are pretty much the same as normal skin cells on the surface of the skin, the thin, flat, layered little fellows called *epidermal keratinocytes*. Their last living function is to separate from each other, a process called *terminal differentiation*. Once these cells are fully differentiated, which is a complex metabolic process, the links between them are dissolved by a protease and they separate from each other and are then free to move in the duct. Together with the hair and the sebum, they flow up the central hollow channel to the surface.

This hollow cellular tube is wrapped in a closely fitted layer of supporting tissues. The first layer just outside the basal cells is actually the extension of the basement membrane. That is the thin layer of tissue between the epidermis and the dermis of our surface skin. Beneath the epidermis, its job is to anchor the bottoms of the basal cells of the epidermis above to the dermis below (Figure 2.3). It then extends down from the epidermis and wraps around the various components of the "pilosebaceous unit," now the FPSU. The horizontal surface basement membrane turns and extends downwards to become the vertical glassy or vitreous layer that wraps around the follicle and the rest of the FPSU.

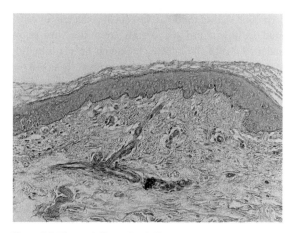

Figure 2.3 The periodic acid–Schiff positive (PAS+) structure that separates the epidermis above from the dermis below is generally homogeneous and well formed, as is the similar material investing vascular and other appendageal structures.

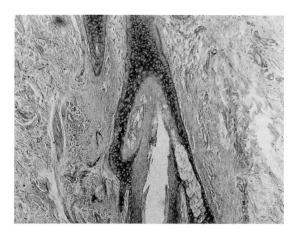

Figure 2.4 Note the well-defined periodic acid–Schiff positive (PAS+) support to the right wall, with no inflammation. On the left, there is marked destructive inflammation from 6 to 9 o'clock, where a sebaceous gland has only a small stump left.

It is continuous because both are produced under the influence of the keratinocyte basal cells above them (Figure 2.4). This glassy or vitreous layer, although it is generally equivalent to the basement membrane, is thicker where it wraps around the pilar unit, lending support. It has a somewhat glassy appearance, hence its name. It is visible on light microscopy with the usual stains but is best demonstrated by using a special technique, the periodic acid–Schiff (PAS) stain. This makes certain substances show up a bright pink (PAS-positive) under the microscope. It makes them easy to see and

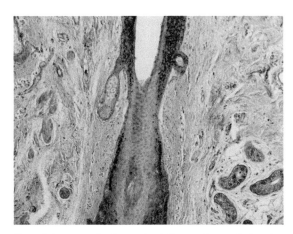

Figure 2.5 Despite the destructive inflammation applied to the sides of the upper portion of this pilar structure, just below the isthmus, there is little to no involvement of the eccrine ducts on the right—hiding effectively behind their periodic acid–Schiff positive (PAS+) protective wrap. Note that the sebaceous glands have been reduced to stumps.

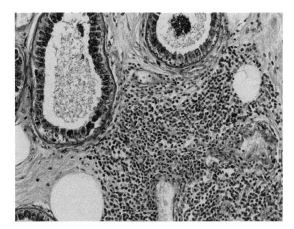

Figure 2.6 These apocrine glands exist in a sea of inflammatory cells, with no suggestion that they are the focus of the activity. There are one or two inflammatory cells beginning to push past the strong periodic acid–Schiff positive (PAS+) protection at 4–5 o'clock on the left and at 6:30 o'clock on the right, substantiating the concept of their secondary involvement.

allows us to estimate or measure the thickness of the basement membrane and its relatives.

The glassy or vitreous basement membrane layer merges into the fibrous root sheath. It is also PAS+ and is composed of thick collagen bundles. This sheath wraps around and contains the follicular portion of the FPSU like a vinyl glove, and extends down to wrap around the pilar and the sebaceous parts as well.

This layer performs two very important jobs. First, the tightness of the wrap provides very significant support to the otherwise weak tubular cellular structures. This wrap limits their expansion and under normal conditions prevents them from overexpanding or simply bursting. The thickness of the wrap is particularly obvious in the eccrine sweat glands and their ducts—they are only one cell thick and would easily burst without this support (Figure 2.5). They have very prominent PAS+ basement membranes. The same is true of the apocrine sweat glands and their ducts (Figure 2.6).

Second, the membrane provides a semipermeable barrier that provides physical separation between the body's "inside" and its "outside." Remember that the basement membrane under the epidermis separates the epidermis, which is considered "non-self," from the underlying dermis, which is considered "self." Material that is enclosed within the glassy membrane is a downward extension of the "non-self" epidermis (Figure 2.7). If you can think of the relationship between these two

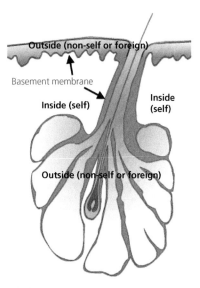

Figure 2.7 The basement membrane (shown as pink under the epidermis) wraps around the whole folliculopilosebaceous unit, like a vinyl glove. Anything above the pink layer, and anything within the vinyl glove equivalent, is considered "non-self" or "foreign" by the inflammatory guardians of the integrity of the inside "self" area.

compartments as "self-inside" and "non-self-outside," it gives you some idea why there is such an inflammatory reaction when the duct bursts, releasing "non-self" materials under the skin into the "self" dermis. If you ever had an ingrown hair, you can now understand why the body reacts to this foreign material. This material, your own hair, is considered by the part of your body beneath the epidermis to be something that was not supposed to ever be in the dermis. It was supposed to be out on the surface of the skin, well beyond the basement membrane and its extensions. This is important in understanding why the immune systems (both innate and adaptive) do what they do. More on that later.

2.5.2 What is going on inside the FPSU?

The three parts of the FSPU are all designed to grow. Each produces its special product, ductal lining cells, hair, or sebum. The growth and replacement of new ductal lining cells, as well as the production of hair and sebum, are turned on by hormones.

Androgens (the male hormones) turn on beard hairs (in both sexes). They also turn on oil glands. And they turn on the ductal lining cells, the keratinocytes that line the central canal of the follicular part of the FPSU. Adding more stimulus (androgens and other hormones) to the system, and then adding more time for the reaction to occur, leads to an increase in production of these ductal lining cells. That increase in production results in effects well beyond what was supposed to happen in nature. That is why *excess* androgen effects produce moustaches and facial hair in women with certain hormonal disorders. And that is why *excess* androgen effects cause the acnes.

Normal levels of androgen working on the follicular part of the FPSU yield a well-regulated production, growth, and elimination of the keratinocytes lining the duct. A finely tuned process called *terminal differentiation* [17] regulates the speed at which new cells, once produced, fulfill their destiny as detached keratinocytes and are lost up the follicular duct.

We know that some human populations that are not exposed to the acnegens in our Western diet do not have acne. That is the baseline I choose to use in providing a rational explanation of acne's development. When androgens and other hormonal acnegens are at normal levels, uninfluenced by unnatural hormone sources, no acne is produced. When the level of acnegenic activity exceeds the threshold of our individual tolerance, increased amounts of hair or sebum or ductal lining keratinocytes are produced.

Increased hair may be a social problem, but hair doesn't generally get stuck in the pores or become ingrown as a result of increased androgens. The reason

is simple—pressure from below, from growth in the hair bulb, pushes the hair shaft to the surface. Likewise, increased sebum production may have sent an earlier generation of women to mirrors to powder their noses, but sebum does not get stuck in the pores. Sebum is a slippery oily liquid at body temperature, and it simply percolates up the follicular canal of the FPSU and onto the surface of the skin. Even when the follicular canal is so choked with keratinous material that a very "tightly inspissated" comedo results, sebum finds its way to the surface [18]. Never in years of "acne surgery" have I ever come across a pool of free sebum "trapped under the skin." "Trapped sebum" as a cause of acne is a misconception that has inappropriately blamed sebum as a cause of acne for well over 50 years. Sebum is a *bystander* in the process of acnegenesis. An innocent bystander as far as comedo formation is concerned, sebum is not innocent of all blame. It feeds the commensal organisms and likely acts like hydraulic fluid in transmitting intraductal pressure—more on that later.

To be clear, there *is* a disease in which sebum *is* trapped under the skin. It is rare, usually runs in families, and has the wonderful name of *steatocystoma multiplex*. But it is not acne, it is not caused by hormones, and it does not respond to the medications that are effective in treating the acnes, not any one of them, not even isotretinoin.

So it is not hair from the pilar area that is plugging the follicular canal—indeed, the hair normally prevents such plugging. And it is not oil from the sebaceous gland plugging up the canal—it is a liquid and doesn't plug anything. That leaves only one other source of trouble. No matter which acne we are discussing, the source of the problem is the little lining cells that are supposed to simply flake off into the canal and disappear up to the surface.

When the ductal keratinocytes don't flake off, they plug the duct, and they cause acne, whether acne vulgaris, acne rosacea, or acne inversa.

So why has this simple and easily observed physical feature not been more widely understood? And why has it not been recognized as the real cause of acne? I think we can blame the "scientific method" in this case. Very early in their investigative lives, scientists learn that they must measure what they wish to study. Thus, for almost 50 years, acne investigators have been measuring what they *could* measure. They could measure sebum production on the surface, or they could count lesions. There are hundreds of papers written about the skin surface lipids and the amount of oil produced by the FPSU. And there are hundreds of acne papers in which comedones have been counted. *Nobody* has measured the weight or volume of the keratinous material caught in the lumen of the FPSU. There were some visually impressive studies done with cyanoacrylate adhesives that demonstrated the plugs to a certain degree, but no assay was ever developed to quantify the weight or volume of the comedo or the microcomedo. Anyone who has ever performed acne surgery or comedo extraction knows the challenge of extracting material of a certain diameter through an orifice with a much smaller diameter. With no ability to accurately and reproducibly measure the keratinous content of the duct, there was no technique to measure the effect of various therapies on the quantity of material trapped in the follicular canal. To do so would have required numerous small biopsies of the pilosebaceous units before, during, and after therapies.

To measure sebum output, a simpler chore, cigarette paper is applied to the study site, held in place for a defined time period, and then removed and weighed to measure absolute weight and so calculate the rate of sebum production. It is sufficiently difficult to recruit study subjects just to wrap cigarette paper onto their greasy foreheads; doing serial biopsies would be a monumental undertaking. It is no wonder that this area has remained uninvestigated, and so it is no wonder that we have remained in the dark. That means that our only option until now has been to observe, postulate, consider, suggest, review, and reconsider the possible mechanisms involved in the development of these tiny early lesions. But perhaps now, with the availability of confocal microscopy, automated serial cross-sectional photography, accurate marker-driven pore location, and almost instantaneous computerized calculation, a system could be designed to quantify comedonal volume. Four matched cohorts of patients previously cleared with isotretinoin could be provided with a zero-dairy, low-glycemic-load diet as a control and three experimental diets: one would be a full-dairy, low-glycemic-load diet; a second would be a zero-dairy, high-glycemic-load diet; and the third, a full-dairy, low-glycemic-load diet. I offer that suggested protocol to better financed and more technologically capable colleagues than I. But I offer one caveat—an attempt to recruit volunteers into such a study, one that involved introducing dairy to a blinded population of patients cleared with Roaccutane attracted only two recruits in 14 months.

So, while we wait for the technical capacity and backing to quantify what we already know, let's look a little deeper into the pore.

Remember the tight PAS + wrapping around the whole FPSU? It fits like a thin, tight, and tough vinyl glove on your hand and fingers. It holds the whole unit firmly together. As the FPSU produces its various products (hair and sebum and ductal keratinocytes), it expands a bit, resistance is created, and just enough pressure is generated to force the contents of the canal, both sebum and keratinocytes, along the path of least resistance toward the surface. If it were not for the glassy membrane and the fibrous root sheath, the whole FPSU would simply expand like the comedones in Favre–Racouchot syndrome. Remember that hair doesn't need any constrictive pressure to head to the surface; it is growing out on its own, pushed from below by the power of cellular reproduction in the hair papilla and the walls of the pilar unit. The same power of cellular reproduction operates within the follicular unit, but the push is centripetal (toward the center). When the center of the tubular structure is filled up and more cells are added, the intraductal pressure must rise, the intraductal keratinocytes become compressed and folded, the duct expands to the circumferential limit imposed by the glassy membrane and root sheath, and there is "pushback" against the constraints of the follicular walls [19]. The pressures are so great that the keratinocytes can be folded back on themselves, as illustrated (Figure 2.8) years ago using electron microscopy [20]. *This* is the source of the pressure that eventually weakens, splits, and ruptures those walls.

That brings us to the very basic question—what leads to the "tipping point" where the ductal keratinocytes stop flaking off and start to form the tiny structure that Plewig called the "follicular filament" [18]? This filament (Figure 1.1A) is the earliest sign of the microscopic keratinocytic plug, just before the formation of the microcomedo. It grows to form the keratinous plug that accumulates within the follicular canal. What starts the life of the plug that slowly grows and expands within the canal until it becomes a force to be reckoned with, a force that can burst that vinyl glove, releasing all that "outside the body" non-self-material into the "inside the body" environment where it causes such trouble? Before we get into the mechanism behind all that, we need to take a further look at the anatomy of the follicular portion of the FPSU as it occurs in acne.

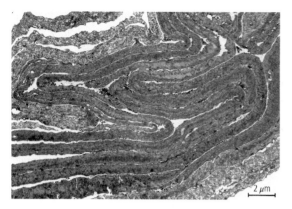

Figure 2.8 The pressure produced within the duct is such that the keratinocytes, unable to separate from each other, are thrown into folds within the strained confines of the follicular duct.

So let's step back a short distance for another look at what we know so far. We have a closed system that has a limit to how much it can expand. We have contents that normally are produced at a steady rate and that can exit the system at the same steady rate, so that there is no real strain on the container's walls. So what can go wrong to challenge the container's walls and lead to their rupture? The first problem worth considering is the increase in output of "product." We know the hair is not part of the problem. Terminal hair is basically a "constant," passing through the canal, always the same diameter, never getting stuck. Even the tiny vellus hairs, supple and soft as they are, normally reach the surface with little or no difficulty. And we know that sebum simply flows out of the follicular canal onto the skin, producing the oily skin we all know is part of acne vulgaris and acne rosacea. Oily skin is not such a constant feature in AI/HS, but there is a reason for that—more later. So that leaves us with the plug in the follicular canal, the distinguishing feature of all the acnes, even when it is invisible.

That leads logically to the next subject, physiology, which gives us an idea of the mechanisms driving the increased amount of material in the follicular canal.

2.6 Physiology

The FPSU makes hair and sebum and a lining for the duct to the surface. What could be simpler? That really is all you need to know, and you could stop right here if it were not for the external factors that convert a well-balanced system to a pathological process.

In the acnes, the normal process of cell renewal in the follicle is overstimulated to the point that it becomes abnormal and comedonal acne is produced. This initial comedonal stage of acne is non-inflammatory acne. In many pores and many patients, it may never get beyond that stage. But when the process expands to involve the immune systems, the characteristics of inflammatory acne appear.

If the cause of the overstimulation is reduced to a normal level, or is eliminated, the pathologic process settles down and the physiologic processes return to normal. If not done in time, the inflammatory epiphenomena take on lives of their own, unless potent therapy and effective secondary prevention are brought to bear. So what drives all this activity, and how does it all work together?

2.6.1 Hair first

Of the three functional units of the FPSU, the pilar unit has the least to do with acne. The area of the body most thickly covered with hair, the scalp, develops true comedones only exceptionally rarely. Each hair is produced on a cyclic schedule, growing under the combined influence of (female) estrogens and (male) androgens. The timing is still a bit of a mystery.

The hair starts in the papilla (hair bulb), the deepest part of the pilar unit. It picks up whatever color its owner's DNA is coded for, from special cells in the papilla and bulb, and then it heads north. Forced upwards from below by new hair cells being continually produced, it is pushed from the pilar unit through the follicular unit on the way to the surface. It starts out in the pilar unit wrapped in two layers called the *inner* and *outer root sheaths*, but it separates from them at the top of the pilar unit. At that point, the now-independent hair shaft acquires a thin and ever-renewing coat of protective and lubricating sebum as sebocytes dissolve around it before the hair heads to the outside world.

2.6.2 Oil second

The sebum that layers onto the hair is produced by the sebaceous glands (Figure 2.9) that are attached to the lower end of the follicular unit at the sebofollicular junction. These glands are narrow-necked structures that look like sacks full of dozens of boring, mostly round, but tightly packed thin-walled cells that are

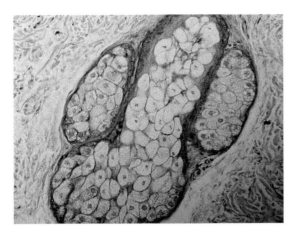

Figure 2.9 This sebaceous gland is cut in cross-section in an area away from the sebofollicular junction and shows a healthy periodic acid–Schiff positive (PAS+) support structure and a minimal population of tissue-resident immunocytes.

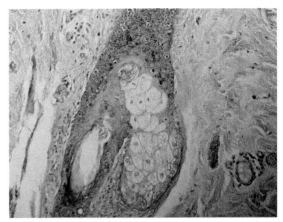

Figure 2.10 The sebaceous unit plugging into the isthmus of the pilofollicular structure. Note there is no free sebum pool—the sebocytes dissolve only upon contact with the hair. Note the inflammation concentrated where minimal periodic acid–Schiff positive (PAS+) material is present at 6–6:30 and 7–9 o'clock and one or two inflammatory cells at 3 o'clock.

almost all fat-laden cytoplasm with only a tiny nucleus. These sebocytes start life as basal cells inside a protective sack of the same basement membrane material that is wrapped around the other two parts of the FPSU.

The basal cells are stimulated into action mainly by androgens, the male hormones, but other hormones and growth factors are all part of the push to grow. When conditions are right (and nobody really knows for sure what the trigger is), a basal cell will divide into two daughter cells. One will stay behind as a basal cell, and the other (now a sebocyte) will be pushed into the body of the gland. There, the sebocytes grow, fill with various lipids (fats, waxes, and oils), and are gradually pushed up to the neck of the gland, near the hair and the follicle. They head toward the *ductus seboglandularis* (sebaceous gland duct). The sebaceous cells are actually pushed toward the exit like people leaving a theatre, jostling for the next free space, but each maintains its walls intact until it actually reaches the "door." As soon as it gets through the sebaceous duct, up against the hair, the sebocyte's wall dissolves, and the oil is released onto the hair in the follicular unit. Even on a microscopic level, there is no "pool" of sebum in the sebaceous duct or anywhere under the skin. The sebocyte remains intact until it actually reaches the hair it is meant to lubricate (Figure 2.10).

Much of the best research in acne has been directed at figuring out what hormone and enzyme systems provide the push to the basal cells to make them produce

either many or few daughter cells (sebocytes), and so regulate the oiliness on the skin surface. This complex subject is coming up in the next couple of sections.

2.6.3 Last but definitely not least: the follicle

The same hormones that push the hair up from the pilar unit and push the sebocytes up to the junction of the follicular unit, where they can burst and lubricate the hair shaft, also have serious work to do in the follicular unit. In fact, they are the *cause*, and this is the *location*, of the first sign of trouble in all the acnes. As the hormones turn on the basal cells that lie just inside the glassy membrane of the follicular unit, daughter cells are again produced, but this time they turn into keratinocytes instead of sebocytes. And instead of heading randomly to the exit, they normally follow a very strict and formal path toward the center of the follicular duct.

When all is going according to plan, each keratinocyte gradually matures from a cuboidal cell to a gradually flattened cell and eventually becomes pancake-shaped as the center of the duct is approached. Internal chemical processes gradually use up the energy provided by the fats and complex sugars. This energy fuels the formation of special proteins that make keratin for the keratinocyte and also forms the protein and complex lipid and sugar junctions between the cells, all needed to complete the maturation and terminal differentiation of the keratinocytes. Residual energy sources then produce proteases that dissolve the junctions between the fully differentiated keratinocytes until they are fully separated into *squames*. These are the residual flat flakes of keratin that normally separate from each other, flake off into the central duct, and mix with the sebum. Suitably lubricated, they slide up to the surface in the space between the follicular wall and the hair shaft, if there is one.

That is how it is supposed to work, and that is how it does work until too much stimulus is added to the system.

2.6.4 Looking deeper

The chemical processes that run in the background, making the physiology work, run through highly complex biochemical reactions that produce equally complex and varied products. Each of the basal keratinocytes and basal hair root cells and basal sebocytes uses its own specialized set of enzymatic reactions, chosen from the huge set of possible reactions the cellular genome can produce on demand.

Just think for a moment—back to the embryology section (Section 2.4). Those few fetal cells that made the buds that formed on the underside of the fetal skin can go on to produce a full beard, or a greasy scalp, or a face and back full of inflammatory acne, or a perineum full of draining acne inversa lesions, or Farrah Fawcett's glorious mane of hair. DNA and hormones are a potent combination.

2.7 Biochemistry

The FPSU produces cells that line the follicle, the hair, the pigments that color the hair, the multiple components of sebum, the cell walls of sebocytes, and the enzymes that run the show.

These products are made up of fats, proteins, and carbohydrates, but the expression and organization of each vary tremendously from tissue to tissue. Let's consider fats first.

Fats can be used for energy, or as a structural material, or they may simply be exported, as sebum. For example, intracellular fat in keratinocytes is used up over their life span to power their metabolic processes. If the terminal differentiation process that leads to keratinocyte maturity is incomplete, lipid is left over unused and

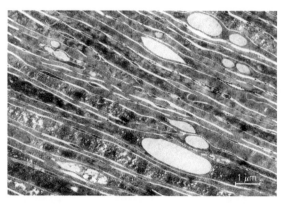

Figure 2.11 The failure of the keratinocytes to achieve terminal differentiation, likely due to anoxia and mediated by hypoxia-inducible factor 1 (HIF-1), leaves behind the lipids that would have been used as structural lipids or as a source of energy to fuel the differentiation.

shows up under the electron microscope as pooled lipid droplets in layers of keratinocytes (Figure 2.11), demonstrating arrested maturity [20]. Other fats are combined with proteins to form complex combinations called *lipoproteins*. These larger molecules are used in cell wall construction and for the creation of the tiny intracellular organelles that are the factories and energy management systems of the cells. The fats that are created for export in the sebocytes are a fairly limited group. They are triglycerides, cholesterol, fatty acids, and squalene. Each has a role to play in acne, but their prime role is lubrication during birth. Their second role is protection of the human skin to prevent its drying out, simply by sealing water into the skin and thereby preventing evaporation from the skin surface.

Proteins come in three sizes, small (peptides with up to 10 amino acids), medium (polypeptides with up to 50 amino acids), and large (proteins with over 50 amino acids). The peptides are usually building blocks for larger proteins. The polypeptides have numerous uses in acne, including a large number of hormones and growth factors. A fairly short example, FoxO1, is the polypeptide nuclear transcription factor that is the prime regulator of the androgen receptor that controls acne [21]. Proteins can be long and strong so they find their main use as structural components like the collagen fibers that wrap around the FPSU to give it strength. They also can be incredibly complex, bent into all sorts of shapes so they can form the flexible, electrically charged, amorphous mass that enzymes are made from.

That leaves the carbohydrates, which generally serve as the prime energy source for the FPSU but also form parts of various structures. One such structural material that is important in all the acnes is glycoprotein (*glucose* is the carbohydrate sugar that is combined with the protein). This is part of the material that makes up the glassy membrane; indeed, the sugar part is what makes the PAS+material stain pink under the microscope [22]. This fibrous web supports the whole FPSU structure, giving it the strength and shape needed to support and anchor hair. It also provides the support that puts the squeeze on sebaceous glands and sebum to keep the oil flowing, and provides support to the follicular tube that takes both hair and sebum to the skin surface.

As elsewhere in nature, "carbs" may be either essential for health in normal amounts, or a cause of disease or disorder in either deficiency or excess.

2.8 Hormones, enzymes, receptors, and the intracrine system

The FPSU, left to itself, would not produce acne. That is the situation in families with congenital absence of 5α-reductase, and also in the Aché and Trobriand tribes whose diets are free of dairy and high-glycemic-load foods. So, where do the hormones come from that cause all this trouble? And why, if these are normal hormones, should we not expect acne as a normal event in everyone during puberty and post-adolescence? And why does acne normally fade when maturity arrives?

Acne is turned on by a cascade of chemical changes that are driven by a host of hormones. Hormones are basically chemical messengers. They are attracted to receptors on the surfaces of enzymes and are modified in various ways while attached to the enzyme receptor, and then these modified (and often more potent) hormones may travel to other enzyme receptors for additional modification. Eventually they travel to the androgen receptor, where they turn on the processes that lead to acne.

The production of dihydrotestosterone (DHT), the potent androgen that drives acne, starts with simple cholesterol, the essential building block of all our steroid-based hormones. Much maligned, cholesterol is the building block for many essential body processes. Our nervous system would not function without it. Its contribution to the reproductive hormones' structure allows us to grow and mature into reproductive human beings. Without cholesterol, we would have evolved in a different direction, if at all.

Through a series of stepwise changes supervised and facilitated by a limited number of enzymes, the cholesterol molecule is neatly converted to pregnenolone (top left) and then to DHT, the most potent androgen and so the most potent acnegen. In the diagram of this cascade (Figure 2.12), the two steps from left to right are the responsibility of 3β-hydroxysteroid dehydrogenase (plus an isomerase) and 5α-reductase; the three steps from top to bottom are mediated by 17α-hydroxylase, 17α-lyase, and 17β-hydroxysteroid dehydrogenase. These are responsible, during the production of cow milk, for the presence of several 5α-reduced molecules that act as precursors of DHT (Section 4.2.4). They are not shown here.

The hormones that drive acne are complex, and they come from different sources. Those from inside the body (from the ovaries, testes, and adrenal glands) are called *endogenous* (Section 4.1). Those from outside of the body are called *exogenous* (Section 4.2). Others are produced within the FPSU itself by the *intracrine system* (see Section 2.8.1).

The exogenous hormones we generally hear about are the "steroid" hormones given to athletes. These are both human and animal hormones, and are used in both human and animal athletes. These are the *anabolic steroids* used to build muscle, strength, endurance, and speed. There are many of them, some natural and some semisynthetic. They may be used singly, or several may be "stacked" together to achieve the results the user desires. The normal human body does much the same with its hormones, but operates with a different and totally natural "stack" to create and grow everything from babies to beards.

But there is another whole world of exogenous hormones out there. Some are present in nature, like those in cow milk, which at least are natural in cows. Some are artificial or manmade (like birth control pills). Some of the chemicals we are exposed to are not really hormones but are environmental pollutants that can mimic the effect of hormones in our bodies. They have the potential to act as hormonal disruptors, another long story. All these chemicals have one thing in common— they are all "keys" to the lock in the androgen (and other) receptors.

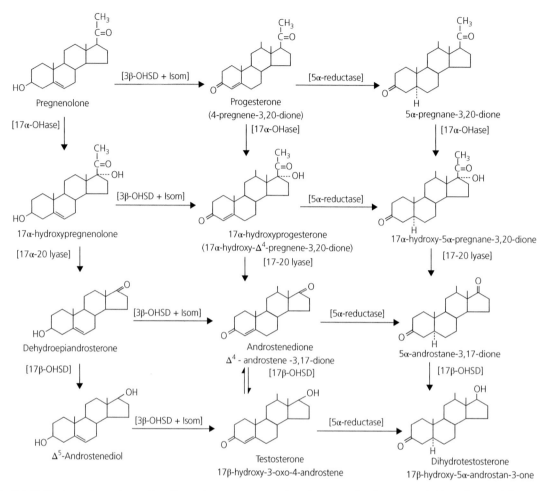

Figure 2.12 The intracrine system utilizes five onsite enzymes to produce the range of androgens needed in and around the folliculopilosebaceous unit and elsewhere in the body. Some may be made directly from cholesterol; others may utilize the androgen precursors in dairy products.

It is important to realize that the keys to the lock are quite varied and have quite varied effects. Imagine a key that fits the keyhole loosely and falls out easily. On the other end, imagine a key that locks into the keyhole permanently and cannot be removed. How about a key that fits lots of different keyholes and can open the door in most of them? Like a master key that can work in many different apartment doors, it has a much broader range of effects. Then consider that some of the loose keys can be pulled away by carrier proteins like sex hormone–binding globulin (SHBG), leaving the keyhole open for another competing hormone that has a greater *affinity* (a stronger pull) to the keyhole. That keyhole, the one that holds the hormone tighter, is said to have a

greater *avidity*. The tighter fitting hormones will stay in the keyhole longer, sometimes forever. Then go one step further and consider that even if the key fits in the keyhole, it sometimes will not turn in the lock. This is the way car keys used to be—you could get in the door with the door key, but even if it fit in the ignition keyhole it wouldn't turn on the ignition. Chemicals with this sort of "chemical look-alike" pattern are used as hormone blockers.

This presents us with a tremendous variation in the effects that various hormones (the keys) have on various tissues. Not only does each hormone sometimes fit in more than one kind of receptor, but it may have effects on that receptor that will vary from antagonism (reversing or blocking the normal effect of the hormone) to neutral (essentially doing nothing, like a key that fits but cannot be turned) to agonism (an agonist is something that positively makes things happen) so the hormone does what it was designed to do. Each action will vary, so, for example, you will see the term *weak agonist*, which means it works, but is not a strong influence. DHT is a 5–10 times stronger agonist in the androgen receptor controlling an acnegenic enzymatic process than is testosterone (T), a weaker agonist.

This process and the whole subject of hormones and receptors would be simple if T and DHT were the only hormones that worked in the androgen receptor, but overlapping functions confuse things. Some receptors will accept a variety of hormones (and other matching chemicals), and some hormones can activate a variety of receptors.

Receptors will also bind things that they were never intended to bind. That includes toxic substances such as dioxins (see Section 5.1) but also some of the drugs we use. To complicate matters further, steroid hormones have the ability to do all sorts of different things, at quite different locations, all related to their attraction to the receptors, the "fit" with the receptors, the "avidity" of the receptors (how hard they hold onto the hormone), the number of competing hormones looking for receptor sites, and other variables. The last variable includes the process regulated by the individual receptor in the individual cell.

For example, dermatologists regularly use spironolactone, a look-alike chemical that blocks androgen receptors and acts as a "competitive inhibitor." It is great for slowing down the plugging of pores and so improving acne in women, but it can also stop or slow hair loss on women's scalps, decrease the amount of unwanted hair on women's faces and bodies, cause breakthrough menstrual bleeding, minimize acne rosacea, reduce leg swelling and lower blood pressure.

PATIENT TIP BOX 2.1

Spironolactone is also a diuretic. Diuretics cause diuresis, the production of more urine, so it is best to time taking it so that a washroom is handy, and not just before starting a long commute. I suggest patients take it when they get home from school or work so the diuretic effect is all over by bedtime. This effect is variable, often as minimal as the effect of a cup of coffee, and may even be unnoticed.

Many steroids have this capacity to stimulate various results in various receptors. The effect we see is therefore not a direct "one-on-one" equation in which one hormonal stimulus produces one result in one tissue. Instead, what we see on a daily basis is the "net" effect of the positives (agonists) balanced against the negatives (antagonists) in every cell in the body.

This variation in response also explains the difference in the effect of different progestins, the active part of birth control pills. While most of the older progestins are somewhat androgenic and tend to make acne worse, the newer ones work the opposite way, both preventing acne and helping acne get better.

In addition to having quite varied impacts depending on the receptors they turn on, all of the hormones that impact our bodies are capable of being changed under the influence of the chemicals and enzymes they encounter in various environments. The major modifiers are the enzymes, folded-up globules of protein that act as catalysts. They speed up chemical reactions, and that changes the shape and function of individual molecules or whole tissue parts. These enzymes are generally single-purpose, specially shaped areas on the cell walls, in the nucleus of the cell, or in the cytoplasm. They are often single but may be part of a small assembly line. Using the complementary electric charges on a single molecule or a portion of a larger molecule, the molecule is attracted into a receptor site on the enzyme's surface. There, a specific reaction can take place that modifies the molecule's structure so that what leaves the enzyme's receptor is slightly different from what arrived.

A single tweak like adding a hydrogen atom onto a specific spot on the testosterone molecule makes the difference between testosterone (T) and DHT. That simple move increases the "maleness" power of the molecule by a factor of 10. Your body's enzymes have thousands of these specialized reactions available. By combining enzymes that add extra pieces to (or nip pieces off) the molecules in Figure 2.12, the six enzymes of the FPSU intracrine system can take a simple cholesterol molecule, run it through a series of enzymes, and produce a cascade of hormones. Eventually DHT is produced. That DHT then moves to another receptor on a protein that is specifically designed to transport it within the cell.

The hormone–receptor combination then actually physically moves (is "translocated") into the cell nucleus. This brings the DHT into position to move to other receptors to turn on various genes, depending upon the kind of cell in which the androgen receptor (AR) is located. This triggers a number of specific processes that are started by creating RNA as a mirror image of DNA. mRNA is produced. This small string of material takes the message to the cell's manufacturing centers, the endoplasmic reticulum, and that leads to production of anything from male beard hair growth to acne (plugging of the pores) to seborrhea (oily skin).

But it is not all about making male hormones. It only takes one more single hydrogen atom added to those Os at the bottom left of the androstenedione (ovary) and T molecules (in the middle of the bottom two rows) to turn those two male molecules into two classic female estrogen molecules, estrone and estradiol, respectively.

The type, number, and location of these enzymes are the factors that determine what a tissue does with the hormones that arrive in its receptors. The enzyme 5α-reductase that normally changes T into DHT, for example, comes in two forms, and these different versions are called *isoenzymes*. Broadly speaking, Type 1 isoenzyme is the one that exists in acne-prone FPSUs and Type 2 is the one in FPSUs that are prone to baldness. Just to confuse the matter, there is actually a mixture of Type 1 and Type 2 and the percentages vary by location.

But that isn't the end of the story. The 5α-reductase (5αR) enzyme sometimes doesn't work at all in some rare situations. There are several family groups around the world whose 5αR enzyme is mutated and doesn't work. There are now 33 different genetic variants of this enzymatic abnormality. The affected children are most often raised as girls but display male characteristics later in their teens. Their genital maturation is delayed because their relatively weak T takes such a long time to do what 10 times stronger DHT does in a short time in normal individuals. This causes serious gender confusion and difficult choices for these teens and their families. For all the negatives, however, there is one slight positive. They do not go bald.

It is obvious from the foregoing that there is a vast menu of possible effects when hormones and enzymes meet. It is no wonder it has taken so long to thoroughly explore the impact of hormones on acne.

2.8.1 The intracrine system

That leads us to some hormone–enzyme interactions that are especially important in human acne. This is the intracrine system, the "onboard" hormone manipulation center that is present in every one of our FPSUs.

I first learned about the enzyme 17β-hydroxysteroid dehydrogenase in the FPSU being able to convert androstenedione to testosterone in a PhD thesis written by a researcher at University of Glasgow in 1970. I cannot recall how I was made aware of the existence of this work, but a trusting librarian wrapped up the university's copy in brown paper and twine and shipped it to me. Being sent from a Scottish university, the postage was "surface mail" and the bound volume took about six weeks to reach me. "The Histochemical Demonstration of Hydroxysteroid Dehydrogenases in Human Skin" is a thesis submitted for the degree of doctor of philosophy in the faculty of medicine by Kenneth Charles Calman in April 1970.

Calman's thesis demonstrated, for the first time of which I am aware, the existence of 17β-hydroxysteroid dehydrogenase in "the lower parts of the secretory ducts" [23]. This location corresponds to the lower end of the follicular portion of the FPSU as described in this book. Indeed, it is within the area I refer to as the *sebofollicular junction*. As has been shown since, this enzyme is an essential part of the intracrine system. Subsequent work by Thiboutot and others has filled in the blanks so we know that all the essential enzymes needed to assist in the production of DHT from various precursors are present within the FPSU [24]. Of particular note, "infrainfundibular keratinocytes have an increased capacity for producing androgens which may play a role in the follicular hyperkeratinization seen in acne" [25].

Calman, now Sir Kenneth Charles Calman, the former Chief Medical Officer of the United Kingdom and now the Chancellor of the University where he did this work, used a fastidious technique to deposit diformazan granules, visible in the accompanying photomicrographs, at the locations of the enzyme. Figure 2.13, taken directly from the thesis, illustrates with some remarkable perspicacity the mechanism of formation of the structural change that is the first invisible sign of the commencement of the acnes. His concept of the overall interaction of steroids and sebaceous glands is summarized in Figure 2.14 and was likewise well ahead of its time.

Thus, local processing of hormones by local enzymes provides a highly efficient upgrading system that takes precursors of T and DHT from the circulating bloodstream and "refines" them to produce the high-potency hormones that drive the acne process. The testosterone and 5α-dihydrotestosterone (5α-DHT or DHT) produced

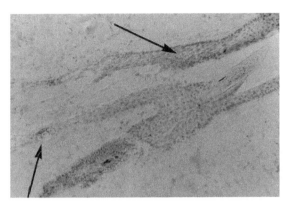

Figure 2.13 The gray dustlike formazan particles sprinkled in the keratinocytes of the ductal wall (top arrow) and concentrated in a sebocyte (bottom arrow) indicate the location of the enzyme 17β-hydroxysteroid dehydrogenase (17β-OHSD in Figure 2.12). From PhD thesis, 1970.

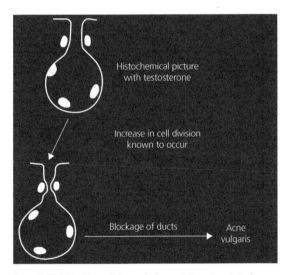

Figure 2.14 This diazo slide made from Calman's original paper illustrates the earliest expression of the present concept of hormonally driven acne. From PhD thesis, 1970.

as a result of the intracrine enzymes' catalytic assistance are on site and immediately available to the androgen receptors in the cell.

It is worth noting that this internal intracellular manipulation is invisible to the clinician's standard laboratory tests. While gross abnormalities may be detected, the use of urine and serum blood tests is far too removed from the action to be of investigative value.

Calman's work set the stage for a series of discoveries that led to Thiboutot's description of the intracrine

system in the sebocytes and the follicular epithelium of the FPSU [23–25]. The word *intracrine* describes the secretion or production of a hormone molecule (polypeptide or steroid) that is subsequently utilized within (*intra*) the same cell. The enzymes that run this cascade are present in the smooth endoplasmic reticulum (SER), a complex of tubules and tiny hollow flattened balloon-like structures attached to the nuclei of metabolically active cells.

For steroids produced within the SER, it is a very short trip to the nuclear androgen receptor. Collecting all the necessary enzymes in close physical proximity facilitates the chances of local conversion of circulating 5α-reduced molecules to DHT. In addition, the intimate transport arrangements provided by the SER's access to nuclear pores will also limit loss of any of the tiny amounts involved, given the nearby availability and avidity of the nuclear androgen receptors.

Androgen receptors rule our lives, from shortly after conception until we pass our genes to the next generation, and beyond. They regulate everything from a baby's rate of growth to the rate of growth of men's prostates in their later years. There is growing evidence that their constant stimulation is involved in the development of cancers of the breast and prostate, but that is another story. Our entire metabolic world is a "net" effect, the result of the pluses against the minuses.

For years, we have believed that to control acne one must selectively minimize the agonist DHT and maximize the antagonists' effects on the androgen receptor. As a result of recent insights, it is apparent that we now need to turn our attention to look at what factors control access to the androgen receptor, an exciting new aspect of acne management. That subject is up next.

2.9 FoxO1 and mTORC1

For an androgenic molecule like T or DHT to turn on the machinery that makes acne (and many other things), it first has to have access to the androgen receptor. This receptor is conceptually similar to a modern vehicle's ignition, which is controlled by an electromagnetic signal from a nearby source (the electronic key) that unlocks the ignition system. The tiny electrical charges on a hormone molecule's surface interact with the complementary charges on the receptor's surface, and that activates the receptor.

In physiology, however, there is one more necessary and carefully controlled step. The keyhole (the receptor) needs to be open and available to the key. Just like in some padlocks, the keyhole cover needs to be moved aside.

No access, no insertion, no ignition, no activity, no acne. So, what governs access? As you might expect, it is a little bit complicated, but it is a step-by-step process that is common to many systems. We owe many thanks to Dr Bodo Melnik for his elucidation of this molecular chain of events [26].

Imagine that the androgen receptor is sitting in the nucleus of an oil gland cell (sebocyte). The receptor has a protective lid on it and that protective lid is in its normal state, which is closed. The scientific word is *repressed*. To open the lid, to expose the receptor, one needs to *de-repress* it. The problem is that there is a small polypeptide molecule sitting on the lid of the receptor, right in the nucleus of the cell. That molecule's single duty in life is to sit on the lid. This keeps the lid closed and the androgen molecule away from the receptor. It "represses" the receptor.

So somehow we need to get that molecule, called FoxO1, off the lid and out of the nucleus. Actually, if we just removed that single one, it would be replaced quickly with another floating about in the area. So we need to get as many of these molecules as possible out of the nucleus. The more FoxO1 molecules we can remove, the more active and receptive the nuclear androgen receptors can become.

It turns out that if we arrange to add a phosphate ion to each FoxO1 molecule (this is called *phosphorylation*), the phosphorylated FoxO1 becomes more soluble and can leave the nucleus. That means it can dissolve in the fluid in the nucleus of the cell and is then able to leave the nucleus and head out into the cell cytoplasm, where it can be broken up. The cytoplasm, which contains many tiny organelles floating in a wet chemical-filled metabolic soup called *cytosol*, fills the rest of the cell. The nucleus is suspended more or less in the middle of the cell, and has pores (like holes in the wall of the nucleus) of various types controlling the entrance and exit of molecules such as phosphorylated FoxO1. So we need something that will attach a phosphate ion onto the FoxO1. The enzyme that does that kind of

work is called a *phosphorylase*, and there are all sorts of these phosphorylase enzymes (called *kinases*) running our body processes.

The specific one that is needed is called Akt kinase. Just to make things interesting, Akt kinase *also* has to be phosphorylated before it can do its job. That is done by another phosphorylase, phosphoinositol-3 kinase (PI3K). Turning on PI3K is done by two molecules that you will hear a lot more about in relation to the cause of acne. One (insulin) regulates sugar levels in our blood and tissues, and the other (insulin-like growth factor 1, or IGF-1) regulates growth. Although the body has a real growth hormone (GH), it is really a signaler and does not actually do the work. GH stimulates the production by the liver of a polypeptide molecule, the hormone called IGF. There are several of these as well, and the one that does the heavy lifting is IGF-1.

Now we can follow the chain of command. Diet induces elevated levels of insulin and IGF-1 (usually both acting at the same time). PI3K is activated. That phosphorylates the second messenger, the Akt kinase, and that phosphorylates FoxO1. That makes the FoxO1 soluble and allows FoxO1 to leave the nucleus, the lid preventing androgens from reaching the receptor is opened up, and the androgen receptor is open for business.

This is the molecular heart of acne. Once the lid on the androgen receptor is lifted, the receptor is de-repressed, and *any* key that can fit in the open lock *and* can turn on the ignition will start the acne process. While the receptor is specifically designed for T and DHT, some other molecules (likely including those found in and derived from milk products) will fit, more or less well, into this receptor. More on this back in Section 2.8.

2.9.1 The next step

The arrival of DHT in the androgen receptor triggers a further chain of events that lead to the metabolic activities that produce acne through the excess production of the keratinocytes that lie at the core of the acnes.

The process is mediated by mTORC1, a nutrient-sensing kinase that regulates growth and metabolism. mTORC1 signaling serves as a "growth checkpoint" (Figure 2.15). mTORC1 surveys the status of growth factors and nutrients in and around cells, especially the

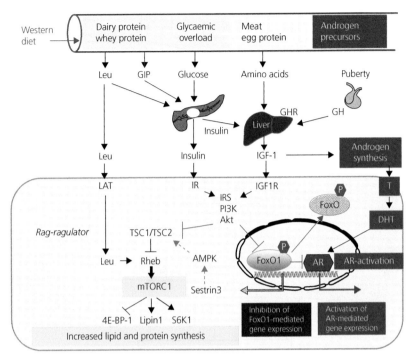

Figure 2.15 Regulation of mTORC1 is the final common pathway to increased lipids (sebaceous) and active protein (ductal plugging cell) activity. From: Potential role of FoxO1 and mTORC1 in the pathogenesis of Western diet-induced acne. Bodo C. Melnik and Christos C. Zouboulis. *Experimental Dermatology*, 2013, 22, 311–315.

availability of essential amino acids. To regulate growth, mTORC1 signaling stimulates gene transcription, translation, ribosome biogenesis, protein synthesis, cell growth, cell proliferation, and lipid synthesis. mTORC1's partner protein Raptor helps mTORC1 to control the G1/S transition and G2/M progression of the cell cycle, and the mTORC1 signaling network further connects various other signaling modules. These sense and relay diverse inputs, especially those related to nutrient, growth factor, and cellular energy status, and report to a central "signaling core." Thus, mTORC1 plays a special role in sensing the cellular nutrients, amino acids, and energy levels important for cell growth and proliferation.

The Western diet stimulates maximal mTORC1 activity in two ways, detailed in Figure 2.16. First, it provides an abundance of essential amino acids and polypeptide hormones from milk and meat proteins. Second, the insulin and IGF-1 stimulation (IIS) provided and induced by dairy protein consumption and high glycemic load further increases mTORC1 activity. After integration of nutrient signals, growth factors, and energy

status, mTORC1 produces metabolic signals and acts as the conductor of the downstream cellular "signaling symphony." The resulting protein and lipid biosynthesis, cell growth, and proliferation coordinated by mTORC1 form an integral part of the pathogenesis of acne that is characterized by increased proliferation of follicular keratinocytes, hyperplasia of sebaceous glands, and increased sebaceous gland lipogenesis [27].

2.9.2 The broad view

Having identified the process at the center of the universe in acne, it is really important to understand four things.

1 The hormones that lead to androgen receptor stimulation are numerous.

2 The access to the receptor is infinitely adjustable because the degree of de-repression varies.

3 Androgen receptor stimulation results in a broad spectrum of downstream effects, from the tiniest vellus hair to the world's worst case of AI/HS.

4 The response to T or DHT varies from person to person. This is called *end organ responsiveness*.

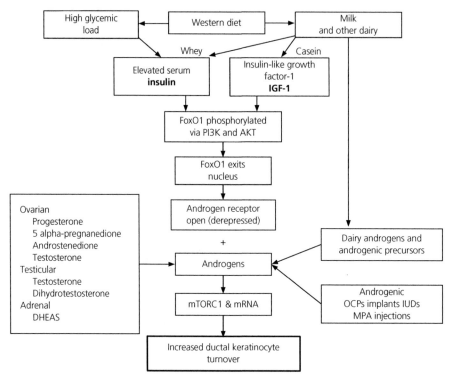

Figure 2.16 The chain of events from diet to plugged duct is simplified here.

Insulin and IGF-1 will be discussed in detail in Sections 4.2.4.1.2 and 4.2.4.1.3. The factors that *modify* insulin and IGF-1 will be discussed under diet (Section 8.3.2).

References

1 Danby FW. Why we have sebaceous glands. J Am Acad Dermatol 2005 Jun;52(6):1071–2.

2 DiLandro A., Cazzaniga S, Parazzini F, Ingordo V, Cusano F, Atzori L, *et al.* Family history, body mass index, selected dietary factors, menstrual history, and risk of moderate to severe acne in adolescents and young adults. J Am Acad Dermatol 2012 Dec;67(6):1129–35.

3 Lindeberg S. Paleolithic diet in medical nutrition—incorporating evolutionary biology in nutritional science. Availble from: http://www.staffanlindeberg.com/TheKitavaStudy.html

4 Cordain L, Lindeberg S, Hurtado M, Hill K, Eaton SB, Brand-Miller J. Acne vulgaris: a disease of Western civilization. Arch Dermatol 2002 Dec;138(12):1584–90.

5 Lindeberg S, Lundh B. Apparent absence of stroke and ischaemic heart disease in a traditional Melanesian island: a clinical study in Kitava. J Intern Med 1993 Mar;233(3):269–75.

6 Thiboutot DM, Strauss JS. Diet and acne revisited. Arch Dermatol 2002 Dec;138(12):1591–2.

7 Glickman FS, Silvers SH. Dietary factors in acne vulgaris. Arch Dermatol 1972 Jul;106(1):129.

8 Hamilton JB, Terada H, Mestler GE. Greater tendency to acne in white American than in Japanese populations. J Clin Endocrinol Metab 1964 Mar;24:267–72.

9 Bamford JT. Rosacea: current thoughts on origin. Semin Cutan Med Surg 2001 Sep;20(3):199–206.

10 Yazici AC, Tamer L, Ikizoglu G, Kaya TI, Api H, Yildirim H, *et al.* GSTM1 and GSTT1 null genotypes as possible heritable factors of rosacea. Photodermatol Photoimmunol Photomed 2006 Aug;22(4):208–10.

11 Palleschi GM, Torchia D. Rosacea in a monozygotic twin. Australas J Dermatol 2007 May;48(2):132–3.

12 Li CR, Jiang MJ, Shen DB, Xu HX, Wang HS, Yao X, *et al.* Two novel mutations of the nicastrin gene in Chinese patients with acne inversa. Br J Dermatol 2011 Aug;165(2):415–8.

13 Cooney CA, Dave AA, Wolff GL. Maternal methyl supplements in mice affect epigenetic variation and DNA methylation of offspring. J Nutr 2002 Aug;132(8 Suppl):2393S–400S.

14 Lyko F, Foret S, Kucharski R, Wolf S, Falckenhayn C, Maleszka R. The honey bee epigenomes: differential methylation of brain DNA in queens and workers. PLoS Biol 2010;8(11):e1000506.

15 Adebamowo CA, Spiegelman D, Berkey CS, Danby FW, Rockett HH, Colditz GA, *et al.* Milk consumption and acne in teenaged boys. J Am Acad Dermatol 2008 May;58(5):787–93.

16 deBeer H. Dairy products and physical stature: a systematic review and meta-analysis of controlled trials. Econ Hum Biol 2012 Jul;10(3):299–309.

17 Gandarillas A. Epidermal differentiation, apoptosis, and senescence: common pathways? Exp Gerontol 2000 Feb;35(1): 53–62.

18 Plewig G. [How acne vulgaris develops]. Hautarzt 2010 Feb;61(2):99–104, 106.

19 Danby FW, Danby DL, Waggoner PS. Pilosebaceous dynamics. 2010. Available from: http://www.acnemilk.com/acne_animation

20 Knutson DD. Ultrastructural observations in acne vulgaris: the normal sebaceous follicle and acne lesions. J Invest Dermatol 1974 Mar;62(3):288–307.

21 Melnik BC. FoxO1—the key for the pathogenesis and therapy of acne? J Dtsch Dermatol Ges 2010 Feb;8(2):105–14.

22 Paulsson M. Basement membrane proteins: structure, assembly, and cellular interactions. Crit Rev Biochem Mol Biol 1992;27(1–2):93–127.

23 Calman KC, Muir AV, Milne JA, Young H. Survey of the distribution of steroid dehydrogenases in sebaceous glands of human skin. Br J Dermatol 1970 Jun;82(6):567–71.

24 Thiboutot D, Knaggs H, Gilliland K, Lin G. Activity of 5-alpha-reductase and 17-beta-hydroxysteroid dehydrogenase in the infrainfundibulum of subjects with and without acne vulgaris. Dermatology 1998;196(1):38–42.

25 Thiboutot DM, Knaggs H, Gilliland K, Hagari S. Activity of type 1 5 alpha-reductase is greater in the follicular infrainfundibulum compared with the epidermis. Br J Dermatol 1997 Feb;136(2):166–71.

26 Danby FW. Turning acne on/off via mTORC1. Exp Dermatol 2013 Jul;22(7):505–6.

27 Melnik BC, Zouboulis, CC. Potential role of FoxO1 and mTORC1 in the pathogenesis of Western diet-induced acne. 2013 May;22(5):311–5.

CHAPTER 3
Pathogenetic mechanisms summarized

The three acnes share several mechanisms that create their specific different appearances, but not all mechanisms are active in all three acnes. That accounts for their morphological variability, so that while plugging of the follicular portion of the folliculopilosebaceous unit (FPSU) is common to all, obvious comedo (visible blackhead and whitehead) development is variable and the ductal obstruction is not clinically visible in some acnes. In addition to the three primary acnes, there are several variants that illustrate exaggeration of one or more of the active pathogenic processes. (See Section 3.4, "Other Variants.")

For all readers, it is necessary for you to know that what follows is a synthesis. Much as I would prefer to write about a fully integrated and proven pathogenesis, science isn't quite there yet. That being so, what you will read here is a mixture of facts and conjecture based on these facts. The challenge, to suggest ethical experiments that successfully test the hypotheses, is considerable.

3.1 Acne vulgaris

Hormones, especially the androgen dihydrotestosterone (DHT), drive the increased production of the keratinocytes that line the follicular portion of the folliculopilosebaceous unit (FPSU). As the lining cells accumulate and grow inwards, the mass created presses outwards against the walls of the follicle. This expansion leads to an increase in pressure within the follicle, and the increase in pressure leads to a lack of oxygen (hypoxia and eventually anoxia). The lack of oxygen encourages the growth of *Propionibacterium acnes*, a bacterium that grows well where there is no oxygen. Indeed, it is the increase in the population of this anaerobic or microaerophilic organism that is the marker that allowed the leap in comprehension linking the lack of oxygen (whether relative or absolute) to the slowing of terminal differentiation described in this chapter. The hypoxia and anoxia appear to have additional effects on keratinocyte metabolism and inflammatory response. (See Section 7.3.)

At the same time as the follicular tube is filling up and plugging, the androgenic hormones are also driving the increased production of sebum by stimulating a marked increase in the production rate of sebocytes. The two major organisms living in the duct can break down the triglycerides (one of the fats in the sebum) into fatty acids for food. This provides nutrition to the *P. acnes* and also to the *Malassezia* yeast in the follicle.

The hypothesis suggests that the lack of oxygen (and other nutrients) caused by the increased pressure impairs the ability of the follicular keratinocytes to undergo terminal differentiation. This is the process through which basal keratinocytes change over their life span from soggy little cuboidal basal cells filled with a metabolically active gel to a thin flat sheet made up mostly of keratin that simply flakes off into the duct at the end of its life. If maturation and differentiation are interrupted, the keratinocyte does not fully mature and does not desquamate. The lining keratinocytes remain attached to each other instead of separating (desquamating). That leads to the continued

Acne: Causes and Practical Management, First Edition. F. William Danby.
© 2015 John Wiley & Sons, Ltd. Published 2015 by John Wiley & Sons, Ltd.

buildup of material in the follicle, and the plug in the pore becomes larger.

At the same time, using electron microscopy, a buildup of lipid-containing vacuoles (little bubbles of lipid) can be seen in the stacked layers of keratinocytes that have stopped differentiating and are piling up in the follicular canal [1]. These lipids likely represent both the source of metabolic energy (that is not being used as energy because there is insufficient oxygen for oxidization) and an unused reserve of the lipid that was intended for incorporation into the lipoprotein end products. In this hypothesis, these lipids are not being used because their metabolism is shut down because of the anoxia.

The androgenic-acnegenic hormones, if not controlled, continue to stimulate the basal cells of this closed follicular system from the outside, producing more and more internal pressure until the walls of the follicles leak or eventually rupture. This takes time, measured in months when young healthy follicles are the target, which is the usual case in teenage acne.

Up to this point, the entire acne production process is due to hormonal stimuli. This is the stage of non-inflammatory acne. Basically, all there is to see at this point is a plugged and swollen follicular unit and a busy oil gland. The bacteria and yeast in the follicular canal, the *intrafollicular flora*, are just innocent bystanders, happy to be consuming the sebum (their preferred food) and multiplying actively.

The leaks and the ruptures that occur at this point in the follicular wall release materials from the follicular canal, including bacteria and yeast and other materials contained within the follicle. These materials, including flakes of keratin in the case of acne inversa [2], leak into the tissue under the surface of the skin, in the upper and mid-dermis. That release of normally intrafollicular contents triggers both of our two immune systems. As these foreign materials interact with the innate immune system, they are termed *stimuli*. When the same materials interact with the adaptive (acquired) immune system, they are called *antigens*. The immune systems awaken, and the fight is on.

The resulting inflammatory cascade lights the fires of inflammation, a molecular and cellular conflagration termed the *inflammasome*. The leaks in the walls of the follicles become a two-way street, allowing some of the inflammatory mediators access to the contents of the duct, leading to intrafollicular collections of inflammatory cells

that push toward the surface as folliculopustules. Most of the inflammation remains outside the FPSU structure, especially in acne inversa. This severe acne variant is distinguished by its failure to discharge to the surface and its failure to subsequently heal quickly, as normally occurs with boils or abscesses due to infection.

Beyond this point, inflammation rules and previously non-inflammatory acne becomes inflammatory, one FPSU at a time.

As Leeming *et al.* state,

> It is probable … that when micro-organisms are present in acne lesions they make a significant contribution to the promotion of inflammation. Indeed it would be surprising if they did not, considering the large number of microbial antigens and metabolic by-products which would be released into the dermis from a colonized acne lesion when ruptured. [3]

The complex interactions that occur have recently been elucidated by Melnik in a remarkable synthesis of the dozens of processes that mediate the inflammasome via Notch1. Acne inversa is the variant explored in his landmark paper, but the same processes are doubtless expressed in the less florid acnes [4]. The basic premise is that the rupture of the FPSU releases *damage-associated molecular pattern* molecules (DAMPs). These fragments bear molecular patterns that identify them as, for example, pieces of yeast or hair or virus. They are recognized as foreign by toll-like receptors (TLRs), and the TLRs turn on the numerous pro-inflammatory cytokines that manage the inflammatory reaction. This inflammation is normally downregulated by Notch signaling, so when Notch signaling is diet impaired, TLR-mediated inflammation is not held in check as it should be, permitting and therefore causing more inflammation.

To add to the problem, Notch1 is also involved in regulation of keratinocyte differentiation. Lack of Notch1 leads to a reduced induction of p21, the earliest regulatory step in the process. Less Notch1 means less differentiation of the keratinocytes and so more ductal plugging.

While control of the effects of excess hormonal stimulation is essential to contain the process and prevent new lesions from forming, hormonal control alone will not provide the anti-inflammatory action needed for an acceptable clinical response and resolution. The object in fighting this fire must be to shut off the fuel supply as well as get to work with fire extinguishers. That means that an essential part of therapy is the total elimination of the intrafollicular flora if possible.

Reversing the whole pathogenetic process once it reaches this stage requires reversal of the hormones, reversal of the follicular plugging, elimination of the bacteria and yeast, and reversal of the inflammation. It is a tall order and not one that can be accomplished with monotherapy. A team attack is essential.

3.2 Acne rosacea

The folliculopapular and folliculopustular forms of acne rosacea are started by the same hormonal stimuli that trigger acne vulgaris. Several local differences lead to a markedly different-looking disorder.

First, the support of follicular walls of the FPSU is, I suspect but cannot prove, slowly weakened by years of exposure to ultraviolet-A (UVA) and UVB light, and the weakness is most prominent at the upper end of the follicular unit where the sun has been strongest and where actinically damaged collagen is commonly seen. (See Section 1.2.) This has two consequences. First, the distribution of acne rosacea is over the convex, sun-exposed parts of the face. Second, the rupture of the follicular wall, with consequent formation of the folliculopapule or folliculopustule, occurs without the development of a visible comedo. It is proposed that these visible plugs do not form because the follicular wall has been so compromised by photodamage from the sun that the leaks and ruptures occur before a visible plug can accumulate. *Demodex* might even find the UV-damaged and dilated follicular orifices more commodious and so an easier place to breed and raise their families.

Second, the flora and fauna in acne rosacea are different from those in acne vulgaris. The hypothesis suggests that the pressure required to induce the apparent anoxia cannot occur because the follicular wall bursts too soon. It follows that there is none of the profound anoxia deep in the follicular duct as is found in acne vulgaris, so enhanced populations of *P. acnes* are not the important players here. Instead, the problem is inflammation induced by a combination of stimuli and antigens from retained vellus hairs, *Demodex* folliculorum, a smaller population of *P. acnes*, and the yeasts, mainly *Malassezia* but occasionally *Candida* species. Early acne rosacea may also differ from later acne rosacea because

antibiotic therapy will change the bacterial and yeast proportions in the intrafollicular cavity. This is because the oral antibiotics, used as anti-inflammatories, reduce the population of *P. acnes* and other bacteria. At the same time, this enhances the population of *Malassezia* that is normally present as an innocent commensal on the face and permits (or encourages) other yeasts such as *Candida*.

As with acne vulgaris, hormonal control alone will not provide the anti-inflammatory therapy needed for an acceptable clinical response in acne rosacea. The intrafollicular flora and fauna must be eliminated as an essential part of therapy. The addition of *Demodex* further complicates an already complex picture. Again, from Leeming, "It is conceivable that the causes of inflammation vary amongst lesions and individuals, and that this variation could explain apparent paradoxes such as the different responses of individual acne patients to various therapies" [3]. Leeming's concept is further illustrated by what seems to be another process underway in acne rosacea when it is being treated with low-dose doxycycline. One of the early selling points used in promoting this low-dose approach was the claim that it was too low to encourage overgrowth of vaginal and vulvar candidiasis [5]. It is reasonable then to suggest that this induces less "biotropic" effect on the *Malassezia* organism as well, inducing *Malassezia* growth to a lesser degree and so tending to allow the cooling of the inflammation without inducing the variant of acne rosacea that requires ketoconazole for control.

Third is the need to avoid sun damage. This is an obvious concern with regard to the damage to the collagenous support tissues of blood vessels as well as the follicles. Such actinic damage induces the actinic telangiectasia that usually accompanies the folliculopustular component of acne rosacea (although it often stands alone). The geographic coexistence of these two damaged tissues underlines the common etiological factor, sun damage. This link is an essential part of the hypothesis here. Thus, effective broad-spectrum sun protection from an early age is highly important to prevent and to minimize cumulative and further damage to both follicular support tissues and the superficial blood vessels in the area.

Unfortunately, a major part of that battle is often lost by the time clinical disease occurs, leaving only prevention of further damage as an option. Physical rehabilitation of the vascular changes with several modalities of selectively destructive laser is possible, but is difficult, time-consuming, and expensive, and it does not return the dilated vessels to normal. The UV damage to the supporting fabric of the follicular canal that may cause marginal dilation (and thus provide the *Demodex* with a more accessible home) is a defect not directly amenable to laser or other repair. Nevertheless, resurfacing and other techniques can provide impressive cosmetic benefit using very selective surface destruction followed by re-epithelialization, and/or microsized scars followed by a healing "tightening effect."

3.3 Acne inversa/hidradenitis suppurativa (AI/HS)

The hormones that activate the other acnes are operative here as well, and their control is essential to slowing the plugging of the follicular portion of the duct. Again, there are regional differences in the way the lesions

evolve. For one, visible open comedones are rare to nonexistent in the early stage of the disease. Comedones do show up as the massively distorted structures called *multiheaded* or *tombstone comedones* later in the disease, but these are end-stage structures, explained elsewhere in this volume.

Obviously, however, there is *something* plugging the pores. Certainly, the hormonal stimulus is operative here and is extensively reviewed elsewhere. The problem is that the follicular plug is in the deeper portion of the follicular part of the FPSU, in the infrainfundibulum, and it is invisible from the surface unless profoundly filled with follicular keratinocytic debris. (See Figure 3.1.)

Building upon work in acne pioneered by the Burkharts [6], recent work in AI/HS points a finger at biofilm formation as a possible contributor [7]. Biofilm is a protective mechanism for intraductal organisms and is an additional attractive explanation for the plugging of the duct. By protecting the organism against contact

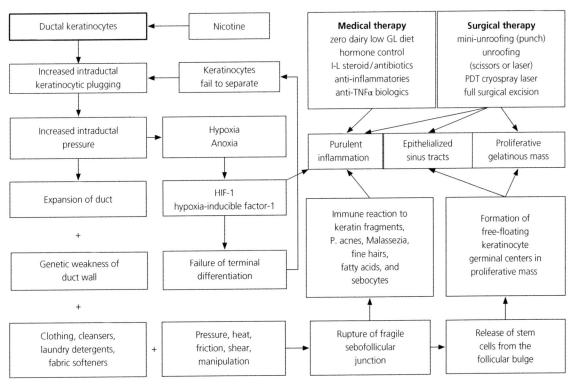

Figure 3.1 The chain of events from keratinocyte excess to medical and surgical management of the plugged and exploded duct is simplified here. Excess keratinocyte production begets the early plug that expands and triggers the anoxia that, likely through hypoxia-inducible factor 1, interferes with terminal differentiation and induces inflammation.

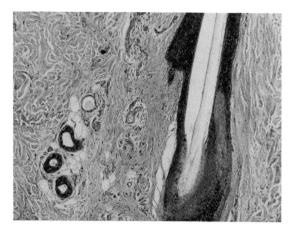

Figure 3.2 The central third of this image shows new scarring and residual inflammation centered on an area where a sebaceous gland has been destroyed, leaving behind the ragged stub of the sebofollicular junction still attached to the isthmus area of the follicle. The nearby apocrine ducts are well protected by their PAS+ (periodic acid–Schiff positive) wrap, while inflammatory cells are still present, attacking the areas of the follicular wall unprotected by PAS+ material at 4–5 and 9–10 o'clock.

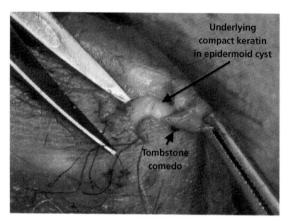

Figure 3.3 Beneath a tombstone comedo. As the sole surviving portion of a folliculopilosebaceous unit that has undergone explosive destruction, the intact residual follicular component, still under the influence of the hormones of growth, continues to produce lamellae of keratin that have difficulty exiting the pore.

with antibiotics and other threats, such a film may facilitate the persistence of *P. acnes* and other film-forming organisms in the follicular duct and thus contribute to the problem. The *Staphylococcus* and *Streptococcus* occasionally encountered in the area, and thought to be innocent, may play a role in this way, protecting themselves and other organisms in the process [8].

If one takes a close look at the general shape and the development of the AI/HS lesions, it is apparent that there has always been a clue to what is really happening under the skin in this disorder. The clue lies in the fact that, unlike acne vulgaris and acne rosacea pustules (and ordinary bacterial and *Candida* folliculitis), the follicular structure in AI/HS does not rupture and discharge vertically to the surface of the skin. Instead, it ruptures at a level deep in the dermis (Figure 3.2). These lesions do not "point" to the surface. They rupture horizontally and then both pyogenic (pus-causing) inflammation and a peculiar gelatinous proliferative mass infiltrate the subcutis, sometimes for significant distances, usually horizontally but to depth as well, along paths of least resistance.

Whether the disorder is in the groin, perineum, or inframammary areas; under pressure areas, like waistbands; or at the site of a *pilonidal cyst*, the rupture occurs deep in the follicular unit. The break occurs at a location

quite the inverse of the very superficial rupture of acne rosacea. In patients genetically predisposed to AI/HS, the same tendency to "burst deep" yields a variant of facial acne that is much deeper and so is much more problematic than usual. (See Figure 3.4.)

Recently, histologic studies have demonstrated in patients with HS/AI that there is a thinning of the normally thick collagenous matrix that supports the structure of the FPSU at the junction of the sebaceous gland and canal with the follicular unit [9]. This may turn out to be the explanation for the "inverse" location of the rupture in this disease, and its tendency to induce aggressive local inflammatory activity that destroys the nearby sebaceous component of the FPSU (Figure 3.2) [10]. It is likely that this is a genetic weakness, but further study is needed [4]. We need these histological findings confirmed, and then we must define the defect, define the gene functionality that is responsible, identify the gene or genes coding for that functionality, and confirm their genomic location. We need to know whether the gene itself is missing or mutated, and we need to know about its heritability. Only then will we have a complete pathogenic trail. But barring "gene therapy," doubtless a few years in the future, the only preventive therapy remains hormonal and dietary.

To complicate matters, but to further explain the clinical picture, the rupture in this location leads to an almost complete destruction of the sebaceous compo-

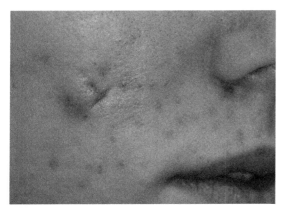

Figure 3.4 As elsewhere, the inverse and deep involvement is a challenge to manage. Surgical I&D (incision and drainage) is best avoided on the face but is sometimes unavoidable, leaving incisional scars, residual activity and epidermoid cystic inclusions.

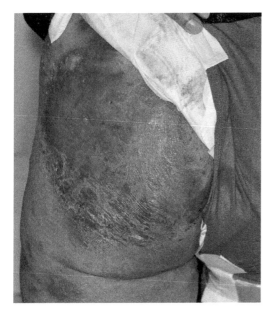

Figure 3.5 AI/HS buttock (1), initial presentation: September 2010. This degree of involvement might attract extensive surgical attention, but that is best avoided.

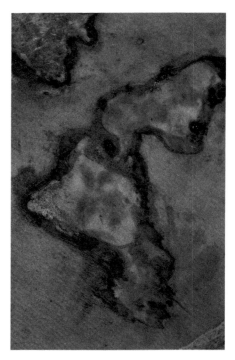

Figure 3.6 AI/HS buttock (2), March 20, 2013: Following confidence building with several smaller areas, this large area on the left hip and buttock was unroofed.

nent and the pilar unit beneath. This leaves behind the intact follicular unit that heals up at its deepest extent. Under continued androgenic stimulation, the follicular infundibular stub becomes the dilated tombstone comedo (Figure 3.3). This destructive explosion appears to release a surviving population of live and aggressive stem cells from the follicular bulge of the ruptured pilar portion of the duct into the underlying dermis [11, 12]. The stem cells are cast free into a nutrient soup of the type that normally nourishes granulation tissue. They appear to create, from within an invasive proliferative gelatinous mass (IPGM), the epithelialized sinuses that are the hallmark of this disease. These sinuses, acting as foreign bodies beneath the surface and trapped in the dermis, perpetuate the inflammation that curses these patients, a curse that sometimes lasts for decades, as in the deep and recalcitrant form of acne that appears on the adult faces of patients with AI/HS (Figure 3.4).

This complex disease, with a complex set of pathogenic activities driving it, requires complex therapy. This includes strict dietary management, hormone control, antimicrobials, anti-inflammatories, physical unroofing of the sinuses (Figures 3.5, 3.6, 3.7, and 3.8) and, in the worst cases, all of the above plus full excisional surgical removal of residua.

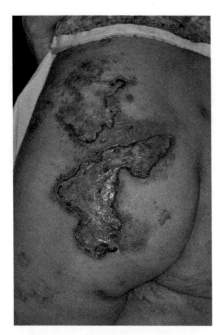

Figure 3.7 AI/HS buttock (3), March 25, 2013: With no dressing other than petrolatum, the wounds are clean and comfortable, causing minimal interference with office work, and without need for analgesia.

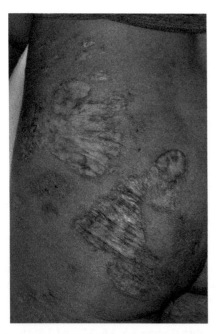

Figure 3.8 AI/HS buttock (4), November 18, 2013: Wounds are clean and dry. Petrolatum is still in use after baths or showers to combat dryness and avoid chafing.

3.4 Other variants

The anatomic and pathogenic factors that contribute to the morphology of the classic three acnes vary in their contribution to the process, not merely by being present or absent but also by varying in degree of activity. Thus, a preponderance of the *Malassezia* yeast induces the picture of *Malassezia* folliculitis, a massive overreaction to the *Malassezia* by the adaptive immune system may be the mechanism that yields Ofuji's disease, involvement of terminal hair follicles in the scalp and the production of an IPGM in the scalp seem to produce dissecting terminal folliculitis, excessive activation of the processes that trigger scarring leads to acne keloidalis, and inhibition of the epidermal growth factor receptors (EGFRs) seems to be responsible for the paradoxical inflammatory flare that clouds the utility of this valuable anticancer modality.

Looking through this lens, one can perhaps see acne vulgaris as due to active production of keratinocytes in otherwise healthy and tight young follicular units, acne rosacea as the variant that occurs when sun damage weakens the top end of the follicular units, and AI/HS as the variant due to an explosion of the follicular unit at the site of congenitally weak support of the sebofollicular junction.

3.4.1 *Malassezia* folliculitis

The skin is host to many organisms, and in acne the one that has been best studied is a normal occupant of the skin that was called *Corynebacterium acnes* in the past and is now renamed *Propionibacterium acnes* (*P. acnes*). Most of the effort to kill bacteria on the skin and down in the pores in acne is directed at this organism. That is what the tetracycline, minocycline, doxycycline, clindamycin, and erythromycin topical and oral preparations are all about. And yet, even when the population of *P. acnes* is reduced to 1/1,000,000th of the original, we still have the inflamed plugged follicles we call *acne*. We also have an increasing population of resistant *P. acnes* that has spread around the world wherever the organism has been exposed to these antibiotics [13].

So, what's going on? Two things at least are at work, and maybe three. First, acne papules are not populated exclusively by *P. acnes*. Cunliffe and his team at Leeds showed 25 years ago that 68% of three-day-old acne papules on the back also contain a yeast called *Malassezia* [14]. This yeast has had a name change over the years—it used to be *Pityrosporum*, but that name was dropped in 1986, the genus was revised in 1996, and there are now 14 recognized species of *Malassezia* [15].

Second, as many patients are aware, taking broad-spectrum antibiotics will often cause "yeast infections" in women's private areas, and even some men get this, especially if they are uncircumcised. This is a different yeast, from a family called *Candida*, but both *Candida* and *Malassezia* grow much faster when the bacteria in the area are reduced by antibiotics. The reason is thought to be the simple fact that less bacteria means more food for the yeast and that leads to more growth of the yeast. The growth of the *Malassezia* yeast down in the pores in acne is not usually recognized by family doctors, pediatricians, and even many dermatologists.

The recognition of the problem is complicated by the fact that this is a silent infection. It does not show up on routine cultures because *Malassezia* is a "picky eater" and needs a certain type of oil in its diet—long-chain (12 to 24 carbon units) fatty acids that are present in abundance down in the plugged pores but are not normally present in the culture medium used in the lab. So if the doctor does a culture of the acne pustules, what shows up are bacteria resistant to the antibiotics that have been used in the past, leading to the use of more and more aggressive antibiotics, and the *Malassezia* usually remains undiscovered. The more antibiotics are used, the more the aggressive antibiotics help the *Malassezia* grow even more. Indeed, it may not be too much of a stretch to suggest that the worldwide induction of antibiotic-resistant *P. acnes* owes more to physicians' failure to recognize *Malassezia* than can be blamed on physicians' overprescribing aimed at the *P. acnes* target itself.

Malassezia folliculitis shows up as a few or hundreds of pinhead to 2 mm folliculopapules and folliculopustules that pretty much all look the same (they are termed *monomorphic*). They are scattered all over the classic acne areas but have a tendency to show up high on the forehead, and at the temples (Figure 3.9). They also extend above the hairline into the scalp where acne comedones are rarely seen (Figure 3.10), and can show up around the periphery of the scalp, at the back of the neck at the hairline, at the nape of the neck (Figure 3.11), and under the jawline. They even show up in the scalp itself where there may be deep, little, itchy pimples and scaling areas and dandruff. Their presentation over the chest, even if only a handful are present, is often confirmatory (Figure 3.12). There are usually no

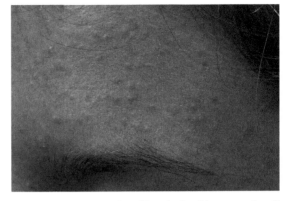

Figure 3.9 Eight weeks of weekly pulsed oral ketoconazole will eliminate the yeast-induced lesions and leave the few closed comedones behind.

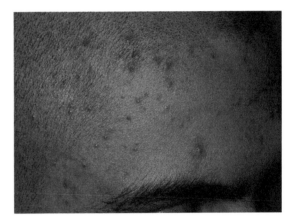

Figure 3.10 While there are a few comedones here, the monomorphous folliculopapules and folliculopustules extending into the scalp make the diagnosis.

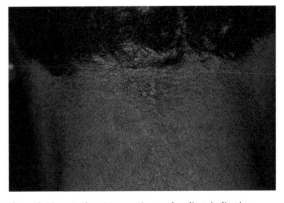

Figure 3.11 Note the pigmentation and scaling, indicating coexisting pityriasis (tinea) versicolor.

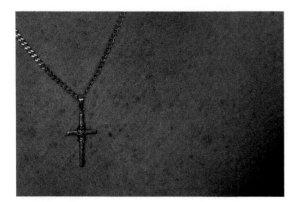

Figure 3.12 A six-month course of doxycycline produced this "antibiotic-resistant acne."

comedones in these areas, or only a few from the original acne. This is often itchy, and the itch is one of the best indications that yeast is present. Any woman who has had yeast vulvitis or vaginitis will confirm that it is one of the itchiest conditions we have to treat. (See Section 8.5.3 for management.)

So, why has this yeast become such a problem? It is likely (and this is speculation) that the "biocides" that are part of our lives, especially the ones in shampoos and soaps to prevent rancidity and improve shelf life [16], have killed or reduced or prevented the growth of competing bacteria in the scalp, and elsewhere on the body surface. There is evidence that the amounts used are in excess of the concentration needed to achieve the goal of adequate shelf life, and this is an area that needs proper investigation [17]. The *Malassezia* yeasts, I suspect, are more resistant to these biocides than the bacteria that are targeted and so are "selected out"; that is why they now survive in higher numbers on our skins and scalps. This may be due in part to their ability to hide down in the follicles, out of reach of the biocides' effects, and then they may repopulate the scalp when the shampoo has been washed away. There is no proof of this idea other than the success I've seen using the fungicidal shampoos for long-term maintenance, on a once-a-week basis, after depopulating both the follicles and the surface with oral ketoconazole.

3.4.2 Eosinophilic pustular folliculitis (Ofuji's disease)

This rare inflammatory folliculitis is currently considered a disorder of unknown cause. It is presented here because I think the case can be made that it is actually a massive immunological overreaction to the *Malassezia* organism, a process mediated by "friendly fire" with eosinophils from the bone marrow set on "full automatic." Essentially, I suspect that Ofuji's syndrome is *Malassezia* folliculitis "gone ballistic."

The evidence is circumstantial; Koch's postulates will never be satisfied for reasons discussed in Section 3.4.1 on *Malassezia*; but there are hints in the several papers published on this disease:

1 The distribution is classically over the "seborrheic areas." No other known pathogen requires the fatty acids that are present in abundance in sebum, and nowhere is there more sebum than in these areas.
2 The profound itch is typical of yeast-mediated infestations such as *Candida vulvovaginitis*.
3 The folliculocentric distribution of the papules and pustules mirrors the pattern seen in the more common *Malassezia* folliculitis. That these form confluent plaques is simply a function of coalescence over time, not an indication that this is primarily a papulosquamous disease.
4 The failure to respond to topical antifungals and to oral terbinafine illustrates both the impossibility of delivering effective anti-yeast doses to the depths of the follicles with topical applications and the limited spectrum of anti-yeast activity of the medications used.
5 The response to anti-inflammatories like indomethacin, antihistamines, dapsone, and topical steroids parallels the mechanism proposed whereby *Malassezia* folliculitis is brought under control. (See Section 6.2.) This consists of a combination of ketoconazole-mediated anti-inflammatory effect and slow but effective elimination of the organism's antigens from the follicular structures.
6 The effectiveness of UVB phototherapy, psoralen–UVA photochemotherapy, and narrow-band phototherapy can all be explained by a combination of the lethal effect of UV light (UVL) on the *Malassezia* organism [18] and the anti-inflammatory effect of UVL on the cellular mediators of inflammation.
7 One reported case developed in a patient who "regularly consumed" body builder's protein shakes, a published and acknowledged trigger of follicular plugging [19].

Although the disorder is generally uncommon, there is extensive experience in Japan [20]. Interestingly, ketoconazole has never been reported among the medications used. It is perhaps time to give it a try.

3.4.3 Dissecting terminal folliculitis

This rather rare disease, most often in the scalp but occasionally on a hairy chest or groin and occasionally on the extremities, is one of the several deep disorders of follicles that have been included in the *follicular triad* and the *follicular tetrad* with acne conglobata, hidradenitis suppurativa, and pilonidal cysts. These all seem to be caused by the same deep inflammatory pattern seen in AI/HS and pilonidal cysts, namely, deeply tracking inflammatory masses that undermine the skin and extend great distances laterally from their tissue of origin. There are numerous synonyms, the most colorful being *perifolliculitis capitis abscedens et suffodiens* (Figure 3.13). No work has yet been done searching for the specific defects seen in the microscopic PAS + (periodic acid–Schiff positive) anatomy of the follicles involved in this variant of these folliculopathies. Nevertheless, there is no reason to suggest a defect different from that in the follicles of acne inversa, especially as these generally are not isolated disorders. The exaggerated feature here is the undermining proliferative mass. It is encountered when attempts are made to perform "incision and drainage" on such lesions.

3.4.4 Acne keloidalis

As the name suggests, this disorder combines the features of both acne and an excessive scarring response. It appears to develop most actively in those of aboriginal African heritage (Figure 3.14). The location is one of the most common sites for development of *Malassezia* folliculitis, which is proposed as the cause of the itch that provides the stimulus to scratch. That scratching trauma, often magnified by manipulation by the patient and his or her physician and/or hairdresser, ruptures the follicular walls and starts the inflammatory reaction. I would not be surprised to see a follicular support defect like the one found in AI/HS underlying this disorder, but that has not been explored. Biopsying an area of hypertrophic scarring risks worsening the problem. The tendency of treating physicians to reach first for an antibiotic may well be responsible for worsening the situation by encouraging the growth of *Malassezia*, and this may be compounded by the use of intralesional steroids in the absence of antifungal therapy. Certainly, there is a tendency to scarring that far exceeds the normal repair process. The overresponsive scarring further compromises the normal architecture of the FPSUs and further drives the process.

My personal approach is to start with full dairy restriction and a low-glycemic-load diet and continue it indefinitely. Ketoconazole 400 mg weekly is introduced first, to control and eliminate the yeast and its associated itch and inflammation. Then, low-dose acitretin or isotretinoin is started as soon as possible, a dose of intramuscular triamcinolone is given in the anterior thigh (1 mg/kg with a maximum of 80 mg) after 10–14 days, and antibiotics (preferably, amoxicillin or cefadroxil) are added at this point if there is evidence of true infection (not just inflammation). Dapsone is also useful as a steroid-sparing adjunctive therapy. Intralesional injection with triamcinolone acetonide 5–20 mg/mL to thick scars is continued until the area is softened. The antibiotic and dapsone are tapered as soon as possible, and ketoconazole is used in maintenance doses indefinitely, usually 400 mg in a single dose monthly.

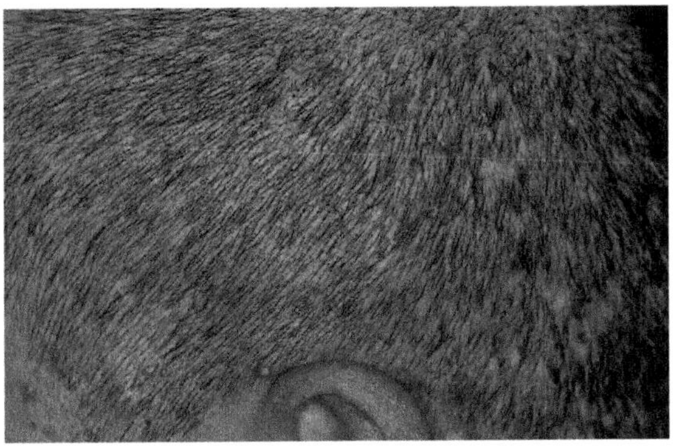

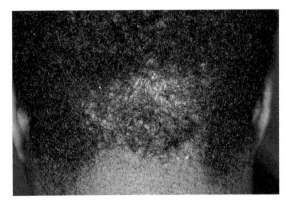

Figure 3.13 Dissecting terminal folliculitis. Note the deep inflammatory nodule and the numerous scars and pustules. This man also had draining nodules in the groin.

Figure 3.14 Acne keloidalis. Classic location with scarring alopecia, inflammatory drainage, and hypertrophic, folliculocentric scars.

3.4.5 Epidermal growth factor receptor (EGFR) inhibitor eruption

Potent inhibitors of the EGFR have been developed as therapeutic agents in the fight against a number of cancers. These agents have several side effects, one of the most difficult being the folliculopapular and folliculo-pustular eruption [21]. This eruption has been called *acneform* by nondermatologists despite the lack of comedones. The folliculocentric distribution of the process certainly produces lesions that look like highly inflammatory acne (Figure 3.15). Despite the fact that this is a drug-induced folliculitis, not acne, the range of therapies offered for this side effect is based on standard therapies for acne. These include benzoyl peroxide, oral retinoids, tetracycline and its derivatives, other topical and oral antibiotics, metronidazole, and topical steroids [22, 23]. An extensive search for a responsible organism did identify "rare incidental ... organisms in the stratum corneum of three patients" that were misnamed as "Pityrosporum" [24]. Despite there being only one case in the literature [25] that truly demonstrates intra- or perifollicular *Malassezia*, I have found low-dose, pulsed, weekly ketoconazole to be exceptionally useful. In the personal case illustrated, initial control was achieved with three weekly doses of 400 mg ketoconazole. Ketoconazole 200 mg weekly was then used as maintenance for nine months, at which point the patient's supply of ketoconazole ran out. She flared within 10 days (Figures 3.16 and 3.17) and was dramatically returned to control within eight days using minocycline and ketoconazole (Figure 3.18). She remained clear on 200 mg of ketoconazole weekly until her death six months later.

A second case with sheets of folliculopapules (but no comedones) presented January 18 on brentuximab (Figure 3.19). She remained on her brentuximab, and ketoconazole therapy alone cleared the lesions by February 8 (Figure 3.20).

Whether ketoconazole works by dislodging *Malassezia*, by permitting its phagocytosis, or as a highly lipophilic anti-inflammatory is worth further investigation, but the response described may be due to a serendipitous combination of all three characteristics of this unusually effective azole.

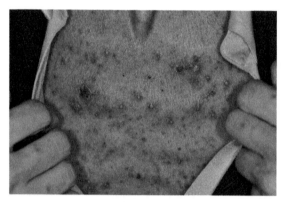

Figure 3.15 EGFR inhibitor eruption. "Acneiform" pattern of eruption due to unknown mechanism.

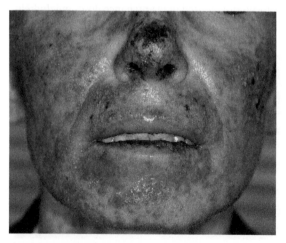

Figure 3.16 EGFR inhibitor eruption. Initial presentation (not shown) cleared and stayed clear with ketoconazole orally while taking erbitux and irinotecan. Ran out of weekly 200 mg ketoconazole and flared over face, trunk, and limbs.

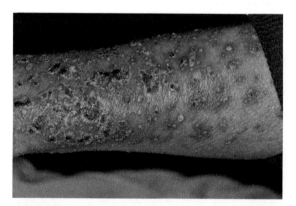

Figure 3.17 EGFR inhibitor eruption. November 2: Same flare, left forearm. Methicillin-resistant *Streptococcus aureus* positive, sensitive to sulfa (patient allergic) and vancomycin (avoiding because of previous diarrhea), and borderline sensitive to tetracycline. Restarted oral ketoconazole and topical neomycin ointment, and added minocycline when cultures available.

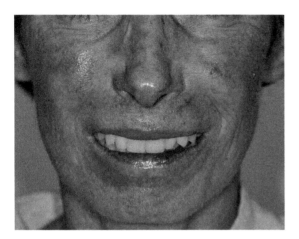

Figure 3.18 EGFR inhibitor eruption. November 10: Cleared and remained clear on 200 mg ketoconazole weekly until deceased five months later.

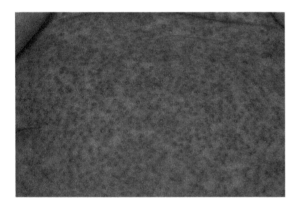

Figure 3.19 EGFR inhibitor eruption. Presented January 16 under treatment with brentuximab with rash on the xiphisternal area of two weeks. Started ketoconazole orally 400 mg in a single dose weekly. Topical petrolatum only.

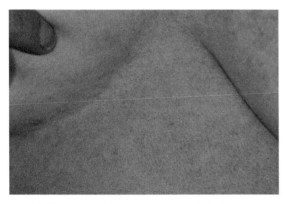

Figure 3.20 EGFR inhibitor eruption. Essentially clear on January 23. Photo shows status on February 6 after a total of four tablets of 200 mg ketoconazole.

Extrait de la *Revue générale de Clinique et de Thérapeutique*
(JOURNAL DES PRATICIENS)

L'ACNÉ EXCORIÉE

DES JEUNES FILLES

ET SON TRAITEMENT

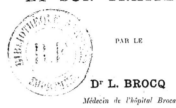

PAR LE

Dr L. BROCQ

Médecin de l'hôpital Broca

Figure 3.21 Brocq monograph of 1898.

3.4.6 Acné excoriée des jeunes filles

The excoriated acne of young women has been a classic presentation since its description by Brocq in his monograph of 1898 (Figure 3.21) [26]. The description of the excoriations, the obsessive opening of lesions with fingernails and household tools from needles to scissors, and the social withdrawal all are familiar. One passage stands out: "most, if not all of these young women demonstrated a ceaseless scratching of their facial acne that proves that they were unable to resist the itching sensations, driven by a sort of imperative need on the order of a mania" (26; author's trans.). Among the therapeutic suggestions, down the list from hydrotherapy, static electricity, and exercise in the fresh air, is the consideration of attention to the possibility of neurasthenia, leading to the suggestion that "le marriage peut-être une diversion des plus salutaires" [26] A salutary diversion, indeed!

Having treated several patients very successfully with ketoconazole, without suggesting marriage, I noted with interest the suggestion, when the seborrhea is especially prominent ("Lorsque la seborrhée est fort intense"), that a sulfur lotion (a mixture of resorcinol, sulfur, glycerin, and camphor in rosewater) should be applied with a cotton ball before retiring. The sulfur and resorcinol doubtless helped reduce the population of *Malassezia*, and possibly suitors as well. Dr. Brocq would have found ketoconazole of much greater value.

References

1 Knutson DD. Ultrastructural observations in acne vulgaris: the normal sebaceous follicle and acne lesions. J Invest Dermatol 1974 Mar;62(3):288–307.

2 van der Zee HH, de RL, Boer J,van den Broecke DG, den Hollander JC, Laman JD, et al. Alterations in leucocyte subsets and histomorphology in normal-appearing perilesional skin and early and chronic hidradenitis suppurativa lesions. Br J Dermatol 2012 Jan;166(1):98–106.

3 Leeming JP, Holland KT, Cunliffe WJ. The microbial colonization of inflamed acne vulgaris lesions. Br J Dermatol 1988 Feb;118(2):203–8.

4 Melnik BC, Plewig G. Impaired Notch signalling: the unifying mechanism explaining the pathogenesis of hidradenitis suppurativa (acne inversa). Br J Dermatol 2013 Apr;168(4):876–8.

5 Korting HC, Schollmann C. Current topical and systemic approaches to treatment of rosacea. J Eur Acad Dermatol Venereol 2009 Aug;23(8):876–82.

6 Burkhart CN, Burkhart CG. Microbiology's principle of biofilms as a major factor in the pathogenesis of acne vulgaris. Int J Dermatol 2003 Dec;42(12):925–7.

7 Kathju S, Lasko LA, Stoodley P. Considering hidradenitis suppurativa as a bacterial biofilm disease. FEMS Immunol Med Microbiol 2012 Jul;65(2):385–9.

8 Vlassova N, Han A, Zenilman JM, James G, Lazarus GS. New horizons for cutaneous microbiology: the role of biofilms in dermatological disease. Br J Dermatol 2011 Oct;165(4):751–9.

9 Danby FW, Jemec GB, Marsch WC, vonLaffert M. Preliminary findings suggest hidradenitis suppurativa may be due to defective follicular support. Br J Dermatol 2013 May;168(5):1034–9.

10 Kamp S, Fiehn AM, Stenderup K, Rosada C, Pakkenberg B, Kemp K, et al. Hidradenitis suppurativa: a disease of the absent sebaceous gland? Sebaceous gland number and volume are significantly reduced in uninvolved hair follicles from patients with hidradenitis suppurativa. Br J Dermatol 2011 May;164(5):1017–22.

11 Gniadecki R, Bang B. Flotillas of lipid rafts in transit amplifying cell-like keratinocytes. J Invest Dermatol 2003 Sep;121(3):522–8.

12 Gniadecki R, Jemec GB. Lipid raft-enriched stem cell-like keratinocytes in the epidermis, hair follicles and sinus tracts in hidradenitis suppurativa. Exp Dermatol 2004 Jun;13(6):361–3.

13 Leyden JJ, Del Rosso JQ, Webster GF. Clinical considerations in the treatment of acne vulgaris and other inflammatory skin disorders: focus on antibiotic resistance. Cutis 2007 Jun;79(6 Suppl):9–25.

14 Leeming JP, Holland KT, Cunliffe WJ. The microbial colonization of inflamed acne vulgaris lesions. Br J Dermatol 1988 Feb;118(2):203–8.

15 Gaitanis G, Magiatis P, Hantschke M, Bassukas ID, Velegraki A. The *Malassezia* genus in skin and systemic diseases. Clin Microbiol Rev 2012 Jan;25(1):106–41.

16 Lundov MD, Johansen JD, Zachariae C, Moesby L. Low-level efficacy of cosmetic preservatives. Int J Cosmet Sci 2011 Apr;33(2):190–6.

17 Lundov MD, Moesby L, Zachariae C, Johansen JD. Contamination versus preservation of cosmetics: a review on legislation, usage, infections, and contact allergy. Contact Dermatitis 2009 Feb;60(2):70–8.

18 Wikler JR, Janssen N, Bruynzeel DP, Nieboer C. The effect of UV-light on pityrosporum yeasts: ultrastructural changes and inhibition of growth. Acta Derm Venereol 1990;70(1):69–71.

19 Silverberg NB. Whey protein precipitating moderate to severe acne flares in 5 teenaged athletes. Cutis 2012 Aug;90(2):70–2.

20 Katoh M, Nomura T, Miyachi Y, Kabashima K. Eosinophilic pustular folliculitis: a review of the Japanese published works. J Dermatol 2013 Jan;40(1):15–20.

21 Abdullah SE, Haigentz M, Jr., Piperdi B. Dermatologic toxicities from monoclonal antibodies and tyrosine kinase inhibitors against EGFR: pathophysiology and management. Chemother Res Pract 2012;2012:351210.

22 Ehmann LM, Ruzicka T, Wollenberg A. Cutaneous side-effects of EGFR inhibitors and their management. Skin Therapy Lett 2011 Jan;16(1):1–3.

23 Hu JC, Sadeghi P, Pinter-Brown LC, Yashar S, Chiu MW. Cutaneous side effects of epidermal growth factor receptor inhibitors: clinical presentation, pathogenesis, and management. J Am Acad Dermatol 2007 Feb;56(2):317–26.

24 Busam KJ, Capodieci P, Motzer R, Kiehn T, Phelan D, Halpern AC. Cutaneous side-effects in cancer patients treated with the antiepidermal growth factor receptor antibody C225. Br J Dermatol 2001 Jun;144(6):1169–76.

25 Cholongitas E, Pipili C, Ioannidou D. *Malassezia* folliculitis presented as acneiform eruption after cetuximab administration. J Drugs Dermatol 2009 Mar;8(3):274–5.

26 Brocq L. L'acné excoriée des jeunes filles et son traitement. Extrait de la Revue generale de Clinique et de Therapeutique 1898;1–15.

CHAPTER 4

The acne hormones

The major stimulus to the development of acne is the male hormone dihydrotestosterone (DHT). It is a member of the family of steroid hormones, specifically one of the reproductive hormones, and in particular the most potent androgenic androgen. Many of these steroid hormones warrant the label of acnegenic because they generate acne. As explained in Sections 2.8 and 2.9, their actions are facilitated by other hormones and growth factors. These hormones are sourced both from within and from outside the human body.

4.1 The endogenous hormones

Endogenous means "generated within" and so this chapter will briefly review the hormones from sources within the body that impact acne, whether positively or negatively.

4.1.1 Androgens and their sources

The androgens are the male hormones. While they are male in effect, they are present in both males and females, with a much higher volume being produced in males. In women there are two sources, the ovaries and the adrenal glands. In males the specialized testosterone-producing Leydig cells in the testicles are the major source. They significantly outproduce the amount and potency of androgens produced by the adrenal glands. In both men and women, although testosterone (T) has a great deal to do with the development of the genital organs in utero, the major activity surrounding sexual maturity is driven by the 5α-reduced testosterone molecule, known as *5α-dihydrotestosterone, dihydrotestosterone*, or *DHT*.

The only difference between testosterone and DHT is the saturation of the double bond at position 5 of the steroid molecule. The double bond disappears, and a hydrogen atom is added at the 5α position, a small change that increases the power of the molecule by 10 times, and that has tremendous consequences. It is DHT that does all the "dirty work" that brings us dermatologists into the lives of our patients. Basically it is responsible for the acnes, for superfluous hair on the upper lip and elsewhere in women, and for balding in both sexes.

In addition to the actual T molecule, there are a number of testosterone precursors (hormones that turn into testosterone) produced by the ovaries and adrenal glands. The overall picture is complex in women, with both testosterone and its precursor androstenedione produced in the ovaries, while dehydroepiandrosterone (DHEA) and its longer lasting sulfate (DHEAS) are produced in the adrenal glands. The percentage produced by each organ will vary somewhat, but the end result is a pool of testosterone and related androgenic molecules circulating in the blood. Some of this T is bound to sex hormone–binding globulin (SHBG), some of it travels free in the plasma (free T), and there is also a small amount of DHT circulating in the blood. There are some daily (diurnal) variations in both sexes. Monthly variations in women depend on the menstrual cycle if it is active. In general the levels are reasonably constant throughout the childbearing years in women. In men, the same is true, but with variations dependent on

Acne: Causes and Practical Management, First Edition. F. William Danby.
© 2015 John Wiley & Sons, Ltd. Published 2015 by John Wiley & Sons, Ltd.

general health, exercise, diet, age, and of course the possibility of supplementation. Supplements, of course, are *exogenous* steroids. They may be used by either sex, and are dealt with in Section 4.2.

4.1.2 Estrogens and their sources

In women, the major source of estrogens is the ovaries. Estrone (E1), estradiol (E2), and estriol (E3) vary both in the amount produced by the ovaries and in their relative potencies. The subject is vast. For our purposes, we will stay with estradiol. It is the prime estrogenic actor in the acne story.

The other source of estrogens, a minor one in women and a major one in men, is peripheral conversion (usually in fatty tissue) from testosterone. With the assistance of the aromatase enzyme, testosterone is transformed to estradiol, and androstenedione to estrone (Figure 4.1).

4.1.3 Progesterone and the progesteroids

The major role of progesterone is the preparation for and promotion of gestation (pregnancy). Because of this, the major source, and it is a cyclic source, is the ovaries. When an ovary releases an egg (ovum), a yellowish collection of cells called the *corpus luteum* (the "yellow body") is left behind at the site of release of the ovum. These cells are the source of the progesterone and other hormones that prepare the lining of the

uterus (the endometrium) for pregnancy. They also stimulate the breasts on a monthly basis to prepare for pregnancy. These are solid monthly reminders that breast tissue and the folliculopilosebaceous unit (FPSU) share a common origin as epidermal appendages and are controlled by the same family of hormones. The increase of facial oiliness at "period time" is familiar to most women. This active oil gland output is caused by the same hormones that produce the breast swelling and sometimes tenderness.

When no pregnancy occurs, the corpus luteum normally simply melts away, and the progesterone and other ovarian hormone levels drop to baseline levels, waiting for another cycle to start. If a pregnancy does occur, the corpus luteum continues producing progesterone and other hormones at levels sufficient to sustain the pregnancy until the placenta can take over that role.

Occasionally, even when no pregnancy occurs, the corpus luteum fails to melt away. This creates a *persistent corpus luteum* or even a corpus luteum cyst, leading to persistent production of these acnegenic hormones. This situation is occasionally identified at ultrasound examination as the cause of an isolated and otherwise unexplained exacerbation of acne. It usually resolves spontaneously.

Progesterone is not the only hormone produced by the ovary in a cyclic fashion. In addition to androstenedione, dehydroepiandrosterone, and testosterone, a

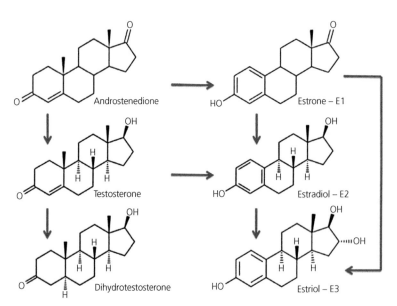

Figure 4.1 Peripheral conversion of androgens to estrogens. The ovaries are the major source of the estrogens in females; these pathways to E1, E2, and E3 are more important in males.

little-known product is 5α-pregnanedione (5α-P) [1]. As an aside, it is important to note that 5α-P is also responsible, in tissue culture, for inducing breast cancer cells to produce increased numbers of estrogen receptors on their cell surfaces, up to two and a half times the normal number, perhaps setting the stage for breast cancer to proceed [2]. In addition, 5α-P is one of the 5α-reduced hormones present in cow milk, another reminder of the common origin of human breasts, cow udders, and the FPSUs. It also provides a basis for speculation that perhaps the FPSUs are stimulated by the same mechanism, 5α-P, priming the human sebocytes to produce estrogen receptors, increasing the sebocytes' response to ingested exogenous dairy estrogens, a subject worthy of laboratory investigation.

While progesterone is a weak acnegen on its own, it also serves as a precursor for a complex cascade of other acnegens. (See Figure 2.12.) It is tempting to consider reducing the progesterone load to minimize acne, but the collateral damage to the androgen cascade and the reproductive system would be unacceptable.

4.1.4 Insulin

Until recently, the only relationship of insulin to the acnes was the known increase in general risk of infection and decreased speed of healing in the acne of diabetics. Insulin's central role in acne has now been recognized and defined [3]. This is not a matter of acne being linked to diabetes, but is instead reflective of the fact that insulin is an important actor in many of our everyday metabolic processes, including those that lead to acne.

Humans evolved to exist on what they found to eat in the world around them. Essentially that included fish and seafood, meat, fowl, eggs, berries, nuts, edible leaves, tubers, fruit, and vegetables. Originally, food was eaten raw. Insulin and insulin-like growth factor 1, both induced by maternal breast milk, were essential stimuli of neonatal growth and development until weaning. Thereafter, insulin served to finely tune plasma glucose levels, the function for which it is best known now.

Eventually, cooking changed previously indigestible complex carbohydrates to a form the human body could more easily digest. The need to handle these simpler carbohydrates made the role of insulin much more important. Insulin's job changed in the face of increasing amounts of dietary glucose. It became the facilitator of the entry of glucose into various cells, for both energy

and storage, thus lowering the level of glucose in the blood. As we learn more of insulin's quiet role in the background before we learned to cook, herd milk cows, and grind grain to fine flour, it is interesting to speculate that insulin has never really evolved as an adequate control mechanism to cope with the vast changes in our diet in the past 15,000 years.

The capacity of each food to produce a rise in blood glucose is measured as the glycemic response. Eating pure sugar produces a very quick rise in blood glucose so the glycemic index (GI) of glucose is high (100), just as the GI of water is low (0). The more easily a carbohydrate-based food is digested and converted to sugar, the higher will be its GI.

One can measure the glycemic response to a fixed weight (usually 100 g) of a solitary food or of a prepared dish by measuring the rise in blood sugar in the hours after the food is consumed, and thus calculate the GI. This then allows one to multiply the GI by the mass/weight of the various components of the food (or of the complete meal) to generate the glycemic load (GL). Small amounts of low-GI foods will have a minimal calculated GL, and large amounts of high-GI foods will yield a very high GL, with an obvious range of response between these two extremes.

This rise in sugar in the blood triggers a rise in serum insulin that is infinitely variable. Because one of the main triggers of androgen receptor receptivity is insulin, this variation translates into a direct but variable relationship between the GI of individual foods, the GL of meals, and the subsequent androgenic response to foods.

Insulin modulates the androgen receptor by inducing the phosphorylation of an intranuclear polypeptide called FoxO1, as described by Melnik [4]. Although it is essentially theoretical, the logical progression of his explanation combined with the experimental documentation of each of the independent metabolic steps are quite compelling. Each link in the argument strengthens the overall explanation he offers, and no logical arguments have been forthcoming to counter his explanations or to suggest alternatives.

Briefly and in summary, insulin and IGF-1 (see Section 4.2.4.1) together synergistically induce a process that de-represses (opens up) the androgen receptor. By so doing, this combination of polypeptide hormones exposes the normally hidden (repressed) androgen receptor, forcing it to become receptive to androgenic molecules. This not only grants access to the endogenous androgens (and their precursors) in both sexes but also welcomes the exogenous androgens and androgenic precursors present in dairy products, plus other exogenous steroid sources such as birth control hormones and even performance-enhancing steroid supplements.

Insulin thus appears to be one of the twin keys to the door that leads to the acnes. Aside from injectable insulin used in the management of diabetes, there is no known exogenous source, the sole exception being very small amounts in dairy-based foods and beverages. The inability to bring an orally administered insulin to market is testimony to the likelihood that the effect (in adults) of orally absorbed insulin is minimal or nil, due to digestion of the insulin molecule.

So, how does all this fit together? Over the past 20 years or so, it has become apparent that, in the group of female patients who have difficulty with acne associated with irregular periods, infertility, ovarian cysts, hirsutism (excess hair), and weight control challenges, there is an additional problem called *insulin resistance*.

This is part of a complex group of metabolic changes that has been given a number of different names, including the cryptic *syndrome X*. The cause of this disorder, usually now referred to as *metabolic syndrome*, is not totally sorted out, but it is important to consider that one of the abnormalities that appears regularly in the fully developed metabolic syndrome, the elevated level of insulin, predisposes to chronic androgen receptor de-repression. Thus, the chronically elevated insulin leads in turn to chronically "available" androgen receptors, leading to the cutaneous and ovarian signs of the disease.

The phenomenon termed *insulin resistance*, through a mechanism that is not yet understood, elevates the circulating levels of insulin to a degree that can be easily measured, allowing fairly easy diagnosis.

Therapy is not so easy. If one does not correct the intake of excessive calories, the insulin level slowly climbs higher. This appears to be part of the link of high-glycemic-load food to the induction and promotion of acne in this special situation. It may also help to explain the results in studies linking acne to high-glycemic-load diet and to elevated body mass index (BMI) [5].

These prolonged elevated insulin levels have the effect of opening the androgen receptors. This means that androgens that previously had been floating in the blood, looking for a place to go, are able to easily access the newly opened androgen receptors, "hook up" with them, and stimulate a host of responses.

Although the most obvious impact of the androgen surge affects the classic hormone-responsive tissues, it is essential to remember that these steroid hormones, besides being involved in reproduction, are also broadly anabolic. This activation of the androgen receptor, through the subsequent activation and direction of *mammalian target of rapamycin complex 1* (mTORC1) (see Section 2.9), stimulates growth of many nonreproductive tissues. That includes muscle and bone, which is why anabolic steroids are used as performance enhancers by many athletes, including race horses.

In turning on the growth of these tissues, androgens contribute to the overall set of body changes that have been referred to in past years as *Stein–Leventhal syndrome*. This is the old terminology for what we now recognize as the collection of prominent markers of *polycystic ovarian syndrome* (PCOS). Although the impact on the acnes is the main subject here, overstimulation of scalp hair growth is also part of the picture and results in female pattern hair loss, for the same reason that men blessed (or cursed) with high testosterone levels tend to early baldness. The same excess of androgen also causes the "superfluous" hair on the face, particularly on the upper lip, and on the trunk, the breasts, the lower abdomen, and the inner thighs in women, all of which are involved to a variable extent in PCOS patients. Although acne is a marker for this disease, there are numerous other tissues impacted as well, particularly the ovaries, all stimulated by an aberrant and interactive testosterone and insulin metabolism.

In Type I (classic early-onset) diabetes, there is a quickly decreasing level of insulin in the early stages of the disease and glucose metabolism is paralyzed by the *lack* of insulin. In the metabolic syndrome, the problem lies elsewhere. The source of insulin in this situation, basically an early manifestation of Type II diabetes, is the pancreas. But in Type II there is too much insulin, and this is most likely a product of dietary insults (outlined in this chapter) that essentially overwhelm insulin's ability to cope, an inability that, as speculated here, may be due to there having been inadequate time for insulin control mechanisms to evolve to handle our calorie-laden modern Western diet.

It appears that whey proteins ingested in milk are a part of the problem. These proteins are the most potent inducers of a polypeptide called *glucose-dependent insulinotropic polypeptide* (GIP) that is secreted in the gastrointestinal tract by neuroendocrine K cells. GIP works together with dietary-sourced essential amino acids derived from intra-gastric hydrolysis (digestion) of whey in milk products. This combination of amino acids and GIP stimulates chronic insulin secretion by pancreatic beta cells, and that is how milk and milk products stimulate the rise in the level of insulin [3]. High-glycemic foods, on the other hand, increase the levels of sugar. While this should be expected to induce more insulin to return the blood levels to normal, chronic hyperglycemia can itself impair pancreatic beta cell function and exacerbate insulin resistance, leading to a vicious cycle of hyperglycemia and causing a worsening metabolic state [6].

The major unanswered question here is the mechanism of insulin resistance. Searching the literature for a solid answer is an exercise in frustration. There are few subjects surrounded by such a high and fuzzy wall of inexplicability.

Several possibilities are being explored, including:

1 A genetic familial (hereditary) abnormality of DNA causing insulin receptor dysfunction. Certainly, a few cases may be explained this way.
2 A mutated DNA causing insulin receptor dysfunction. Again, this is likely causing only a tiny part of the massive obesity epidemic we are facing.
3 Antibodies directed against the insulin receptor, damaging its ability to function. This is an explanation from yesteryear when allergic reactions and "insulin resistance" were due to antibodies to the pork and cow insulins that were used in the past. This was *immunological*, not biochemical, insulin resistance.
4 Epigenetic changes in intracellular DNA could induce the insulin receptors to dysfunction. The inciting factor has to be something *common* (because tens of millions are affected), and if it is an epigenetic influence it has to be something potentially reversible. That limits the field, and the most likely candidate is something to which we are all exposed, likely every day, some with more exposure (or more sensitivity) than others. It needs to be something simple and ubiquitous. Food is a tempting consideration. "Natural" food (the food we consumed over the millions of years while we humans evolved) would be, on the basis of these several million years of experience, an unlikely candidate as the cause of a sudden epidemic. And this most certainly is a sudden epidemic. That narrows the field to only a few considerations, the most likely being the dairy and high-glycemic foods of our modern era, the foods that are now considered to comprise the Westernized diet and that were not present during the millions of years of our early evolution.

While it is tempting to speculate that the most highly consumed "unnatural" foods and their derivatives might be at fault, is there any reasonable alternative to the likely culpability of milk and dairy products, with or without a high-glycemic-load diet? What alternatives exist for consideration? Pesticides, fungicides, antibiotics, and other industrial and agricultural chemicals are possibilities, but the molecular mechanisms that link our modern diet to this group of conditions is becoming more readily understood and better explained year by year. In simple terms, the new chemicals are poisons and are likely to *inhibit* biologic processes. Our modern food, on the other hand, is producing disease by over-stimulating normal metabolic processes.

In a thorough discussion of the effect of diet on the most common disorder elevating the general population's insulin levels, the metabolic syndrome, Unger and Scherer state,

> Based on evidence reviewed here, it seems that prevalent forms of metabolic syndrome and type 2 diabetes mellitus (T2DM) result from unremitting caloric surplus complicated by failure of adipocytes to maintain protection against lipotoxicity. If one imagines the US population to be unwitting volunteers in the largest (300 million subjects) and longest (50 years) clinical research project in history, the specific aim of which was to determine if the deleterious effects of sustained caloric surplus in rodents also can occur in humans, the outcome of the project becomes clear—after 50 years of exposure to an inexpensive calorie-dense diet high in fat and carbohydrates, 200 million subjects are overweight and over 50 million have metabolic syndrome. The failure of healthcare providers and pharmaceutical industries to contain the pandemic suggests that elimination of "bargain basement" calories will be required to "price obesity out of the market." Unfortunately, this would have profound socioeconomic implications: how do we tax excessive calories while at the same time guaranteeing sufficient access to high quality foods for the underprivileged? [7]

Whatever the cause, weight loss and a low-glycemic-load diet plus a zero-dairy diet minimize the risk, and can reverse the process. Studies of severe caloric restriction (600 calories per day for weeks) have recently shown promise in returning diabetics' serum insulin levels to normal [8], but such a restrictive diet will be a tough sell to the general public.

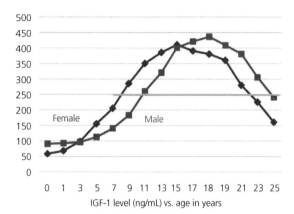

Figure 4.2 The green line at the 250 level gives a remarkably accurate "acne threshold" for both the prevalence and the timing of acne vulgaris.

4.1.5 Growth hormone and insulin-like growth factor-1

The other molecule that leads to de-repression of the androgen receptor is insulin-like growth factor 1 (IGF-1). It is produced by the liver as a result of stimulation by growth hormone (GH) from the pituitary. Together with insulin, as detailed in Section 2.9, IGF-1 triggers the de-repression of the androgen receptor, setting the stage for the development of acne. Just as was shown with insulin, the blood level of IGF-1 can be raised by ingestion of milk, and the casein component has been demonstrated to be responsible [9]. Other than therapeutic injection of GH for dwarfism, there is no known exogenous source.

There is a very close relationship between the incidence of acne and the level of IGF-1 during puberty and adolescence. This far more closely approximates a reasonable causal relationship of acne to IGF-1 than has ever been demonstrated to any androgen (Figure 4.2) [10]. What's more, recent work demonstrates that IGF-1 deficiency prevents the occurrence of acne [11].

In summary, insulin and IGF-1 are the "dynamic duo" in the chain of events that lead to the acnes. Controlling the endogenous stimuli that lead to their elevation is one-half of the battle for control of the forces that cause the acnes.

4.2 The exogenous hormones

Any hormone that originates outside the body, whether or not it is identical to an endogenous hormone, must be considered exogenous. The list is long, and growing.

1-Androstenediol	Methasterone
1-Androstenedione	Methyldienolone
Bolandiol	Methyl-1-testosterone
Bolasterone	Methylnortestosterone
Boldenone	Methyltestosterone
Boldione	Metribolone
Calusterone	Mibolerone
Clostebol	Nandrolone
Danazol	19-Norandrostenedione
Dehydrochlormethyltestosterone	Norboletone
Desoxymethyltestosterone	Norclostebol
Drostanolone	Norethandrolone
Ethylestrenol	Oxabolone
Fluoxymesterone	Oxandrolone
Formebolone	Oxymesterone
Furazabol	Oxymetholone
Gestrinone	Prostanozol
4-Hydroxytestosterone	Quinbolone
Mestanolone	Stanozolol
Mesterolone	Stenbolone
Metenolone	1-Testosterone
Methandienone	Tetrahydrogestrinone
Methandriol	Trenbolone

Figure 4.3 This list comprises the exogenous anabolic androgenic steroids, the man-made or man-modified hormones used to enhance performance (or to treat some diseases). Some of the endogenous anabolic androgenic steroids (androstenediol, androstenedione, dihydrotestosterone, dehydroepiandrosterone [DHEA], and testosterone) may also be used by injection and are then considered exogenous.

4.2.1 Anabolic steroids

These are the steroids that are taken by or given to body-builders and athletes in order to produce superior performance (Figure 4.3). The word *anabolic* comes from the Greek word *anabole*, meaning "that which is thrown up; a mound." Certainly, mounds of muscles (and medals) can be created, using what is essentially too much of a good thing. The general public and news readers are generally unaware that anabolic steroids are the normal everyday growth stimulants in our mothers' milk, the food that starts each of us on the road from infancy to maturity.

4.2.1.1 Mothers' milk

Let's start with a little-known fact. Anabolic steroids were part of your first meal. Our mothers' milk contains anabolic steroids. They are an essential part of the stimulus to growth that turns a baby into a self-sufficient individual. They are totally natural, easily absorbed, impressively effective, uniquely tuned to the species of the mother, and, depending on your mother's diet,

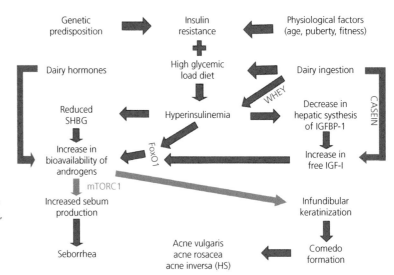

Figure 4.4 The final effector, mammalian target of rapamycin complex 1 (mTORC), gives the green light to growth, causing the plugged pores that are at the root of all acnes plus the seborrhea that accompanies some varieties.

probably "organic." Nobody injected your Mum with steroids or growth hormone to make her produce more milk. These anabolic steroid hormones are provided in nature as part of what is intended as a *temporary* source of complete nutrition. Milk is indeed nature's "perfect food," but it wasn't intended to be continued after the offspring had learned to adapt to a full childhood and adult diet.

As Melnik has written, "We have to appreciate that milk is a species-specific endocrine signalling system that activates a central signalling node in cellular metabolism for stimulation of growth and cell proliferation." Furthermore,

> The endocrinological changes in milk signalling are … comparable to the endocrinology of puberty. Both periods of growth, the milk-driven period of neonatal growth and growth hormone-driven puberty are associated with elevations in IGF-1, insulin and insulin resistance. [12]

In all mammalian species, the nutrient-sensitive kinase mTORC1 integrates nutrient signals, such as glucose (adenosine triphosphate/energy status of the cell), essential amino acids (predominantly leucine availability), and growth factor signals (insulin, IGF-1, and fibroblast growth factors [FGFs]).

Puberty-induced growth and milk-induced neonatal growth are driven by the same insulin and IGF-1 signal transduction pathways, which ultimately upregulate mTORC1 signaling to make things grow. FPSU overgrowth is highly likely to occur as the result of being

overstimulated through this pathway, but although the "high glycaemic load pathway to mTORC1 in acne appears to be established, … the nutrient signalling of high milk/dairy protein consumption awaits further experimental confirmation" (Figure 4.4) [13].

We have all seen nature films in which the mother deer or cow is chasing away her growing offspring, discouraging further nursing as part of the weaning process. Weaning is natural; it is nature's plan. Humans are the only species who consume the milk of other species, or who encourage house pets to do the same. I occasionally remind teenaged patients that, if Mother Nature intended them to be still drinking milk, they would have a closer relationship with their maternal parent.

There are a number of substances in mothers' milk that stimulate growth, but only some of them are exogenous steroidal hormones. These are dealt with in Section 4.2.4. Milk contains numerous nonsteroidal hormones and growth factors [14] plus the fats, proteins, and carbohydrates that provide the energy and material for growth. But once a human baby or other young mammal is capable of consuming and digesting a standard diet, weaning in nature (and in civilization) should occur, despite the ability of some of us to consume milk over our entire lifetimes, and despite the temptations of ice cream sundaes and artisanal cheeses.

The accident of nature that led to the genetic mutation that codes for lactase persistence arose several millennia in the past, apparently in what is now Central Europe.

This permits individuals who would be otherwise lactose intolerant to continue to consume lactose-containing milk. It is argued that this mutation allowed early humans to take advantage of domesticated cattle and so survive in early Europe. While this may be considered a successful adaptive gene, it can be argued that this is really not a survival gene. If it were, drinking milk to ensure the propagation of the species would improve fertility or provide some reproductive advantage. As for drinking milk universally enhancing fertility, this is clearly not the case—millions of lactose-intolerant and milk-allergic individuals avoid milk and other dairy products and have babies every year. In fact, infertility was 85% higher in women who consumed two or more servings of low-fat dairy milk compared with those who consumed one or less servings per day. High-fat daily milk consumption gave opposite results [15]. Not all adaptations that human evolution has brought us are to our benefit, nor are we physicians free of blame, exposing our patients to man-manipulated hormones as we trade the loss of a natural, organic, and hormone-free existence for the expediency of effective birth control. Life is a trade, with costs, savings, risks, and benefits vying for consideration.

4.2.1.2 Muscle makers
The provision of anabolic steroids to athletes is a huge business. There is a vast array of steroids available. They are used singly and "stacked" in various combinations both orally and by intramuscular injection. A few minutes spent on the Internet will enlighten you more than I intend to do here. I am personally surprised that we see so few patients with acne triggered by nonprescription use of these potent molecules. I suspect this is because the users are aware that acne is a known side effect, and those who suffer from acne either stop the use of steroids on their own or prefer to avoid contact with dermatologists and other physicians who are known to be critical of such practices. On the other hand, the few patients I have seen with this problem actually improved while spending time on my waiting list, having already made their decision and having already discontinued the drugs. In general, the anabolic steroid users tend to be in their 20s and 30s, so they may be protected to some extent by their lower post-adolescent endogenous levels of IGF-1. But sometimes the chemically induced acne gets seriously out of hand, producing truly horrendous and destructive variants of

acne [16]. The dermatologist's role has generally been to clean up the residual. Only once (so far) has a resistant personal case of acne proven to be due to continued use of steroids. The confession occurred only after several months of frustration on my part. The message to physicians is clear—keep asking, and forbid whey and casein!

4.2.2 Oral contraceptive hormones
Our world has been seriously rocked by the invention and introduction of this class of medications, particularly those used as oral contraceptives. We are now experiencing the fourth generation of "the Pill," and there may be more to come.

4.2.2.1 Oral estrogens
The original birth control pill (BCP) was intended to be a progestagen (progestin)-only preparation. Estrogens were not originally intended as part of BCPs. Curiously, an estrogenic substance, mestranol, was found as a contaminant during the development of the strongly progestagen/progestin-dominant preparation that was eventually to be marketed as Enovid®. The mestranol was found to prevent breakthrough bleeding and so, once an optimal dose had been established, the original preparation as sold contained 150 µg mestranol (the estrogen) and 9850 µg norethynodrel (the progestin/progestagen) for a total hormone dose of 10,000 µg or 10 mg, a much higher dose than is prescribed today. During the five decades since, the estrogen used has been generally standardized and is usually ethinyl estradiol (EE2). The dose has gradually been reduced as low as 10 µg per tablet. While this lower dose is usually sufficient estrogen to have the desired effect in preventing breakthrough bleeding, it does not provide the major contribution to acne control of the former higher doses. Where acne control is a consideration, higher doses of estrogen are needed, especially in young women weighing 55 kg (110 lbs.) or more. The dose of the EE2 needs to be raised for this population or they will risk an unacceptable incidence of breakthrough bleeding (as was the case with the original BCP before the mestranol was added). There is limited flexibility available in choosing doses for "the pill," but the subject deserves consideration by the prescriber.

Just as women vary by weight, they vary by age. Acne is not a disease restricted to women younger than 35 years of age. In the past decade, one of the many results of the scare induced by the Women's Health Initiative in the United States (and similar initiatives elsewhere) has been the re-emergence of what is best termed *acne climacterica*, or menopausal acne. As women's natural endogenous estrogen production fades around the late 40s and early 50s, testosterone's effect becomes more and more dominant, being relatively unopposed by less and less estrogen. This androgen-dominant environment causes a variant of late-onset acne. Sometimes insult is added to injury, and hirsutism, androgenic alopecia, and numerous nondermatological complaints are added to the mix. Exogenous bio-identical estradiol administered as a patch is the safest, and most easily regulated, way of handling this estrogen deficiency. Bio-identical micronized progesterone, available as oral Prometrium® or as a generic, is used at the same time to support the health of the uterus, if it is still present. These bio-identical estradiol patch and oral progesterone preparations are preferred because they avoid the use of nonhuman and manufactured equivalents. Careful counseling and coordination with primary care physicians, gynecologists, and endocrinologists are advised. Fortunately, papers showing the advantages of hormone replacement therapy (HRT), when commenced early and when composed of less troublesome molecules, are beginning to appear [17]. Updated guidelines for HRT and reconsideration of the data that led to tens of millions of women (and their doctors) being frightened away from HRT are now available [18, 19] and should in time make this growing and multifaceted problem less common. Meanwhile, see the "Warnings" at Section 8.6.1.1.

4.2.2.2 Oral progestins

The original progestin used in BCPs was norethynodrel. Over the years, a trend to less androgenic progestins has made BCPs less acnegenic but there are still many androgenic progestins in use, including levonorgestrel, dl-norgestrel, and desogestrel.

In choosing oral contraceptives with a view toward managing acne, the least androgenic progestin possible is needed, and is best combined with a reasonable dose of estrogen. The 20 µg dose, the "low dose" of the estrogen ethinyl estradiol, in the product containing 3 mg drospirenone, is normally sufficient for women weighing less than 50 kg (110 lbs.). Over that weight, we prefer to see the 30 µg dose used. The same general approach is used in other products containing different progestins (Table 4.1 and Figure 4.5).

Table 4.1 Progestins vary, the more androgenic make acne worse, the less or non-androgenic prevent and clear acne.

Progestin	Progestational activity (relative to 1 mg of norethindrone	Androgenic activity (relative to 1 mg of norethindrone
Norethindrone 1 mg	1.0	1.0
Norethindrone acetate 1 mg	1.2	1.6
Ethynodiol diacetate 1 mg	1.4	0.6
Levonorgestrel 1 mg	5.3	8.3
Dl-norgestrel 1 mg	2.6	4.2
Norgestimate 1 mg	1.3	1.9
Norelgestromin 1 mg	1.3	1.9
Desogestrel 1 mg	9.0	3.4
Drospirenone 1 mg	1.5	0.0

Source: Dickey RP. Individualizing oral contraceptive therapy. OBG Management Supplement October 2000:5.

4.2.2.3 Extended cycles

In suppressing acne, extended cycles of drospirenone-based BCPs have been particularly useful but others can be used in a similar fashion. Instead of repeated 21/7 cycles, multiple 21-day courses can be taken sequentially. By taking the active tablets from four packages of BCPs and using four of the 21-day cycles in a row, one can achieve an 84/7 cycle. This gives excellent persistent unbroken androgen blockade and a three-month interval between menses. Young women divide almost instantly into two camps when offered this option. There are those who say, "Neat! Where do I sign up?" and those who say, "No way, Doc, that's too weird." Those who wish to try it need to know that there is a 15% incidence of occasional breakthrough bleeding with the "extended" program, and for them we can always offer a return to the regular cycle. Providing prescriptions for *both* options at the time of discussion (with a supportive handout—see Section 12.6 and Figure 4.5) gives the patient both the time to consider and discuss the options and the option to revert to the standard routine if desired. To complicate matters, the packaging for drospirenone comes as either 24/4 (20 µg EE2) or 21/7 (30 µg EE2). If you're using the low-dose product, you will have a 96-day (24 × 4) extended cycle, and the higher dose product will yield an 84-day (21 × 4) cycle, with a 7-day break between each, for a total cycle time of 103 or 91 days, respectively. Packaging and availability will vary by country and by insurance. Pharmacists

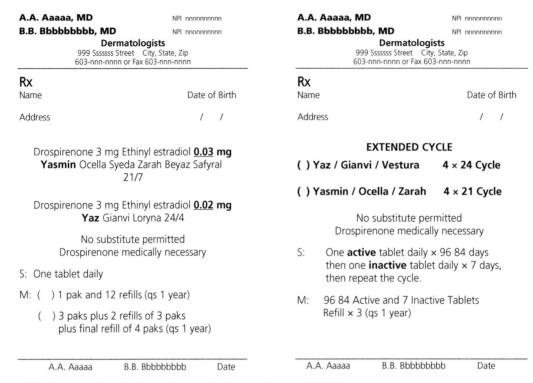

Figure 4.5 Patients appreciate the choice of the standard versus the extended BCP regimen.

generally need education, supportive information, and sometimes documentation.

Studies over the last 10 years of the products containing drospirenone have suggested an increased risk of clotting disorders (venous thrombo-embolisms, or VTEs) during the early years of therapy. The effect seems to fade over 2–3 years of use, for reasons that are not fully understood. Research in this area appears almost monthly, and "When the newest OCs containing drospirenone were compared with non-drospirenone-containing OCs … VTE risk did not significantly increase (OR 1.13; 95% CI 0.94, 1.35)" [20]. This is a 13% increase in risk and was not statistically significant. However, "Among the carriers of genetic blood clotting mutations G20210A (a Prothrombin II anomaly) and Factor V Leiden (FVL or R 5062), OC users showed a significantly increased VTE risk compared with non-users (OR 1.63)" [20]. This is a significant 63% increase in risk. Whenever there is a family history of VTE or arterial occlusive problems such as strokes or heart attacks in women in the family under the age of 55, testing for these mutations (also called *anomalies*) and the

option to avoid drospirenone (or all sources of oral estrogens) needs to be seriously considered. To add to the confusion, there are now data that show an increased risk of VTEs in patients on BCPs with blood types A, B, or AB [21].

There is an additional and unwelcome layer of confusion and fear generated by the lay press occasionally reporting these studies in a sensational fashion. It should be remembered that the frequency of VTEs in women aged 15–49 using nonhormonal contraception is 3 per 10,000 woman-years and that increases to 12 during pregnancy and to 30 in the months after delivery. There is a threefold increased risk of VTE (to nine) in current users of OCs with norethisterone, levonorgestrel, or norgestimate and a sixfold increased risk (to 18) with desogestrel, gestodene, drospirenone, or cyproterone acetate, and in users of the contraceptive vaginal ring, compared with nonusers [22].

The most recent large US-based study reported much lower rates for nonfatal VTEs of 1.25/10,000 woman-years for levonorgestrel and 3.08/10,000 for drospirenone. The consensus is that drospirenone doubles the risk but

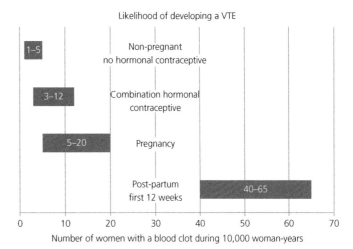

Figure 4.6 If every women were to be tested, before starting hormonal contraceptives, for factor V Leiden, prothrombin II, and blood type—and if a clinical trial to check on the efficacy of 81 mg acetylsalicylic acid were to show a protective effect—lives could be saved. Meanwhile, personal and family history is all we can rely on.

the absolute medical risk is still low [23]. It can be kept low by prescribing BCPs only to ideal candidates who do not smoke, are under age 35 years, have normal blood pressure, have no family history of VTEs, and have no family history of myocardial infarcts or strokes under age 55. Testing for clotting anomalies and blood type might be considered but is not yet the standard of care.

The legal risk is another consideration entirely. At the time of writing, the best overall option for acne sufferers needing BCPs seems to be the oral contraceptive containing norgestimate, a progestin that balances fairly low androgenicity and a lower risk of VTE than drospirenone [22]. Other options are available, and the data in Figure 4.5 should be used to select progestins as appropriate. If additional androgen blockade is required, supplemental spironolactone can always be considered.

With the lay press and lawyers maintaining a constant vigilance on behalf of patients and prospective clients, it is important that the risks of VTE events be kept in perspective. The risks of pregnancy and the postpartum period far exceed the risks posed by combination hormonal contraceptives, and until there is universal monitoring for genetic predisposition to clotting, there will always be a baseline of patients developing VTEs with no obvious risk factors (Figure 4.6).

4.2.3 Other exogenous birth control hormones

There are many reasons to avoid oral medications. Patient preference is often cited, as is "inability to take pills." Forgetfulness is another reason. Incompetence is

a fourth. One of the best reasons for avoiding the oral route is to avoid the first pass of estrogens absorbed from the stomach and routed via the portal vein to and through the liver. This is where the changes in circulating proteins that predispose to thrombosis (clotting factors VII, IX, X, and X complex; and decreased antithrombin III and anti Xa) are actually induced by orally administered estrogens [24]. See "Warnings" at Section 8.6.1.1. Several devices have been marketed that can assist the consumer in avoiding the direct transport of oral estrogens to the liver.

4.2.3.1 Implants

The original subcutaneous implant (Norplant®) contained the androgenic progestin levonorgestrel but no estrogen. It worked reasonably well, but was eventually withdrawn because of menstrual and other problems, one of which was acne. The latest is Implanon®, which contains 68 mg of etonogestrel, a progestin related to norgestimate that is significantly less androgenic than levonorgestrel. The cost of insertion and removal is considered by many to be prohibitive, but the good news is that there is only one "rod" that needs to be inserted. This implant lasts three years, it contains no estrogen, and it has a very low failure rate of less than 1%. In an online patient review of this product, there was no mention of increased acne in 729 entries (http://www.drugs.com/comments/etonogestrel/)—and I've personally seen no acne associated with its use, so far. A new version called Nexplanon® is visible on X-ray and is inserted with a redesigned appliance that facilitates shallow insertion, patient-touch assurance of its location, and easier removal after 3 years.

4.2.3.2 Intrauterine devices

When the intrauterine hormone-containing contraceptive devices first arrived on the market, the general message was that they acted locally on the uterus and there was no systemic effect. The original (Progestasert®) contained only molecular progesterone, a very weak acnegen, but it was discontinued in 2001. I can find no reported instances of associated acne in the literature, but it was not widely used. The units now available in the United States are the levonorgestrel-containing 5-year (52 mg) Mirena® introduced in 1990 and the new 3-year (13.5 mg) Skyla®. Mirena® was originally marketed with the message that there was no systemic absorption. Wikipedia contained in 2012 the statement, of questionable authorship, "With the use of the Mirena the hormones are localized to the uterine area unlike oral contraceptives" [25]. Evidence to the contrary did not take long to show up: the product insert now states, "Only small amounts of the hormone enter your blood," and most dermatologists are now aware that Mirena® presents a problem with acne vulgaris. This association now extends to acne inversa/hidradenitis suppurativa (AI/HS) in a few personal cases. The reduction in levonorgestrel dose from 18 mcg/day in Mirena® to 14 mcg/day in Skyla® may reduce the risk of acne somewhat, especially near the end of the three years when the dose will be down to 5 mcg/day, but the incidence of acne in clinical trials was 13.4% [26].

4.2.3.3 Intravaginal devices

The NuvaRing® is a flexible, 4 mm thick, 54 mm (2 in.) diameter ring, composed of ethylene vinyl acetate copolymers and magnesium stearate. Each contains EE2 and etonogestrel. A new ring is inserted into the vagina and retained for three weeks each month. This combination of medications, delivered through the vaginal wall, avoids most of the first pass of the estrogen EE2 through the liver, a worthwhile and novel approach. The progestin is the same low-androgenicity etonogestrel used in the insert Implanon®. The acne side effect profile should be less, but the EE2 is still associated with increased clotting problems in women [22]. See the "Warnings" at Section 8.6.1.1.

4.2.3.4 Topicals: the patches

Ortho Evra® contains 0.75 mg EE2 and 6.0 mg norelgestromin in each weekly patch. This combination, delivered through the skin, avoids the first pass of the estrogen EE2 through the liver, a worthwhile approach to minimize clotting risk, but the constant level of EE2 delivered to the blood is higher than with a comparable oral birth control pill. The progestin is etonogestrel, fairly low in androgenicity, so the acne side effect profile should be less but the EE2 still presents a theoretical, albeit lower, risk of clotting problems.

For postmenopausal replacement of estradiol deficiency, important in cases of acne climacterica, there is a collection of bio-identical estradiol (E2) patches marketed. The shapes, sizes, adhesives, and doses provide a wide selection. These are used to provide a minimum amount of estradiol, just enough to relieve and prevent the symptoms of natural estradiol deficiency. Compared to the 0.75 mg of EE2 weekly in an Ortho Evra® contraceptive patch, the E2 content of these bio-identical patches ranges from 0.39 to 1.56 mg *twice* weekly. That means that the Ortho Evra® contraceptive patch is roughly dose equivalent to the lowest dose E2 replacement patch. The highest dose E2 replacement patches surprisingly deliver almost five times as much estradiol as the Ortho Evra®, but no progestin. See the "Warnings" at Section 8.6.1.1.

4.2.3.5 Intramuscular (depot) injections

The potent semisynthetic progestin medroxyprogesterone acetate (MPA or Depo Provera®) is an effective contraceptive and can be given intramuscularly once every three months with a 3% failure/annual pregnancy rate. Its major advantage is its effectiveness in the handicapped or noncompliant. Unfortunately, it is highly androgenic, almost equal to DHT in vitro [27]. It has been responsible for AI/HS plus many cases of rather recalcitrant acne and should be avoided in the acne-prone. It also carries warnings related to loss of bone mass. The oral form, used in postmenopausal HRT, was associated with increased risk of breast cancer in the Women's Health Initiative study [19].

4.2.4 Dietary sources of hormones

Milk contains a vast array of totally natural bioactive chemicals. Each sip of milk provides you with numerous growth stimulators and regulators [14]. The following list is a compilation, and some of the names have changed over the years.

1 Steroid hormones
  estradiol
  estriol
  progesterone
  testosterone
  androstenedione
  17-ketosteroids
  corticosterone
  20α-dihydropregnenolone
  5α-pregnanedione
  5α-pregnan-3β-ol-20-one
  5α-androstene-3β,17β-diol
  5α-androstanedione
  5α-androstan-3β-ol-17-one
  20α- and 20β-dihydroprogesterone
  dehydroepiandrosterone (DHEA) acyl ester
2 Pituitary hormones
  prolactin (PRL)
  growth hormone (GH)
  thyroid-stimulating hormone (TSH)
  follicle- stimulating hormone (FSH)
  luteinizing hormone (LH)
  adrenocorticotropic hormone (ACTH)
  oxytocin
3 Hypothalamic hormones
  thyrotropin-releasing hormone (TRH)
  somatostatin
  PRL-inhibiting factor
  PRL-releasing factor
  luteinizing hormone–releasing hormone (LHRH)
  gonadotropin-releasing hormone (GnRH)
  growth hormone–releasing factor-like activity
  neurotensin
4 Thyroid and parathyroid hormones
  triiodothyronine (T3)
  thyroxine (T4)
  reverse triiodothyronine (rT3)
  calcitonin
  parathyroid hormone/parathormone (PTH)
  PTH-related peptide (PTHrP)
5 Gastrointestinal peptides
  vasoactive intestinal peptide
  Y peptide, *now* neuropeptide Y (NPY)
  substance P
  gastric inhibitory peptide (GIP)
  cholecystokinin
  gastrin
  pancreatic polypeptide

  bombesin
  neurotensin
  somatostatin
6 Growth factors
  insulin-like growth factors 1 and 2 (IGF-1 and IGF-2)
  IGF-binding proteins (IGFBP)
  nerve growth factor (NGF)
  epidermal growth factor (EGF)
  transforming growth factors alpha (TGFα) and beta (TGFβ)
7 Growth inhibitors
  mammary-derived growth inhibitor (MDGI)
  macrophage-activating factor (MAF)
  platelet-derived growth factor (PDGF)
8 Others
  prostaglandins PGE and PGF2α
  cyclic adenosine monophosphate (cAMP)
  cyclic guanosine monophosphate (cGMP)
  delta sleep–inducing peptide (DSIP)
  transferrin
  lactoferrin
  β-casomorphins
  erythropoietin
  vitamin D
  relaxin
  insulin
  and numerous uncharacterized nucleotides.

Some of the hormones are the anabolic steroids mentioned in Section 4.2.1, and some are 5α-reduced hormones. It is worth pointing out that potent androgens impact numerous receptors in babies' muscles and bones, not just the FPSU [28]. Some of the milk hormones are polypeptides, the type of molecule one would expect to be digested into multiple amino acids and used for nourishment [29]. Fortunately, the acidic stomach contents cause the casein in milk to "curdle" or "clot" at pH 4.6. A protective coat of aggregated and folded casein molecules forms the casein micelle [30, 31]. This is believed to create a three-dimensional space that allows the relatively fragile polypeptide hormone molecules to pass intact to the alkaline intestine where the casein unfolds, releasing the intact polypeptide hormones and growth factors for absorption. Some of these compounds, such as the nucleotides, have no demonstrated connection to the drive to stimulate growth. They likely serve functions not yet recognized, given that nature rarely intentionally wastes resources. One recent suggestion is that the passage of single-stranded RNA may be part of milk's role in evolution [32].

4.2.4.1 The impact of diet on acne

The story of the dietary impact on the acnes is gradually evolving. My original theory in the early 1980s was that the steroid hormones naturally present in dairy products were the sole stimulus to acne. Milk had not been under serious suspicion as a cause of acne since the late 1940s, with one unpublished exception [33]. The concept that diet might be a cause of acne was reintroduced by Cordain in 2002 [34]. Acne was labeled a "disease of Western civilization" and was blamed on our high-glycemic-load diet. It was not noted in the original publication that both tribes studied were consuming no dairy products, but further inquiry led to the fact that dairy simply was not available in any quantity to the Kitavan people in Papua, and the Aché in Paraguay considered drinking the milk of another species "abhorrent."

This work led to several studies, designed in Australia, to investigate the role of high- versus low-glycemic-load diets in acne vulgaris [35–37]. The work of Smith and Mann took this approach, and they were able to demonstrate a definite difference in the impact on acne of their two diets. The group that consumed a high-glycemic-load diet continued with acne, with no definite improvement. The low-glycemic-load diet was associated with a statistically significant decrease in acne activity [36]. A close look at these diets reveals that the high-glycemic-load diet was also higher in dairy content than was the low-glycemic-load diet, which provides further evidence that it is not just glycemic load but also the dairy content that is important. These papers formed the basis for the growing acceptance of the role of a low-glycemic-load diet in reducing the activity of acne vulgaris.

Professor Jennie Brand-Miller, an Australian biochemist and another member of the Lindeberg–Cordain investigative team, subsequently designed a larger study comparing the impact on facial acne of diets with glycemic indices of 51 (low) and 61 (high), but the differences between the diets did not reach significance [38]. Subsequent glycemic-load experiments by Kwon did achieve statistical significance, thus making the point about the influence of glycemic load [39], but much greater statistical significance was achieved with reference to dairy consumption in the Italian study by Di Landro, whose team demonstrated an odds ratio of 2.20

Table 4.2 Changes in growth and dairy consumption in Japan, 1950 and 1975.

12-year-old girl in Japan	1950	1975
Weight (lbs.)	71	90
Height (in.)	54	58.5
Dairy intake (lbs. per year)	5.5	117.4
Age at first period	15.2	12.2

for acne patients who drank three or more 250 mL portions per week of skim milk [5]. The effect is even more apparent in a culture with a traditional diet that is less dairy oriented than those of the United States and Italy. A Malaysian study demonstrated that the frequency of milk ($p < 0.01$) and ice cream ($p < 0.01$) consumption was significantly higher in acne cases compared to controls. The odds ratio for one serving of milk per week was 3.99, and that for one serving of ice cream per week was 4.47 [40]. Melnik's theoretical work has effectively knit together the impact of these two very different but synergistic stimuli [41, 42].

The abhorrent attitude of the Aché tribe toward the consumption of milk was echoed for generations in the Japanese population, perhaps because of lactase deficiency. This large and homogeneous Asian population, with a previously highly standardized diet based mainly on steamed rice and fish, was subject to very slow change over centuries. The Western influence that started in the mid-sixteenth century with the introduction of tempura by Jesuit priests slowly changed the diet over two or three centuries. Beginning in the first quarter of the twentieth century there was a gradual introduction of dairy, and the substitution of wheat for rice and meat for fish changed the Japanese diet, particularly the amount of fat. The change accelerated in the years following the close of the Second World War with a remarkable 20-fold increase in per capita dairy consumption over 25 years. Table 4.2 illustrates the unequivocal changes in the population's postwar metrics [43].

It is apparent that future clinical trials investigating acne must take both dairy intake and glycemic load into consideration. Indeed, the effect of these two components of diet has now been so well demonstrated that the design of any clinical trial looking at the cause of acne, or indeed the effect of any acne therapy, must take into consideration adequate control for dairy and glycemic load to avoid the risk of dietary confounding.

Imagine the confounding impact of requiring that an antibiotic under investigation for acne therapy be taken with milk to avoid gastric irritation.

4.2.4.1.1 The ice cream salesman's son

Early in my years in private practice, about 1975 or so, I was referred the oldest acne patient I had ever seen. He was 61 years of age.

His back was a veritable moonscape, but it was not just old scars. He had active, fresh, and very inflammatory nodular and comedonal acne on top of the scars. He had had the problem for half a century, starting at age 11, and he had almost run out of available follicles to get involved.

The dietary history was a landmark learning experience for me, and he was one of the original patients who pointed me toward the dairy link.

It so happened that this man's father worked for the local dairy and was the local ice cream salesman and deliveryman. He would set out from the dairy in the morning in a horse-drawn wagon with insulated bags containing ice and the cardboard-wrapped bricks of ice cream. There was no refrigeration of note in 1925 or so, and that meant the trick was to get the ice cream sold, delivered, and into the buyers' ice boxes before the end of the day to avoid melting. Any ice cream left over at the end of the day was soft and could not be refrozen and sold, so it went home to the ice cream salesman's family where it supplemented his income and the family food supply as a perquisite of his job.

The son, later my patient, developed an early love of ice cream from this exposure. During the period from his teens to the time I met him at age 61, he generally consumed a "brick" of ice cream every day of his life. That was the equivalent of an Imperial pint, or 568 mL. As a teen he had the worst acne of anyone he knew. His doctors over the years were basically unable to help him with anything other than X-ray to the facial area, which was scarred as a result but it was not as active as his back, chest, and shoulders. The back and chest were too great an area to irradiate, and he was basically denied any social life by the severity of his disorder.

When I told him I wanted him to stop all his dairy intake, and in particular the ice cream, his eyes widened and then filled with tears and he broke down and sobbed. It was my turn to be dismayed! He calmed down and was willing to try life without ice cream, so I loaded him up with tetracycline for a few months to cool things down and after a year all the active lesions were gone.

Once he was clear, I never saw him again. I have wondered for years whether he returned to the ice cream in spite of the acne. It was really his only friend and comfort.

4.2.4.1.2 Reproductive hormones

The list of hormones present in milk (and presumed to be present in milk derivatives) is impressive and includes all classes of the steroid reproductive hormones. Work on estrogens has shown significant amounts in milk, and it is worth noting that milk labeled *organic* had higher levels of estrogens and progesterone [44]. There are lower levels of total combined estrogen metabolites in goat milk than in cow milk, but the differences are unlikely to be clinically significant [45]. Of particular note are the truly anabolic androgen precursors of 5α-DHT, the 5α-reduced molecules that include:

5α-pregnanedione

5α-pregnan-3β-ol-20-one

5α-androstene-3β, 17β-diol

5α-androstanedione

5α-androstan-3β-ol-17-one [46].

Modern analytic techniques needed to identify additional analogs (chemical brothers and sisters) and measure these related androgens in dairy products have not yet been used to bring these older data up to date [47].

These molecules, when they arrive in the FPSU, are available to the enzymes of the intracrine system, which consists of the entire set of enzymes necessary for direct conversion to more potent androgens, on site right within the FPSU. Whether these molecules, bearing the 5α-reduction "handle," are a suitable or perhaps even an enhanced "fit" for the androgen receptors is unknown. Likewise, whether they are indeed androgenic agonists in their own right, even without conversion to DHT, is presently unknown. These areas of research should be high priority for study. Meanwhile, speculation suggests that the capacity of these structurally similar molecules for inducing androgenic effects will be significant.

4.2.4.1.3 Insulin

Insulin's presence in milk, if the insulin is indeed absorbed directly rather than being destroyed by digestion, will translate into a de-repressive effect on androgen receptors throughout the newborn's body. That, of course, is the object of the exercise in infants—milk is designed to open the androgen receptor for business so that the anabolic phase of infant growth can commence. It is believed by some that the polypeptide insulin molecule is protected on its journey through the low pH of the stomach by folded casein molecules, arranged in micelles as described above, and is then released into and absorbed from the upper bowel of the neonate. At the same time, the degree to which human milk stimulates growth and promotes intestinal health is variable, nonlinear, and likely synergistic in ways that will need further exploration [48].

It appears that the important role of raising the level of insulin and initiating the chain of anabolic events is filled by yet another polypeptide, GIP. Hydrolyzed whey protein–derived essential amino acids (from maternal milk) are the most potent inducers of GIP. It is secreted by enteroendocrine K cells, specialized endocrine cells of the gastrointestinal tract. GIP stimulates the secretion of insulin by pancreatic beta cells. This molecule's task, once its production is stimulated by absorbed whey in mother's milk, is to raise the level of insulin in the newborn's body [49]. This insulin, working in concert with IGF-1 (see Section 4.2.4.1.4), magnifies the speed of FoxO1 elimination from the cellular nucleus of androgen-responsive cells (Section 2.9), thereby activates the androgen receptor, and so permits the natural maternal anabolic steroids in milk to get to work growing the newborn.

4.2.4.1.4 Insulin-like growth factor 1 (IGF-1)

IGF-1 is insulin's coworker in the de-repression of the androgen receptor, and its presence in milk is part of the anabolic push for growth. There is debate, as with insulin, whether it survives the acid environment of the stomach, but there is good reason to trust that nature has provided a protective mechanism through casein envelopment, as described in this chapter. It matters little whether it is itself absorbed from milk and is thus exogenous or, alternatively, milk's casein content stimulates its endogenous production (or both). Either way, once it becomes available as a trigger or co-trigger of the FoxO1 phosphorylation process, the anabolic steroids can get to work.

4.2.4.1.5 Growth factors and androgens combined

The reader will appreciate that this is an immense field and, while the important points are presented here, a full discussion is beyond the scope of this book.

I hope that the points have been adequately made that:

- Reproductive steroidal and polypeptide hormones, endogenous or exogenous, alone and synergistically, drive acne development.
- Exogenous hormones consumed during puberty stimulate acne.
- Milk is species specific and custom designed to make babies grow.
- Milk and other dairy, consumed during puberty and adolescence when IGF-1 is naturally at its peak, will lead to a marked increase in incidence of acne.
- Other sources of exogenous acnegens include body-building injectables plus oral, injectable, and "wearable" androgenic progestins used for birth control.
- Acne can be prevented, minimized, or cleared by stopping exogenous hormones.

4.2.4.1.6 Dairy intolerance

During "question periods" after lectures I have given, the subjects raised most often concern lactose intolerance, milk allergy, "organic" milk, and "hormone-free" milk.

This seems as good a place as any to discuss them. All humans prior to about 15,000 years ago became lactose intolerant after weaning, but it didn't really matter back then, because there was essentially no lactose in their natural diets after weaning. As a result of a chance mutation, this changed for many of us whose ancestors were from what is now Central Europe. While those of African and Asian heritage tend to life-long lactose intolerance, to varying degrees, we who harbor the mutant trait for lactase *persistence* can consume this substance well past the time of life when it would be wise to stop. Lactose intolerance, while uncomfortable, does have the benefit of signaling sufferers that something is wrong with what they are eating! Perhaps the abhorrence of milk displayed by the Paraguayan Aché reflects a cultural rejection based on this discomfort. As presumed descendants of the Bering Sea bridge migrants, it is likely that they lack lactase persistence.

Milk *allergy* is something else again. Books have been written! Again, nature seems to be trying to send us a message. Acne is not *caused by* milk *allergy*, but if you have **both** *a milk allergy and acne* and you stop milk because of the allergy, you can guess what happens to the acne. It fades away at the same time as the allergy, and so it is wrongly thought to be *caused* by the allergy. There is no present science in the world literature to suggest that milk allergy itself *causes* acne. I personally suspect it has the capacity to flare acne that has already been induced by the mechanisms being discussed here, but that is another story, for another time.

4.2.4.2 Carbohydrate load versus dairy load

Cordain's work suggested that the low glycemic load might play a decisive role in the absence of acne in his study population.

We know that every diet contains elements from various food groups and types. Each food, depending on how much sugar is generated when it is digested, is given a rating called a *glycemic index*. If you look at each food in a meal, then assign a glycemic index to each, and then multiply the glycemic index number by the weight of that specific food in the meal, you get a number that will give you the glycemic load of that food in that meal. By adding the glycemic load of each food type, you can get an overall rating of glycemic load of the entire meal and the entire diet of similar meals. A low-glycemic diet consists of multiple low-glycemic-load meals, and those meals are composed of low-glycemic-index foods.

In general, the foods that cause high-glycemic-index ratings are those that contain highly refined carbohydrates. The classic is the sugar *glucose* for which the index is named, and it has a glycemic index of 100, as you would expect. Water would have a glycemic index of zero, because it contains no glucose whatsoever. Highly refined white flour and anything made from it such as white bread, cakes, and cookies all show up at the upper end of the glycemic index along with white potatoes and non-Basmati rice. All will push sugar up in the blood quickly, causing insulin to be released. This elevated insulin level is one of the two factors that open the androgen receptor, activating it to accept the androgenic molecules that stimulate growth in tissues that are dependent on androgen signaling. This is one of the major links between diet and acne.

So, in summary, the high-glycemic-load diet appears to have a *single* acne-promoting effect. It raises the insulin level. While this *predisposes* to the development of acne, examination of the glycemic variable alone,

without reference to ingestion of steroidal and other hormones, shows to date only nonsignificant or barely significant results [39, 50].

On the other hand, milk and the dairy products made from milk appear to have a more potent, three-pronged effect.

First, milk and milk products (especially those containing whey) raise the insulin level, but by a mechanism unrelated to lactose or glucose or the attempted reduction of hyperglycemia [51].

Second, milk and milk products (especially those containing casein) raise the level of IGF-1 [9]. These two polypeptides, insulin and IGF-1, working in concert, stimulate the two kinases that phosphorylate and so flush FoxO1 out of the nuclei of androgen-responsive cells, thus exposing the androgen receptor. This process is called *insulin/insulin-like growth factor-1 signaling*, or IIS [42].

Third, milk and milk products contain numerous growth factors, mostly polypeptide hormones plus a group of anabolic steroid hormones. These androgenic steroids become available to the newly opened androgen receptors as a result of IIS, and the fire is lit.

That dietary cascade effectively opens the gate, not only to the androgenic acnegens (or acnegenic androgens) from the ingested milk and other dairy products, but also to those anabolic and acnegenic androgens from the endogenous gonadal (ovaries and testicles) and adrenal (stress gland) sources, and to the androgenic progestins in BCPs and other contraceptive devices. This hormonal cascade, triggered by exogenous stimuli against which the body cannot defend, falls on FPSUs that have not yet evolved any protective mechanism. The FPSUs are therefore defenseless against the onslaught of both endogenous and exogenous androgens that trigger the proliferative activity that is the driving force of the acnes.

Over time, it is becoming clear that the trigger to acne is *neither the steroid hormones alone nor the high-glycemic-load diet alone. It is both.*

The impact falls not only on the FPSUs, however. In nature, maturity occurs in the fullness of time under IGF-1's gradual influence. There is usually no added hormonal push after weaning. Only in humans is this extra stimulation provided by the introduction of milk, other dairy products, and the additional push provided by high-glycemic-load foods.

The enablers that facilitate this process are:

- The polypeptide GIP, which raises the level of insulin in the blood after the ingestion of whey polypeptides in milk
- IGF-1, which is raised in the blood after the ingestion of milk, especially the whey portion
- The natural anabolic steroids present in human milk
- The elevated levels of insulin and subsequent secondary insulin intolerance induced by excessive intake of a high-glycemic-load diet and the casein fraction of dairy foods.

This hormonal messaging system evolved over millions of years to stimulate fast growth in breastfed infants. Human breast milk may be considered a milder version of the super-enriched material called *royal jelly* in the world of the honeybee. In nature, the hormonal growth-stimulating cascade closes down to a great extent after weaning, and the rate of growth is slowed in childhood until the onset of puberty. That second growth spurt is brought on by naturally increased levels of IGF-1. This endogenous pubertal IGF-1 comes from natural sources at this time of life, reactivating the growth system to enable the push to sexual and reproductive maturity. This requires the full engagement of all the reproductive hormones, so the system that slowed down upon weaning is activated a second time by IGF-1.

The addition of the high glycemic load and the dairy-laden components of the Western diet (WD) adds an unexpected stimulus, the IIS, which perverts and accelerates the natural process of growth and maturation (Figure 2.16).

It is no surprise that we see the consequences expressed in susceptible girls as early acne, early breast development, and early menstruation. Susceptible boys show early acne and enhanced height. Early sexual maturity (up to two years earlier than 40 years ago) has now been described in boys as well as girls [52]. Less well described is a feature that I observe daily in patients, and that has become so common that I suspect it is going largely unnoticed—a prominent, bulky, well-padded muscularity shared by members of both sexes. This may occur alone, or as a forerunner to or in combination with obesity. Longer term, this is producing a nation plagued by the metabolic syndrome and its associated obesity. These changes, likely mediated by the same hormonal influences [53, 54], are to me a more worrisome and life-threatening concern than the acnes dealt with here.

References

1 Backstrom T, Andersson A, Baird DT, Selstam G. The human corpus luteum secretes 5 alpha-pregnane-3,20-dione. Acta Endocrinol (Copenh) 1986 Jan;111(1):116–21.

2 Wiebe JP, Beausoleil M, Zhang G, Cialacu V. Opposing actions of the progesterone metabolites, 5alpha-dihydroprogesterone (5alphaP) and 3alpha-dihydroprogesterone (3alphaHP) on mitosis, apoptosis, and expression of Bcl-2, Bax and p21 in human breast cell lines. J Steroid Biochem Mol Biol 2010 Jan;118(1–2):125–32.

3 Melnik BC. Evidence for acne-promoting effects of milk and other insulinotropic dairy products. Nestle Nutr Workshop Ser Pediatr Program 2011;67:131–45.

4 Melnik BC. FoxO1—the key for the pathogenesis and therapy of acne? J Dtsch Dermatol Ges 2010 Feb;8(2):105–14.

5 Di Landro A., Cazzaniga S, Parazzini F, Ingordo V, Cusano F, Atzori L, et al. Family history, body mass index, selected dietary factors, menstrual history, and risk of moderate to severe acne in adolescents and young adults. J Am Acad Dermatol 2012 Dec;67(6):1129–35.

6 Li Y, Xu W, Liao Z, Yao B, Chen X, Huang Z, et al. Induction of long-term glycemic control in newly diagnosed type 2 diabetic patients is associated with improvement of beta-cell function. Diabetes Care 2004 Nov;27(11):2597–602.

7 Unger RH, Scherer PE. Gluttony, sloth and the metabolic syndrome: a roadmap to lipotoxicity. Trends Endocrinol Metab 2010 Jun;21(6):345–52.

8 Lim EL, Hollingsworth KG, Aribisala BS, Chen MJ, Mathers JC, Taylor R. Reversal of type 2 diabetes: normalisation of beta cell function in association with decreased pancreas and liver triacylglycerol. Diabetologia 2011 Oct;54(10):2506–14.

9 Hoppe C, Molgaard C, Dalum C, Vaag A, Michaelsen KF. Differential effects of casein versus whey on fasting plasma levels of insulin, IGF-1 and IGF-1/IGFBP-3: results from a randomized 7-day supplementation study in prepubertal boys. Eur J Clin Nutr 2009 Sep;63(9):1076–83.

10 Melnik BC, Schmitz G. Role of insulin, insulin-like growth factor-1, hyperglycaemic food and milk consumption in the pathogenesis of acne vulgaris. Exp Dermatol 2009 Oct;18(10):833–41.

11 Ben-Amitai D, Laron Z. Effect of insulin-like growth factor-1 deficiency or administration on the occurrence of acne. J Eur Acad Dermatol Venereol 2011 Aug;25(8):950–4.

12 Melnik BC. Diet in acne: further evidence for the role of nutrient signalling in acne pathogenesis. Acta Derm Venereol 2012 May;92(3):228–31.

13 Inoki K, Ouyang H, Li Y, Guan KL. Signaling by target of rapamycin proteins in cell growth control. Microbiol Mol Biol Rev 2005 Mar;69(1):79–100.

14 Koldovsky O. Hormones in milk. Vitam Horm 1995;50: 77–149.

15 Chavarro JE, Rich-Edwards JW, Rosner B, Willett WC. A prospective study of dairy foods intake and anovulatory infertility. Hum Reprod 2007 May;22(5):1340–7.

16 Kraus SL, Emmert S, Schon MP, Haenssle HA. The dark side of beauty: acne fulminans induced by anabolic steroids in a male bodybuilder. Arch Dermatol 2012 Oct 1;148(10): 1210–2.

17 Schierbeck LL, Rejnmark L, Tofteng CL, Stilgren L, Eiken P, Mosekilde L, *et al.* Effect of hormone replacement therapy on cardiovascular events in recently postmenopausal women: randomised trial. BMJ 2012;345:e6409.

18 de Villiers TJ, Gass ML, Haines CJ, Hall JE, Lobo RA, Pierroz DD, *et al.* Global consensus statement on menopausal hormone therapy. Climacteric 2013 Apr;16(2):203–4.

19 Manson JE, Chlebowski RT, Stefanick ML, Aragaki AK, Rossouw JE, Prentice RL, *et al.* Menopausal hormone therapy and health outcomes during the intervention and extended poststopping phases of the Women's Health Initiative randomized trials. JAMA 2013 Oct 2;310(13): 1353–68.

20 Manzoli L, De VC, Marzuillo C, Boccia A, Villari P. Oral contraceptives and venous thromboembolism: a systematic review and meta-analysis. Drug Saf 2012 Mar 1;35(3):191–205.

21 Sode BF, Allin KH, Dahl M, Gyntelberg F, Nordestgaard BG. Risk of venous thromboembolism and myocardial infarction associated with factor V Leiden and prothrombin mutations and blood type. CMAJ 2013 Mar 19;185(5):E229–37.

22 Lidegaard O, Milsom I, Geirsson RT, Skjeldestad FE. Hormonal contraception and venous thromboembolism. Acta Obstet Gynecol Scand 2012 Jul;91(7):769–78.

23 Jick SS, Hernandez RK. Risk of non-fatal venous thromboembolism in women using oral contraceptives containing drospirenone compared with women using oral contraceptives containing levonorgestrel: case-control study using United States claims data. BMJ 2011;342:d2151.

24 DiCarlo F. [Action of drugs in relation to the administration route]. Minerva Endocrinol 1989 Jan;14(1):41–4.

25 Wikipedia. S.v. IUD with progestogen [Internet; redirected from s.v. Mirena]. 2012 [cited 2012 Feb 20]. Available from: http://en.wikipedia.org/wiki/Mirena

26 Bayer. Skyla package insert [Internet]. 2013 [cited 2013 Dec 6]. Available from:http://dailymed.nlm.nih.gov/dailymed/lookup.cfm?setid=9f44ff35-e052-49cd-a1c2-0bfd87d49309

27 Luthy IA, Begin DJ, Labrie F. Androgenic activity of synthetic progestins and spironolactone in androgen-sensitive mouse mammary carcinoma (Shionogi) cells in culture. J Steroid Biochem 1988 Nov;31(5):845–52.

28 Belvedere P, Gabai G, Dalla VL, Accorsi P, Trivoletti M, Colombo L, *et al.* Occurrence of steroidogenic enzymes in the bovine mammary gland at different functional stages. J Steroid Biochem Mol Biol 1996 Nov;59(3–4):339–47.

29 Lonnerdal B. Human milk proteins: key components for the biological activity of human milk. Adv Exp Med Biol 2004;554:11–25.

30 Liu Y, Guo R. Ph-dependent structures and properties of casein micelles. Biophys Chem 2008 Aug;136(2–3): 67–73.

31 McMahon DJ, Oommen BS. Supramolecular structure of the casein micelle. J Dairy Sci 2008 May;91(5):1709–21.

32 Irmak MK, Oztas Y, Oztas E. Integration of maternal genome into the neonate genome through breast milk mRNA transcripts and reverse transcriptase. Theor Biol Med Model 2012;9:20.

33 Fisher JK. Acne vulgaris; a study of one thousand cases. JK Fisher; 2006 [cited 2014 Aug 13]. Available from: http://www.acnemilk.com/fisher_s_original_paper

34 Cordain L, Lindeberg S, Hurtado M, Hill K, Eaton SB, Brand-Miller J. Acne vulgaris: a disease of Western civilization. Arch Dermatol 2002 Dec;138(12):1584–90.

35 Smith R, Mann N, Makelainen H, Roper J, Braue A, Varigos G. A pilot study to determine the short-term effects of a low glycemic load diet on hormonal markers of acne: a nonrandomized, parallel, controlled feeding trial. Mol Nutr Food Res 2008 Jun;52(6):718–26.

36 Smith RN, Mann NJ, Braue A, Makelainen H, Varigos GA. The effect of a high-protein, low glycemic-load diet versus a conventional, high glycemic-load diet on biochemical parameters associated with acne vulgaris: a randomized, investigator-masked, controlled trial. J Am Acad Dermatol 2007 Aug;57(2):247–56.

37 Smith RN, Mann NJ, Braue A, Makelainen H, Varigos GA. A low-glycemic-load diet improves symptoms in acne vulgaris patients: a randomized controlled trial. Am J Clin Nutr 2007 Jul;86(1):107–15.

38 Reynolds RC, Lee S, Choi JY, Atkinson FS, Stockmann KS, Petocz P, *et al.* Effect of the glycemic index of carbohydrates on acne vulgaris. Nutrients 2010 Oct;2(10):1060–72.

39 Kwon HH, Yoon JY, Hong JS, Jung JY, Park MS, Suh DH. Clinical and histological effect of a low glycaemic load diet in treatment of acne vulgaris in Korean patients: a randomized, controlled trial. Acta Derm Venereol 2012 May;92(3):241–6.

40 Ismail NH, Manaf ZA, Azizan NZ. High glycemic load diet, milk and ice cream consumption are related to acne vulgaris in Malaysian young adults: a case control study. BMC Dermatol 2012;12:13–8.

41 Melnik BC, Zouboulis CC. Potential role of FoxO1 and mTORC1 in the pathogenesis of Western diet-induced acne. Exp Dermatol 2013 May;22(5):311–5.

42 Melnik BC, Schmitz G. Are therapeutic effects of antiacne agents mediated by activation of FoxO1 and inhibition of mTORC1? Exp Dermatol 2013 Jul;22(7):502–4.

43 Kagawa Y. Impact of Westernization on the nutrition of Japanese: changes in physique, cancer, longevity and centenarians. Prev Med 1978 Jun;7(2):205–17.

44 Vicini J, Etherton T, Kris-Etherton P, Ballam J, Denham S, Staub R, et al. Survey of retail milk composition as affected by label claims regarding farm-management practices. J Am Diet Assoc 2008 Jul;108(7):1198–203.

45 Farlow DW, Xu X, Veenstra TD. Comparison of estrone and 17beta-estradiol levels in commercial goat and cow milk. J Dairy Sci 2012 Apr;95(4):1699–708.

46 Belvedere P, Gabai G, Dalla VL, Accorsi P, Trivoletti M, Colombo L, et al. Occurrence of steroidogenic enzymes in the bovine mammary gland at different functional stages. J Steroid Biochem Mol Biol 1996 Nov;59(3–4):339–47.

47 Yeung A, Sheehan J. Hormone concentrations in milk and milk products [letter from FDA Center for Food Safety and Applied Nutrition]. Washington, DC: US Food and Drug Administration; 2012.

48 Donovan SM, Odle J. Growth factors in milk as mediators of infant development. Annu Rev Nutr 1994;14:147–67.

49 Salehi A, Gunnerud U, Muhammed SJ, Ostman E, Holst JJ, Bjorck I, et al. The insulinogenic effect of whey protein is partially mediated by a direct effect of amino acids and GIP on beta-cells. Nutr Metab (Lond) 2012 May 30;9(1):48.

50 Reynolds RC, Lee S, Choi JY, Atkinson FS, Stockmann KS, Petocz P, et al. Effect of the glycemic index of carbohydrates on acne vulgaris. Nutrients 2010 Oct;2(10):1060–72.

51 Hoyt G, Hickey MS, Cordain L. Dissociation of the glycaemic and insulinaemic responses to whole and skimmed milk. Br J Nutr 2005 Feb;93(2):175–7.

52 Herman-Giddens ME, Steffes J, Harris D, Slora E, Hussey M, Dowshen SA, et al. Secondary sexual characteristics in boys: data from the pediatric research in office settings network. Pediatrics 2012 Nov;130(5):e1058–68.

53 Melnik BC. Permanent impairment of insulin resistance from pregnancy to adulthood: the primary basic risk factor of chronic Western diseases. Med Hypotheses 2009 Nov;73(5):670–81.

54 Melnik BC. Milk—the promoter of chronic Western diseases. Med Hypotheses 2009 Jun;72(6):631–9.

CHAPTER 5

Exogenous acnegens and acneform eruptions

True acne vulgaris requires comedones for diagnosis, acne rosacea does not, and acne inversa can cause hugely destructive lesions even when the obstruction in the follicle is invisible to the naked eye. Chemical toxins, medications, bacteria, yeasts, parasites, friction, and maceration all trigger other "acneform" disorders presenting as inflamed follicles. *Folliculitis* is the accurate term, and these lesions should be labeled as such. Although the tendency of non-dermatologists to label such eruptions as *acneform* has the advantage of acting as a sort of shorthand that conveys a mental picture of the disorder, the term causes etiological and diagnostic confusion.

5.1 Chemicals and medications

The most infamous "acnegen" is 2,3,7,8-tetrachlorod-ibenzo-*p*-dioxin (TCDD), the poison that disfigured then-presidential candidate Victor Yushchenko of Ukraine with severe chloracne (Figure 5.1). This chemical is slowly eliminated, a small part of it in sebum [1]; and, despite receiving an estimated 2 mg of TCDD, he survived and eight years later he was planning a return to politics.

Numerous medications produce acneform reactions. Litt's *Drug Eruptions and Reactions Manual* lists 210 such medications from acamprosate to zonisamide [2]. The most acute form of these eruptions is induced by the epidermal growth factor receptor (EGFR) inhibitors (see Section 3.0.4.5). With the mechanism of causation in doubt, management of this new arrival is not yet standardized. Variants of anti-acne and anti-inflammatory therapy are in use [3, 4].

There are new androgens in the pipeline with potential therapeutic applications. Two do not require 5α-reduction to exert their maximal androgenic effects: dimethandrolone (7α,11β-dimethyl-19-nortestosterone) and 11β-methyl-19-nortestosterone [5]. Will these new androgens, with no 5α-reduction, be acnegens? We don't know yet.

5.2 Endocrine imitators and disruptors

Our modern world is contaminating itself at a remarkable rate. Signs of this contamination have been showing up for years, and it is a wonder that the effects have not been far worse than have been noted to date. Everyday exposure to everything from pesticides through plastics to phytoestrogens in soy may be seen as a threat. Extensive documentation to date has but scratched the surface of the problem. Regulation of potential threats faces truly daunting economic, social, and legal hurdles. We are living with endocrine-disrupting chemicals (EDCs), we are learning about their effects [6], but they do not seem to be impacting acne in humans to a noticeable or measurable degree.

On the other hand, because many are estrogenic and therefore anti-androgenic, one wonders whether the possibility exists that such artificial endocrine disruptors may actually be beneficial in the acnes! The scare tactics surrounding the question of phytoestrogens and soy

Acne: Causes and Practical Management, First Edition. F. William Danby.
© 2015 John Wiley & Sons, Ltd. Published 2015 by John Wiley & Sons, Ltd.

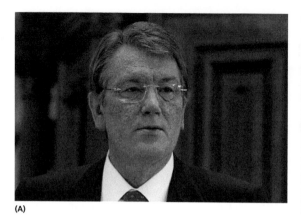 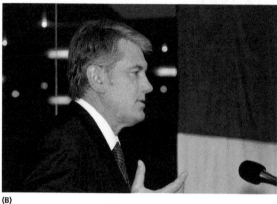

(A)   **(B)**

Figure 5.1 Victor Yushchenko (A) after TCDD exposure, and (B) at 5 years. (A) By Muumi (own work) [CC-BY-SA-3.0 (http://creativecommons.org/licenses/by-sa/3.0/)], via Wikimedia Commons. (B) By http://www.flickr.com/photos/maiakinfo/3664435519/ JürgVollmer/maiak.info [CC-BY-SA-2.0 (http://creativecommons.org/licenses/by-sa/2.0)], via Wikimedia Commons.

must be tempered by the fact that *all* plants contain phytoestrogens, although some more than others. After all, phytoestrogens are to growing plants what human estrogens are to growing humans, essential chemical messengers guiding reproductive life.

5.2.1 Environmental contamination

The presence of herd animals on the land, the use of hormones agriculturally, and hormone use in human medicines like birth control pills result in hormones showing up in groundwater [7] and downstream in the silt of the waterways that drain our cities and country-side. Several river outflows in the United Kingdom have been studied, and significant levels of androgens found [8]. The impact is on the fertility of fish, not something we notice every day, and fish don't suffer from acne, so this is also not seen as a threat. Furthermore, the water-ways studied flow into the sea, so although they are not sources of human drinking water, the concentration of these hormones in the sea will doubtless inexorably increase. One wonders what would show up in a study of the Great Lakes of North America, where much of the hormone-containing water is recycled and consumed by millions before being flushed to the sea.

5.3 Foods

All that we consume can impact our health, usually positively but sometimes negatively. There is nothing more natural than mothers' milk for babies, but dairy products are now consumed by hundreds of millions for whom they were not intended. The tendency of consumers to seek "all-natural" or "organic" products is a step in the right direction, but the *all-natural* label can apply to poison ivy as well as to broccoli. And any food that contains toxins from whatever source, even unknowingly, obviously loses its "organic" designation despite claims on the label.

There are also a few normally innocent compounds that can be troublesome. This includes the acnegens in foods we consume every day. Defining them is a challenge, but we can start by noting that numerous ecologic and migrant studies demonstrate increased prevalence of acne vulgaris with a more "Western" lifestyle and diet. Steiner saw no acne in Okinawans and noted, "Milk from goats or cows was used only by those who were ill and by babies whose mothers had insufficient milk. Cheese was repellent to the Okinawans" [9]. Robinson's food diary study named milk as the most common exacerbant reported [10]. Fisher's personal study of over 1000 consecutive acne patients implicated milk [11]. Never published, it is now at http://www.acnemilk.com. On the simple-carbohydrate side, Bendiner reported,

Acne vulgaris now scars the hitherto renowned complexions of the Eskimo [*sic*] and the evidence leaps at one from even the most casual glance at the faces of the youngsters who seem constantly to be nibbling at candy bars or drinking soda pop out of a can. Indeed, the whites have swamped the Eskimo in a mass of sugar and carbohydrates.

Shelves of the Hudson Bay Trading Company stores are heavily stocked with a glittering variety of chocolates, gumdrops, potato chips, sodas. These readily absorbable carbohydrates have flooded the system of a people totally unused to them and highly vulnerable to their effects, Dr. Shaeffer [*sic*] has pointed out [12]. Eskimos lack the white's ability to stabilize their blood sugar levels. Consequently their systems react by over-stimulating their production of insulin, as well as growth hormones, gluco-corticoids, and catecholamines. Canadian doctors draw little comfort from the fact that the Eskimo young people are growing taller. [13]

Anderson fed subjects milk, nuts, cola drinks, and chocolates (whatever his individual subjects—medical students—claimed had worsened their acne), but no acne flares were noted [14]. Unfortunately, the trial was only 7 to 10 days long, far too short to demonstrate a dairy effect. Clinical experience shows that acne normally takes a minimum of two months to develop but it can take years, depending upon individual thresholds. There are, however, no blinded and controlled "feeding studies" that provide accurate documentation. Recruiting study subjects to volunteer to try for *more* acne (or *any* acne if they have none) is an obvious social and ethical challenge.

Among aboriginal hunter-gatherers, Bechelli noted a 2.7% prevalence of acne in Amazonia [15], and Cordain found no acne whatsoever in either the Kitivan islanders of rural Papua New Guinea or the Aché tribe in Paraguay [16]. The latter considered the consumption of dairy "abhorrent."

5.3.1 Iodine and bromine

Two related chemicals, salts called *bromides* and *iodides*, cause bromism and iodism, respectively, when consumed in excess. These toxic disorders show similar folliculitic eruptions (bromoderma and iododerma). These look superficially like acne, so they are termed *acneform*. Close inspection reveals no comedones, eliminating the diagnosis of acne vulgaris, but the clinical similarity is close enough to generate confusion with acne rosacea. That led researchers to question whether iodine, bromine, iodides, or bromides could actually *cause* acne. Oral iodine therapy in acne vulgaris failed to produce pustular exacerbations [17]. Indeed, generations of dermatologists have used a saturated solution of potassium iodide (SSKI) as an anti-inflammatory to manage several inflammatory skin diseases. Despite exposing patients to thousands of times more iodide than the amount present as iodine in either milk or seaweed, they generated no true acne.

The misconception that iodine causes acne lives on, but two comments are warranted, in fairness and for completeness. Iodide and bromide supplementation can worsen preexisting folliculitis and, because acne is basically a folliculitis, this link is understandable. Second, acne rosacea can only be distinguished from bromo-derma or iododerma by history because acne rosacea is basically an inflammatory folliculitis, without comedones, in the same general facial distribution as these disorders and is essentially indistinguishable clinically from rosacea fulminans.

Concern that iodine is present in sufficient amounts in milk to cause such problems can be laid aside. The doses of iodine in milk are so low, and therefore so safe, that in some countries with agricultural iodine deficiencies, the regulatory authorities rely on the iodine in milk, from the washing of the cows' teats prior to milking, to supplement the national diet. The same result is achieved with iodized salt elsewhere [18].

5.3.2 Chocolate

Dermatologists have heard patients link acne and the ingestion of chocolate anecdotally for years. I've probably heard the story a few hundred times, although it is usually now preceded by "I know you don't believe this, doctor, but chocolate breaks me out." A 1969 research paper linking chocolate and acne [19] has been criticized on several fronts: for using non-identical fats in the two chocolate bars, a lack of adequate controls, the use of combined comedo and pustule counts rather than separating pustule counts (the pustular flares would presumably indicate worsening), the small sample size (five patients) in one part of the study in which normal subjects were fed special chocolate bars daily for a month, and the overall short length of the trial (six weeks) when it takes significantly longer to form comedones. This trial, despite being discredited by numerous critics, led in the popular press to 30 years of misinformation—the myth that diet doesn't cause acne. Unfortunately, many physicians and, incredibly, many dermatologists have accepted the myth unquestioningly, despite the valid scientific criticism.

Indeed, the question of chocolate's influence on acne refused to die despite the science. That led Berman and a research team at the University of Miami to look at the problem anew [20]. They took care to avoid dairy in the chocolate that was used, they described a folliculopapular flare of acne in the test subjects, and they reported a positive correlation. The timing was far too short (a single dose of chocolate given to 10 subjects, with reviews at four and seven days) for the lesions to have been due to comedo development. It is suggested, pending further study, that the chocolate flared preexisting subclinical acne.

5.3.3 Casein and whey

About seven years ago, I treated a small group of men approximately 40 years of age, each of whom had realized that he was getting "out of shape." Each headed off to the gym in search of his youthful silhouette, and each of these five patients came to me seeking help with their acne, a problem they had thought they had left behind 20 years previously. It was certainly not the sign of youth they were seeking!

In addition to the exercise and general dietary instructions, these men had been introduced to "protein powder" supplements. I had them stop all food supplements containing casein and whey protein: in body-builder protein powder supplements (Figure 5.2), as well as "instant breakfast" and "snack bar" products. All cleared within a few months.

During a question period after a lecture in India, during which I did not mention this subject, a petite female dermatologist got to her feet. She mentioned that she had been seeing several "young men with recent acne who go to the gymnasium and are encouraged to consume protein supplements." She wondered if there was something in the protein food and drinks causing acne, and I was happy to support her perspicacity. To hear such independent confirmation, halfway around the world, before anything on the subject had appeared in the literature, was a fascinating and confirming experience.

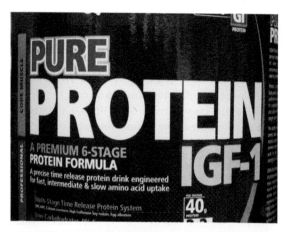
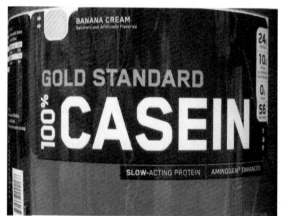
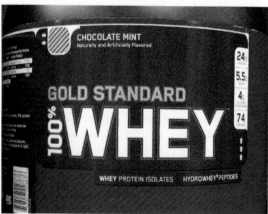
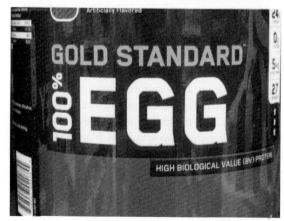

Figure 5.2 One out of four (the egg protein) isn't bad!

Subsequently, five independent cases have been reported [21], and I see cases regularly.

An effort will need to be made to rule out steroid "doping" of these products, a risk in the body-building environment. Unfortunately, the US Food and Drug Administration (FDA) has never investigated hormones in dairy products, and as of July 2012, a letter indicates that the FDA has no plans to do so [22].

We now know that consuming whey stimulates elevations in insulin, casein ingestion stimulates elevations of IGF-1 [23], and these two dairy components, found together or separately in such protein supplements, are the twin stimuli to de-repression of the androgen receptor [24], as Melnik has pointed out so eloquently (see also Section 2.9).

5.4 Photodamage, glycation, and the acne and aging processes

As discussed in Section 1.2, the pathogenesis of acne rosacea, like that of Favre–Racouchot syndrome, is based upon the contribution of sun damage to the collagen-based support structures wrapped around the FPSU. It is now apparent that a process called glycation may contribute to the photodamage of collagen in acne rosacea and, more importantly, to the apparently poor support of the follicular structures in patients with acne inversa/hidradenitis suppurativa (AI/HS).

How could that be? Basically, glycation is the permanent cross-linking of collagen fibrils by glucose molecules. This cross-linking, a process that is ultraviolet enhanced in sun-exposed areas but is also active in non-light-exposed areas, prevents the normal and regular renewal and repair of structural collagen, locking in the damage and making it either difficult to repair or indeed irreparable [25]. A chronic and increasing weakening of these structural supports occurs, particularly in those individuals with compromised metabolic states, insulin resistance, and chronic hyperglycemia. Hyperglycemia breeds elevated levels of glucose in the skin. No surprise there, although it is rarely spoken of. That means that sugar, the raw material for glycation, is instantly available in our "super-sized" and chronically hyperglycemic society. All that is needed is the addition of sunlight, real or artificial. This represents another link the acnes have to metabolic syndrome (also called *syndrome X*).

5.5 Smoking and nicotine

There is new evidence that another exogenous substance, nicotine, has an influence on two of the acnes. Convincing epidemiological evidence of a link between smoking and post-adolescent acne now exists [26]. Based on work on nicotine in other species, this appears to be due to the ability of nicotine to activate non-neuronal acetylcholine receptors, causing increased keratinization of the follicular infundibulum. Hana's study gives us the "first hints for a causative role of the non-neuronal cholinergic system in the pathogenesis of HS (acne inversa) by promoting infundibular epithelial hyperplasia and thus follicular plugging" [27]. A randomized controlled trial to actually prove causation is unlikely to be conducted, however, given that it would require researchers to introduce smoking or highly addictive nicotine to previously nonsmoking bearers of the AI/HS gene! Based on this suggestive evidence and considerable experience-based medicine, nicotine avoidance must be an essential part of AI/HS management. Patients with AI/HS have major problems complying with advice to stop this highly addictive substance. Substitution with an alternate nicotine source such as patches or gum is obviously not appropriate. Counseling these patients is an ongoing challenge, because "cutting down" simply doesn't do the job.

References

1 Geusau A, Tschachler E, Meixner M, Papke O, Stingl G, McLachlan M. Cutaneous elimination of 2,3,7,8-tetrachlorodibenzo-p-dioxin. Br J Dermatol 2001 Dec;145(6):938–43.

2 Litt J. Drug eruption reference manual. 17th ed. London: Informa Healthcare USA; 2012.

3 Bachet JB, Peuvrel L, Bachmeyer C, Reguiai Z, Gourraud PA, Bouche O, *et al.* Folliculitis induced by 3.0.4.53.0.4.5R inhibitors, preventive and curative efficacy of tetracyclines in the management and incidence rates according to the type of EGFR inhibitor administered: a systematic literature review. Oncologist 2012;17(4):555–68.

4 Gerber PA, Meller S, Eames T, Buhren BA, Schrumpf H, Hetzer S, *et al.* Management of EGFR-inhibitor associated rash: a retrospective study in 49 patients. Eur J Med Res 2012 Jan 30;17(1):4.

5 Attardi BJ, Hild SA, Koduri S, Pham T, Pessaint L, Engbring J, *et al.* The potent synthetic androgens, dimethandrolone (7alpha,11beta-dimethyl-19-nortestosterone) and 11beta-methyl-19-nortestosterone, do not require 5alpha-reduction

to exert their maximal androgenic effects. J Steroid Biochem Mol Biol 2010 Oct;122(4):212–8.

6 Schettler T, Solomon G, Valenti M, Huddle A. Generations at risk: reproductive health and the environment. Cambridge, MA: MIT Press; 1999.

7 Cai K, Elliott CT, Phillips DH, Scippo ML, Muller M, Connolly L. Treatment of estrogens and androgens in dairy wastewater by a constructed wetland system. Water Res 2012 May 1;46(7):2333–43.

8 Thomas KV, Hurst MR, Matthiessen P, McHugh M, Smith A, Waldock MJ. An assessment of in vitro androgenic activity and the identification of environmental androgens in United Kingdom estuaries. Environ Toxicol Chem 2002 Jul;21(7):1456–61.

9 Steiner P. Okinawa and its people. Sci Mon 1947 Mar;64(3):233.

10 Robinson H. The acne problem. South Med J 1949 Dec;42(12):1050–60.

11 Fisher JK. Acne vulgaris; a study of one thousand cases [Internet]. JK Fisher; 2006 [cited 2014 Aug 21]. Available from: http://www.acnemilk.com/fisher_s_original_paper

12 Schaefer O. Pre- and post-natal growth acceleration and increased sugar consumption in Canadian Eskimos. Can Med Assoc J 1970 Nov 7;103(10):1059–68.

13 Bendiner E. Disastrous tradeoff: Eskimo health for white civilization. Hospital Practice 1974;9:156–89.

14 Anderson PC. Foods as the cause of acne. Am Fam Physician 1971 Mar;3(3):102–3.

15 Bechelli LM, Haddad N, Pimenta WP, Pagnano PM, Melchior E Jr, Fregnan RC, et al. Epidemiological survey of skin diseases in schoolchildren living in the Purus Valley (Acre State, Amazonia, Brazil). Dermatologica 1981;163(1):78–93.

16 Cordain L, Lindeberg S, Hurtado M, Hill K, Eaton SB, Brand-Miller J. Acne vulgaris: a disease of Western civilization. Arch Dermatol 2002 Dec;138(12):1584–90.

17 Gaul L, Underwood G. Oral iodine therapy in acne vulgaris; failure of iodine, or the equivalent of iodized salt, to produce pustular exacerbations. Arch Derm Syphilol 1948 Oct;58(4):439–43.

18 Danby FW. Acne and iodine: reply. J Am Acad Dermatol 2007 Jan;56(1):164–5.

19 Fulton JE, Jr., Plewig G, Kligman AM. Effect of chocolate on acne vulgaris. JAMA 1969 Dec 15;210(11):2071–4.

20 Block SG, Valins WE, Caperton CV, Viera MH, Amini S, Berman B. Exacerbation of facial acne vulgaris after consuming pure chocolate. J Am Acad Dermatol 2011 Oct;65(4):e114–15.

21 Silverberg NB. Whey protein precipitating moderate to severe acne flares in 5 teenaged athletes. Cutis 2012 Aug;90(2):70–2.

22 Yeung A. FDA measurement of hormone concentrations in milk and milk products [personal communication]. Communication to F.W. Danby, 2012 Jul 2.

23 Hoppe C, Molgaard C, Dalum C, Vaag A, Michaelsen KF. Differential effects of casein versus whey on fasting plasma levels of insulin, IGF-1 and IGF-1/IGFBP-3: results from a randomized 7-day supplementation study in prepubertal boys. Eur J Clin Nutr 2009 Sep;63(9):1076–83.

24 Melnik BC, Schmitz G. Role of insulin, insulin-like growth factor-1, hyperglycaemic food and milk consumption in the pathogenesis of acne vulgaris. Exp Dermatol 2009 Oct;18(10):833–41.

25 Danby FW. Nutrition and aging skin: sugar and glycation. Clin Dermatol 2010 Jul;28(4):409–11.

26 Capitanio B, Sinagra JL, Bordignon V, Cordiali FP, Picardo M, Zouboulis CC. Underestimated clinical features of postadolescent acne. J Am Acad Dermatol 2010 Nov;63(5):782–8.

27 Hana A, Booken D, Henrich C, Gratchev A, Maas-Szabowski N, Goerdt S, et al. Functional significance of non-neuronal acetylcholine in skin epithelia. Life Sci 2007 May 30;80(24–25):2214–20.

CHAPTER 6
Follicular flora, fauna, and fuzz

The inflammatory reaction that causes the trouble in all the acnes is directed at a limited number of foreign materials. Remember that *foreign* is defined as anything that is not supposed to be in the dermis, and the dermis is that part of the skin that is below (on the dermal side of) the basement membrane. And remember that the basement membrane runs horizontally under the epidermis but dives deep and wraps around the epidermal appendages, all of them, from sweat glands to hair bulbs. It is thin in some areas, thicker in others. It follows the contours of the folliculopilosebaceous unit (FPSU) like a vinyl glove on your fingers. It provides support to the appendages. It anchors the epidermis to the dermis. It is a semipermeable barrier, allowing limited amounts of water, chemicals, and a few mobile cells to cross into and out of the epidermis and the appendages. (See Figure 2.7.)

A recently described chemical messenger system, hypoxia-inducible factor 1 (HIF-1), may be responsible for the two processes that are active at this point in the process of acne development. HIF-1 appears to be able to induce "hyperproliferation and incomplete differentiation of epidermal keratinocytes" [1]. It is also "a major regulator of cellular adaptation to low oxygen stress" and "plays an important role in cytokine production by keratinocytes and in neutrophil recruitment to the skin" [2]. Thus, it may stimulate the overgrowth to bursting and recruit inflammatory cells to migrate to the area in response to the anoxic stress.

Once the barrier is broken, foreign material that is located in the ducts of the FPSU becomes "visible" to the body's immune systems. This can happen if the immune cells find their way through a split in the basement membrane into the follicular duct, or if the materials inside the duct find their way out through a leak. Either way, the immune systems recognize the foreign material, and this is the first trigger to inflammation. If and when the immune reactions proceed, the duct leaks even more and often ruptures, and greater volumes of materials in the duct find their way out into the dermis. There they trigger the numerous inflammatory processes of the innate and adaptive immune systems, and so the battle intensifies.

To cool and clear acne, we must know all the materials stuck down in the duct that are causing the inflammation. Then we can plan to eliminate each and every one of them.

6.1 *Propionibacterium acnes* (*P. acnes*)

Bacillus acnes, the "acne bacillus," was first described by Gilchrist in 1900. It was renamed *Corynebacterium acnes* in 1909 and later *Propionibacterium acnes* (*P. acnes*). There are 22 members of the *Propionibacterium* family, but *P. acnes* (which comprises several strains) appears to be the only important one in acne. As such, it has been the target for elimination by dermatologists for decades. But there is a problem. Simply overwhelming the population of *P. acnes* with antibiotics doesn't usually clear acne. This simple fact should have given us a hint, decades ago, that something else was going on. More on that below.

Acne: Causes and Practical Management, First Edition. F. William Danby.
© 2015 John Wiley & Sons, Ltd. Published 2015 by John Wiley & Sons, Ltd.

6.1.1 Normal role of *P. acnes*

While it has been generally accepted that *P. acnes* is a normal organism on everybody's skin (a *commensal*), that is not the whole story. Recently, with a simple but sophisticated technique, Bek-Thomsen showed that *P. acnes* seems to have exclusive rights of occupancy to the FPSU. His work shows that no other organism can make that claim [3]. Furthermore, it was suggested that this relatively harmless organism actually has a role as a gentle guardian of the integrity of the FPSU, a concept that has found support elsewhere [4]. So how does such a protective role really work?

Imagine that *P. acnes* is sitting quietly in a follicle. It is a facultative anaerobe. That means it can survive and multiply in a very low-oxygen (or no-oxygen) environment. Normally, the follicle is well oxygenated so *P. acnes'* motor is simply "idling in neutral." If there is a minor injury to the duct, like a scratch or a rub, a little bit of *P. acnes* antigen may leak out of the duct. Or, much less likely, perhaps a wandering dendritic cell bearing toll-like receptor 2 (TLR2) may gain access to the ductal lumen. If such contact is made between *P. acnes* and the innate immune system, the inflammatory cascade gets to work, and normally this initiates activities that repair the damage. One must remember that such low-grade "inflammation" is really designed to return the physical structure of the duct back to normal. The inflammatory system we work so hard to suppress is not *all* "destruction"—its reparative function is usually ignored, and many of the medications we use will actually compromise this function. Topical steroids, for instance, cause thinning of the skin in hand eczema, a thinning that takes months of steroid avoidance to repair.

Barring serious abnormalities (like the overstuffed duct with weak walls in acne inversa), the repair is quickly completed and everything goes back to normal. *P. acnes'* role as an immune sentry has been fulfilled. Only if things go terribly wrong is there a hot, destructive inflammatory reaction resulting in permanent damage.

6.1.2 Pathogenic role of *P. acnes*

We are much more familiar with *P. acnes'* role as a pathogen, a bad actor that needs to be eliminated in order to cure the disease. Over the past 60 years, we have brought to bear tetracycline, erythromycin, doxycycline, minocycline, lymecycline, azithromycin, sulfa drugs with and without trimethoprim, clindamycin, clarithromycin, ampicillin, amoxicillin, ciprofloxacin, and even rifampicin. Despite this aggressive attack, we still see the term *antibiotic-resistant acne*, and that term usually addresses only acne vulgaris. If you add acne rosacea, then metronidazole, neomycin, fusidic acid, mupirocin, azelaic acid, and retepamulin are on the list. Take one step further to acne inversa/hidradenitis suppurativa (AI/HS), and we see that escalation to the "nuclear option" includes long-term systemic rifampicin, moxifloxacin, and metronidazole [5]. It is hard to believe that any bacterial infection could survive that onslaught, and yet only 16 of 28 patients with HS/AI achieved complete remission with up to 12 months of this aggressive triple-antibiotic therapy. We have not yet learned what will occur when the medications are stopped in those temporarily fortunate 16 successfully treated patients. But we can guess.

What happens to change *P. acnes* from a mild-mannered commensal to a "pathogen" able to destroy faces and backs and psyches? And why does our most aggressive antibiotic therapy not work? There are likely four factors at work that bear on *P. acnes*, and one that has been roundly ignored despite posted warnings.

First, *P. acnes* shifts out of neutral and really gets to work only in an anaerobic (no-oxygen) or a microaerophilic (low-oxygen) environment. So, how does one achieve such an anoxic environment in a healthy teenage face, full of life and the vigor of youth, well vascularized, and supplied with adequate nutrients and all the metabolic systems needed to sustain and repair all normal processes? The answer is possibly, but not proven, that there is simply too much of a good thing available. As described in detail in Section 2.9, increased insulin-like growth factor 1 (IGF-1) and increased insulin and exogenous androgens, added to endogenous steroids and endogenous pubertal IGF-1, overstimulate the follicular ductal keratinocytes. A traffic jam occurs in the follicle: pressure within the confines of the follicular duct compromises the availability of nutrients, especially oxygen. The lack of nutrients diffusing into the area interferes with normal metabolic processes within the keratinocytes. The concurrent anoxia provides a wonderful place for *P. acnes* to flourish. Nourished anaerobically by the fatty acids of the sebum, *P. acnes* multiplies mightily, to the point that the colonies are large enough to be easily visible in microscopic sections. When the overstressed follicle leaks or ruptures, the population of *P. acnes* will have increased by several orders of magnitude, becoming a very potent stimulus of the innate immune system. That is what lights the fire in acne vulgaris.

Second, *P. acnes* has the genomic capacity to support a large number of functions. These enzymatic abilities are not much in evidence when the organism is "idling" quietly in the duct, but under the conditions of anoxia that occur in the compressed confines of the crowded and distended duct, the organism is capable of springing to life at full anaerobic throttle, and the broad panel of metabolic options that the genotype can support apparently become selectively deployed. This shows up as a change in the organism to a fully active reproductive phenotype, triggered by the provision of the anaerobic or microaerophilic environment that the organism prefers. This can be expressed in many destructive ways [6]. These include virulence-associated and fitness traits such as transport systems and metabolic pathways, and the encoding of possible virulence factors such as dermatan–sulphate adhesin, polyunsaturated fatty acid isomerase, iron acquisition protein HtaA, and lipase GehA. The authors argue "that the disease-causing potential of different *P. acnes* strains is not only determined by the phylotype-specific genome content but also by variable gene expression" [6].

Third, it isn't really all *P. acnes'* fault that such a mess is created. While the genome offers considerable potential for havoc, there is also the reaction to the numerous materials that are explosively released into the dermal and subcutaneous world beyond the basement membrane. These are both the immediate stimulants of the innate immune system and the antigens that the slower acting, yet very potent, adaptive immune response will need to identify, react to, and neutralize.

Fourth, the blame for stimulating the immune systems needs serious recognition as a shared responsibility. Not only has the other major intraductal organism been inexplicably ignored, but also the attempts to eradicate this bacterial activity have done wonders to increase the impact of another actor, *P. acnes'* silent partner, the yeast *Malassezia*.

6.2 *Malassezia* species

Malassezia yeasts were first recognized by Louis-Charles Malassez in 1874, and Sabouraud named the yeast *Pityrosporum malassez* in 1904. It was not until 1988 that the taxonomists adopted *Malassezia* as the genus name and combined the ovale and orbiculare forms as *Malassezia furfur*. There are now 14 species characterized:

M. furfur
M. pachydermatis
M. sympodialis
M. globosa
M. obtusa
M. restricta
M. slooffiae
M. dermatis
M. japonica
M. yamatoensis
M. nana
M. caprae
M. equina
M. cuniculi [7].

They are found widely among sebum-secreting animals other than humans. Relationships between specific animal species, specific yeast species, the diseases they induce, and even their geographic human variations are being worked out, but *M. globosa* seems to be the major contributor to dandruff.

Malassezia requires a specific lipid for growth and reproduction, so it is demonstrably lipophilic. Indeed, its need for long-chain fatty acids of carbon chain length greater than 10 (C12–C24) is so profound that positive cultures can be obtained only by adding a source of this material to the culture medium. An olive oil overlay of the Sabouraud culture medium is commonly used. (See Figure 1.8.)

While there are several rare *Malassezia* infections reported in immunocompromised patients, the major widely recognized clinical presentations of *Malassezia* are as tinea (pityriasis) versicolor (Figures 6.1 and 6.2) and *Malassezia* folliculitis (Figures 6.3, 6.4, 6.5, 6.6, and 6.7). This yeast's papulopustular involvement in atopic dermatitis (particularly of the head and neck—see Figures 6.8 and 6.9) [8], in psoriasis (particularly in the scalp—see Figures 6.10 and 6.11) [9], in seborrheic dermatitis [9], and in acne [10] is far from being generally recognized and treated in the general dermatologist's office or clinic.

6.2.1 Normal role

So far, there has been no adaptive or physiologically important role assigned to the *Malassezia* organisms. We know that "M. globosa uses eight different types of

Figure 6.1 *Malassezia* growing on the surface is unrecognized by the immune system at first, whether here on the skin surface or down in the pores. Once recognition occurs, this surface infection can become quite itchy and may become pale pink or red.

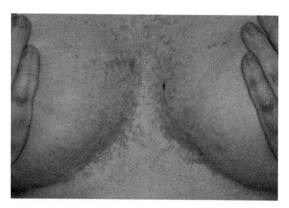

Figure 6.2 The pink inflammation of active *Malassezia*-induced tinea versicolor.

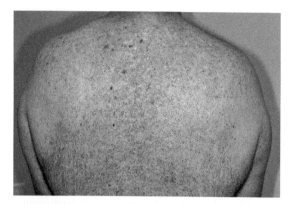

Figure 6.3 Once *Malassezia* in the pores is recognized by the immune system, an impressive immunological follicular inflammation starts.

Figure 6.4 The eruption is most active over the central back, where the sebaceous activity is at its highest.

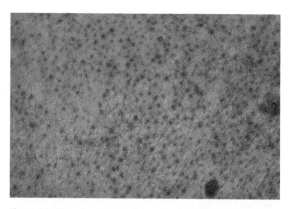

Figure 6.5 Note that the skin between the folliculopapules is totally normal—no dry itchy scaling, asteatotic eczema, or atopic or contact dermatitis.

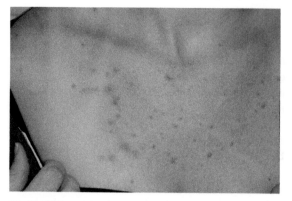

Figure 6.6 The pattern is folliculopustular on this central and lateral chest.

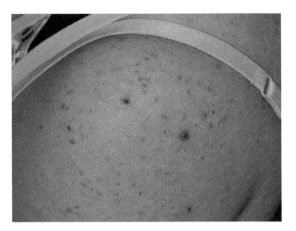

Figure 6.7 The pattern has become folliculopustular on this left shoulder, and the itch is manifested as early excoriations.

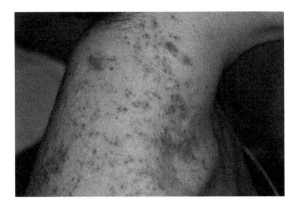

Figure 6.8 The typical folliculopapules over the right shoulder and clavicle are often ignored, or misdiagnosed as bacterial, leading to antibiotics that make matters worse.

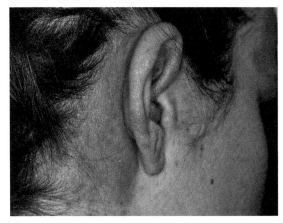

Figure 6.9 Same patient as 6.8. The extension of the atopic dermatitis combined with the small folliculopapules from the neck and the forehead into the scalp, with no evidence of psoriatic scale, suggest the combination diagnosis. The failure of oral antibiotics and topical steroid scalp lotions and creams solidifies the case.

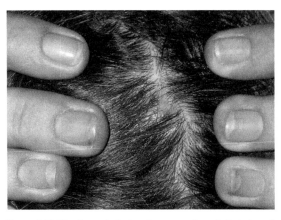

Figure 6.10 Distal onycholysis points toward psoriasis; itch and response to ketoconazole point to the inciting microbiological stimulus to trauma and Koebnerization.

lipase, along with three phospholipases, to break down the oils on the scalp" [11], but it is not suggested that the species has evolved as a grooming aid for humans. It is more likely that this important human pathogen has evolved with an adaptive capacity that ensures its survival on hosts no matter what different types of lipids it encounters on different skin surfaces. Even more important to the pathogenesis of acne, these lipases and phospholipases are added to those produced in the follicular duct by *P. acnes*, further increasing the irritation in the duct by the fatty acids produced by the breakdown of sebum triglycerides. It has been speculated for decades that the fatty acids produced by these lipases actually threaten the integrity of the lipid-containing duct wall.

Whether the lipases and phospholipases are themselves a threat to the duct wall remains to be seen.

6.2.2 Immunogenicity

Several components of *Malassezia* with the ability to induce immunoglobulin E have been defined and characterized to the point of sequencing over the past 20 years, and clinical experience confirms a strong association of the yeast and pruritus. Itch is one of the most intractable aspects of atopic dermatitis, but it is also part of the symptomatology of seborrheic dermatitis,

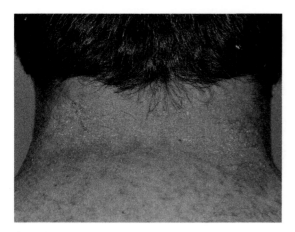

Figure 6.11 Psoriasis descending the back of the neck, with folliculopapules and folliculopustules on the upper back.

seborrhea capitis, some tinea (pityriasis) versicolor cases, and *Malassezia* folliculitis. Specific treatment provides welcome relief, but persistence is required. As Faergemann has written, a single dose of 400 mg ketoconazole orally every month is effective [12].

6.2.3 Pruritogenicity

Importantly, itch is present in about 25% of cases of acne rosacea and in about the same proportion of acne vulgaris, particularly on the face [13]. What causes this intolerable itch? I strongly suspect but cannot prove that *l'acné excoriée des jeunes filles* (Section 3.4.6) is in reality acne vulgaris colonized with *Malassezia*, to which the patient is allergic. Indeed, most acne patients who are drawn to mindlessly (or mindfully) manipulating their lesions likely do so as a result of attention being drawn to the lesions by itch. If history taking includes an inquiry into previous vulvovaginal yeast infections, a negative history is decidedly rare, and a single episode "a long time ago" is the most common story by far. I hear the story daily and suspect that earlier exposure to the antigens in *Candida*, the better known yeast, is the "sensitizing dose" that leaves the patient with an immune system primed to recognize the *Malassezia* invading the follicles in both acne vulgaris and acne rosacea.

6.2.4 *Malassezia* in the acnes

In 1988, Leeming, Holland, and Cunliffe published what I consider to be the most significant and the single most ignored paper in all the work ever done on acne, "The

Microbial Colonization of Inflamed Acne Vulgaris Lesions" [14]. Did the misspelling of Cunliffe's name as Cuncliffe [*sic*] lead to the paper being missed in literature searches, or was it simply not recognized as a seminal piece of work? Whatever the reason, this paper has languished in almost complete obscurity.

The study was simple and elegant. Punch biopsies (3 mm) from the upper back of acne patients with 1-day-old and 3-day-old papules were carefully examined microscopically and cultured. This revealed that biopsies of 3-day-old acne papules hosted a 68% colonization rate by *Malassezia furfur*. "None [of the patients] had received antimicrobial treatment for at least 4 weeks" [14], but details of earlier treatment are not provided.

In addition to the 68% yeast count, "*Propionibacterium acnes* … constituted a colonizing population in only 71% of papules and was completely absent in 20% of papules" [14]. Two explanations suggest themselves. First, perhaps previous courses of antibiotics selectively sterilized 20% of the pores of detectable *P. acnes*; or, second, the suggestion that *P. acnes* is necessary for the production of a simple acne papule may need to be reconsidered. As the authors opine, "The isolation of papules which were not colonized by micro-organisms is at variance with hypotheses stating that inflammation in acne vulgaris is invariably initiated by microbial activity" [14]. It would appear that sterile follicles can indeed produce both non-inflammatory and inflammatory papules. Of note, this does support the anoxia/hypoxia/HIF-1 hypothesis (see Section 7.3) and certainly calls into question the role of *P. acnes* as the prime mover in acnegenesis.

Perhaps a follicle swollen by hormonal overstimulation could leak and release intrafollicular materials (such as the keratin fragments found in acne inversa infiltrates) into the neighboring tissues, stimulating inflammation? This possibility, championed in Section 3.3, was not missed by these authors, who wrote, "Our results suggest that other components of comedones, such as keratins and lipids, should also be considered as potential inflammatory initiators" [14]. That possibility is further considered in this chapter.

Acne rosacea's flare by *Malassezia* has been all but ignored in the literature, yet I recognize it as a factor two or three times a month.

There is no evidence that *Malassezia* plays any role in acne inversa. That may be partly due to the destruction of the sebaceous glands (see Figure 3.2) and the subsequent lack of sebum to attract the yeast.

6.3 Staph, Strep, and Gram-negative organisms

We live in a sea of microorganisms. Positive cultures as used in modern clinical medicine are more often than not an attempt to confirm the obvious, and to satisfy the community standard of care. Truly obsessive searches for our commensal bacterial friends and potential enemies (now called our *microbiome*) have demonstrated hundreds and indeed thousands of species living on and in us [15].

So, it is no surprise when a patient who has been on antibiotics, often in a less-than-optimal dose or following an incomplete regimen, then develops a secondary infection with a "new" or resistant organism. If one kills off all the "easy-to-kill" germs, that leaves the "hard-to-kill" ones behind. And if one kills off all the resident bacteria, any of the millions of women who have suffered the pruritic (itchy) tortures of vulvovaginal candidiasis can tell you that the yeast will be delighted to take over both the space and the unused nutrients left by the departed bacteria. Far too many women know all about this.

Given the vast population of organisms, all the cultures looking for staph and strep and Gram-negative organisms are going to be positive for *something*. But is the bacterial organism that is found really the organism responsible, or is it just a local survivor? Certainly, you can eliminate pretty much all common bacteria if you choose the nuclear option (broad-spectrum antibiotics), but are you really helping clear the cause of acne? If you ignore the fact that you are inducing a growing population of *Malassezia*, and ignore the inflammation that this yeast has triggered, and ignore the vicious, destructive, and self-perpetuating immunological fires that have been set alight, the problem will persist. If not appropriately treated, *Malassezia* will disappear only when the sebaceous glands are gone (as happens in AI/HS) or when there is no more lipid for the *Malassezia* to feed upon (as with isotretinoin therapy). When the stimuli or antigens fueling the immune systems are gone, only then will the fires burn out.

A far better option from the patients' point of view is the early elimination of the yeast. Learn how to do this in Section 8.5.3.

6.4 *Demodex*

Mixed in with the entire bacterial and yeasty flora (the flowers), there is really only one little bit of fauna (an animal, but a very small one). Meet the rather amazingly well-adapted little pore mites called *Demodex folliculorum*. They are cousins of scabies, the cause of probably the itchiest rash you can suffer. *Demodex* can also be really itchy, and because the mites are active on your skin at night, you may wake up in the morning with scratches on your face you never knew you caused. While *Demodex* is mostly a problem with acne rosacea, it can be a problem with acne vulgaris as well, but it plays no known role in HS/AI. The tight acroinfundibulum and the lack of sebum ensure this.

The *Demodex* mites normally live head down in the pore, enjoying your sebum (skin oil) as food during the day. The males back out of the pores at night and wander on your skin in search of a mate, then return to the pore before you wake up to shower them off. There may be several in a pore at various stages of development, from eggs to larvae to juveniles to adults. Only if the patient becomes allergic to the mites do they cause any difficulty. They cause redness, swelling, itching, and often little, tiny, easily broken pustules (Figure 6.12).

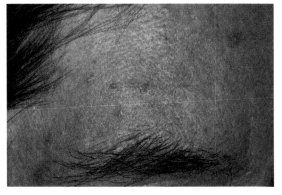

Figure 6.12 Two questions must be asked at every visit: "What is in the pustules at this point?" And "What will be needed to get rid of them?"

PRACTICAL TIP BOX 6.1 FINDING DEMODEX

This is easy to do, the hardest part often being to find a pustule that has not been ruptured. I prefer to use the corner of a glass microscope slide coverslip as a combination pustule breaker and sampling device (Figure 6.13).

If you use a scalpel blade it will cost more, some of the valuable material you want to examine under the microscope will stick to the blade, and you are going to need a coverslip anyway. Those of you who have extracted a scabies mite from her location under the skin know that mites will stick to stainless steel for reasons that have

never been explored. The coverslip is held gently because it is fragile, and a 45° angle is used to open the pustule with a corner of the coverslip. Then the pus and other material are collected in one single action. This is then transferred to a standard glass microscope slide by simply wiping both sides of the corner of the coverslip onto the center of the slide. The coverslip is then laid on top of the sample area, and a drop or two of 10% potassium hydroxide (KOH) is placed at the edge of the coverslip. The KOH moves by capillary action under the coverslip, and the slide can be examined immediately.

The mites are distinctive and easily detected under the low light usually used for KOH examinations. Various forms can be seen, such as the baby *Demodex* larva (Figure 6.14) and the molting *Demodex* (Figure 6.15). The rest of the slide usually shows nothing but pustular debris.

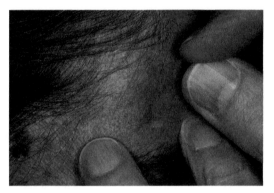

Figure 6.13 Here, a microscopic slide "coverslip" is used to sample a pustule's contents.

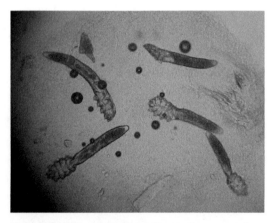

Figure 6.14 All from a single pustule, at various ages and stages. A small cap-shaped newborn larva is at top left.

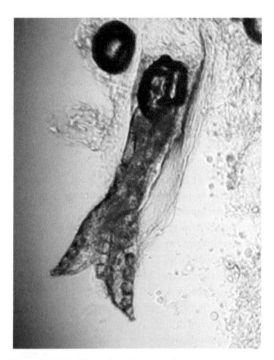

Figure 6.15 The life cycle includes molting.

This is the easiest place to find *Demodex*, either alive before treatment is initiated or after treatment when the dead ones are being pushed out of the pores.

Fortunately, there are several treatments available. (See Section 8.5.3.)

PRACTICAL TIP BOX 6.2 INGROWN HAIRS

Dealing with an ingrown hair is best done by flipping the free end of the ingrown hair out of its trapped location under the skin, but at the same time leaving it still attached. That way, the excess hair above the skin can be neatly cut short and the follicle can then regrow around the hair, using the hair as a stent. If this is in a shaving area, it is safe to shave a few days later. Plucking is to be avoided because, when the new hair grows in, it may not be able to find its way to the surface if the follicle is damaged.

6.5 Vellus hairs

Just about everyone has had an ingrown hair at some time. They can be really annoying, tender, and sore; and if they actually become infected, then there are bacteria under the skin, not just the hair. The treatment is simple (see Practical Tip box 6.2).

Once the hair is flicked out, everything cools down really quickly. Even with no antibiotics. So that approach will look after big (terminal) hairs, but what about the tiny little "peach fuzz" hairs that our FPSUs grow and that get caught and all wrapped up in a ball of ductal keratinocytes in a plugged pore? Well, these little fellows can also cause inflammation, and the place I've seen this most is in the very superficial folliculopustules of acne rosacea. Sometimes, when I use the microscopic slide cover technique to check for *Demodex*, I find nothing but a tiny hair stuck in the pore. No *Demodex*, just the hair (Figure 6.16). One can prevent these little plugs in the pores by including a gentle comedolytic in the anti-rosacea routine. More details at Section 8.4.1.1. As for HS/AI, ingrown hairs are occasionally found in the contents of unroofed HS/AI lesions, and more often in pilonidal cysts.

In summary, inflammatory acne is basically the result of the immunological responses to materials normally safely contained within the follicle; follicular flora,

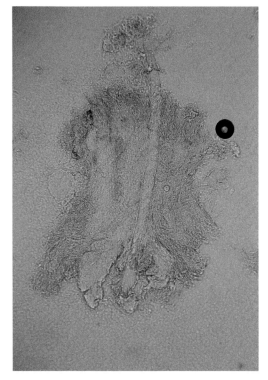

Figure 6.16 This little hair and its surrounding plug were the only foreign material in this pustule.

fauna, and fuzz. These materials, released from the ruptured duct into the dermis, are eventually eliminated by macrophages and foreign body reactions, eventually either clearing the area of foreign material and allowing healing or producing the sinuses and scars characteristic of the various acnes.

References

1 Kim SH, Kim S, Choi HI, Choi YJ, Lee YS, Sohn KC, *et al.* Callus formation is associated with hyperproliferation and incomplete differentiation of keratinocytes, and increased expression of adhesion molecules. Br J Dermatol 2010 Sep;163(3):495–501.

2 Leire E, Olson J, Isaacs H, Nizet V, Hollands A. Role of hypoxia inducible factor-1 in keratinocyte inflammatory response and neutrophil recruitment. J Inflamm (Lond) 2013;10(1):28.

3 Bek-Thomsen M, Lomholt HB, Kilian M. Acne is not associated with yet-uncultured bacteria. J Clin Microbiol 2008 Oct;46(10):3355–60.

4 Naik S, Bouladoux N, Wilhelm C, Molloy MJ, Salcedo R, Kastenmuller W, et al. Compartmentalized control of skin immunity by resident commensals. Science 2012 Aug 31;337(6098):1115–9.

5 Join-Lambert O, Coignard H, Jais JP, Guet-Revillet H, Poiree S, Fraitag S, et al. Efficacy of rifampin-moxifloxacin-metronidazole combination therapy in hidradenitis suppurativa. Dermatology 2011 Feb;222(1):49–58.

6 Brzuszkiewicz E, Weiner J, Wollherr A, Thurmer A, Hupeden J, Lomholt HB, et al. Comparative genomics and transcriptomics of Propionibacterium acnes. PLoS One 2011;6(6): e21581.

7 Gaitanis G, Magiatis P, Hantschke M, Bassukas ID, Velegraki A. The Malassezia genus in skin and systemic diseases. Clin Microbiol Rev 2012 Jan;25(1):106–41.

8 Zhang E, Tanaka T, Tajima M, Tsuboi R, Kato H, Nishikawa A, et al. Anti-Malassezia-specific IgE antibodies production in Japanese patients with head and neck atopic dermatitis: relationship between the level of specific IgE antibody and the colonization frequency of cutaneous Malassezia species and clinical severity. J Allergy (Cairo) 2011;2011:645670.

9 Schwartz JR, Messenger AG, Tosti A, Todd G, Hordinsky M, Hay RJ, et al. A comprehensive pathophysiology of dandruff and seborrheic dermatitis—towards a more precise definition of scalp health. Acta Derm Venereol 2013 Mar 27;93(2): 131–7.

10 Hu G, Wei YP, Feng J. Malassezia infection: is there any chance or necessity in refractory acne? Chin Med J (Engl) 2010 Mar 5;123(5):628–32.

11 Juntachai W, Oura T, Murayama SY, Kajiwara S. The lipolytic enzymes activities of Malassezia species. Med Mycol 2009;47(5):477–84.

12 Faergemann J. Pityriasis versicolor. Semin Dermatol 1993 Dec;12(4):276–9.

13 Emerson R. Incidence of itch in acne vulgaris and acne rosacea [personal communication]. Communication to F.W. Danby, 2011 Jul 5.

14 Leeming JP, Holland KT, Cunliffe WJ. The microbial colonization of inflamed acne vulgaris lesions. Br J Dermatol 1988 Feb;118(2):203–8.

15 Chen YE, Tsao H. The skin microbiome: current perspectives and future challenges. J Am Acad Dermatol 2013 Jul;69(1): 14355.

CHAPTER 7
The inflammatory response

Acne is either non-inflammatory or inflammatory. Classic comedones (the plugs in the pores) show no significant inflammation during their early development whether these are open comedones (blackheads) or closed comedones (whiteheads). There is no inflammation until the immune systems recognize a problem. From that instant until all is returned to normal, acne is inflammatory, even though the inflammation may be so subtle as to be invisible.

The body has two separate and very different types of immunity, one that is present at the time of birth (innate or inborn immunity) and a second system that adapts to new threats and acquires new responses as a result (adaptive or acquired immunity). This chapter examines the innate and adaptive immune responses and their effects on the acnes.

7.1 Innate immunity

The innate immune system is the "first responder." It developed during our evolutionary process when our primordial ancestors' bodies needed to learn to neutralize or get rid of anything that penetrated their "skin" very quickly, or else they would die. The innate immune system developed over millions of years and it can respond to all sorts of different foreign materials and threats, from jellyfish to splinters and from ingrown hairs to viruses.

This is the defensive system we are all born with. That means it can get to work immediately. This detection and reaction system works fast because there are millions of "sentry posts" just under the skin. They are continuously alert for any strange "foreign" material and can respond instantly, releasing a cascade of chemical messengers that either provide instant response or call for additional help. The sentries that are the backbone of the innate immune system are the *toll-like receptors*, or TLRs. Each type of TLR (and there are 13 in humans) has evolved to respond to defined stimuli. Some are quite specific and respond to only one stimulus. Others respond to more than one stimulus, and sometimes two or more TLRs will respond to the *same* stimulus. The combinations are complex and beyond the discussion here, but there are some general rules to illustrate the point. Bacterial lipoproteins (what bacterial cell walls are made of) are recognized by TLR1 and TLR2. Yeast wall materials (like *Malassezia*) trigger TLR2 and TLR6, but those two are also turned on by bacterial lipoproteins (*Propionibacterium acnes* again). Some viral material turns on TLR4; other viral material does the same for TLR7, TLR8, and TLR9; but TLR9 also triggers a reaction to bacterial material as well [1]. Experimental work in acne has specifically confirmed that both TLR2 and TLR4 are activated by *P. acnes*, while TLR2 responds to *Malassezia* [2].

Once the TLR "receptor" sees a threat it recognizes, it pushes the panic button and a vast number of events take place. In general, two types of messengers are produced, cytokines (the *cell* movers) and chemokines (the *chemical* movers).

The cytokines send a message to cells, like the white blood cells called *polys* (polymorphonuclear leukocytes, or PMNLs), to come to help get rid of the invader. There is a crossover here with the adaptive immune system

Acne: Causes and Practical Management, First Edition. F. William Danby.

(see Section 7.2) because some of the cytokines will call for help from lymphocytes and others involve even more complex combinations of cells.

The chemokines cause a vast array of chemical responses, from something as simple as releasing histamine to the complex chemical cascade that causes clotting.

As a well-coordinated system, evolved over millions of years, the innate immune system does its best to identify, isolate, neutralize, and eliminate the foreign material. If the body needs more weapons than are available to the innate system alone, it has the capacity to call for further help: the body has evolved the additional ability to adapt itself to any new threat, threats for which the innate system has not evolved an instant response. This second level of defense is the adaptive immune response.

7.2 Adaptive (acquired) immunity

The second kind of immunity is called *adaptive* because it needs to learn to adapt. *Acquired immunity* is an older term, but the meaning is the same. The newly learned immune response is acquired by adapting to the new situation. It has to learn *how* to fight the invader. Adaptive immunity has to take a look at the new invader, and the mechanisms involved actually take tiny bits of it to a local lymph node. Lymph nodes are those glands that become inflamed and swollen, like those under your jaw and in your neck when you have a sore throat. Your body has lots of them scattered about, sitting quietly waiting for the adaptive immune system to bring them evidence of trouble.

Each lymph node has two possible ways of responding to these microscopic and molecular-sized pieces of foreign matter, called *antigens*. It can develop an antibody (a kind of custom-made protein that circulates in the blood to find, match up with, and neutralize invaders like viruses) or it can train certain types of specialized white blood cells called *lymphocytes* to recognize, kill, or immobilize the invader. That takes time, sometimes just a few days but often a week or more if the immune system has never "seen" this invader before. The adaptive immune system is always slower to get going than the innate system when something new shows up. Even when it has already learned (from prior exposure) what the invader is, it may take a day or two to get up to speed, but some responses are almost instant. Think about peanut or penicillin allergy, which can onset in

minutes with devastating effects. A longer delay is to be expected for some invaders if the original exposure was a long time ago. The innate system is faster because it doesn't need to process the invading materials again to figure out what the material or foreign invader is. The innate immune system already knows how to react.

Whatever the response of the immune systems, the results are always after the fact in acne. There has to be a trigger. A small population of an organism like *P. acnes* or *Malassezia* sitting quietly down in the follicular duct, out of reach of the innate and adaptive immune systems, is not by itself enough to cause acne. If it were, we would all have acne, all the time. The same is true of other things found naturally in the follicular units of the folliculopilosebaceous units (FPSUs). *Malassezia* live on all of us, as do *P. acnes* and *Demodex* and many *hundreds* (no exaggeration!) of other kinds of organisms. If the "acne bacillus" (*P. acnes*) were the real primary cause of acne vulgaris, all we would need to do is eliminate *P. acnes*. It has taken over 60 years to realize that killing *P. acnes* is not enough to clear this disease. We are just now learning that our attempts may have done more harm than good [3, 4].

7.3 Inflammation as the primary acnegen

A tremendous amount of work has been done looking at the cause of inflammation in the acnes and the mechanisms by which inflammation is produced [5]. This has led to the identification of a large number of inflammatory mediators (messengers) present in various stages and forms of the disease. These are triggered by the cytokines, the group of chemicals produced by the inflammatory cells of both immune systems. Some of these molecules are cytokines all by themselves; others trigger additional cytokine and chemokine activity. Cytokines are basically messengers, rather as hormones are messengers. Chemokines are specialized cytokines that tell specific cells, usually lymphocytes, what to do and where to go. Usually the message is that the cell is needed elsewhere to do battle, and to come quickly. But nature likes a balance, so there are other chemokines and cytokines that are inhibitory.

Questions have been raised concerning the influence of the immune system on the initiation of the process that leads to acne. Specifically, "What is the message that turns on the increase in production of the keratinocytes in the follicular unit, causing the plugging that leads to acne? Could the keratinocytes be turned on by certain cytokines, independent of the stimulatory effect of hormones?" There is a specific cytokine, interleukin 1 (IL-1), actually produced by epidermal keratinocytes that may be involved [6]. This has led Zouboulis to wonder, "Is acne vulgaris a genuine inflammatory disease?" [7]. Experimental work by Baroni showed that there is another messenger, IL-8, whose DNA shows up in cultures of *Malassezia*-infected keratinocytes and that "TLR2 mediates intracellular signaling in human keratinocytes in response to Malassezia furfur" [2]. Watanabe showed that "Malassezia stimulates cytokine production by keratinocytes, the cytokine production needs the presence of Malassezia, and there are differences in ability to induce cytokine production by human keratinocytes among Malassezia yeasts" [8].

So there is evidence of interleukins lurking in the keratinocytes' neighborhood. But some of the keratinocytes examined were surface epidermis dwellers, not ductal keratinocytes, and there may be a difference. Why are these messengers present? Are they not just doing what they are supposed to be doing, responding to *Malassezia* in the follicular duct when the *Malassezia* is recognized by the TLR? Do they actually have the ability on their own to start the ductal keratinocytes growing? My personal sense is that, if that were the case, there would be acne everywhere, in everybody, throughout our lives. Fortunately, true acne seems to occur only in those FPSUs primed by hormones, usually of exogenous origin but sometimes because of an abnormal and excessive endogenous source. Suggesting that the presence of inflammatory mediators like IL-1 means there is preexisting inflammation is like suggesting that the presence of white blood cells in the blood means there is septicemia.

The gentlemanly argument pitting the hormone-driven theorists against the inflammation-driven theorists may now be solvable because there now seems to be a pathway, mediated by hypoxia-inducible factor 1 (HIF-1), that stimulates *both* ductal keratinization and inflammation. The hypothesis is that the hypoxia is caused by excessive intraductal pressure, induced in turn by excessive keratinocyte production, which is turned on by components of the Western diet [9]. HIF-1 appears to be able to induce "hyperproliferation and incomplete differentiation of epidermal keratinocytes" [10]. It is also "a major regulator of cellular adaptation

to low oxygen stress" and "plays an important role in cytokine production by keratinocytes and in neutrophil recruitment to the skin" [11]. Thus, it may mediate the overgrowth to bursting, and recruit inflammatory cells to migrate to the area, both in response to the anoxic stress.

There is no doubt that the interleukins are there. We know that their list of post-inflammatory responsibilities includes the stimulation of keratinocyte multiplication needed to repair a damaged area [12, 13]. In the *normal* course of events, in a process such as repair, the activity is regulated so it shuts down when the repair is accomplished. The acnes, to the contrary, are characterized by the *failure to shut down* ductal keratinization even when far too many ductal keratinocytes are produced. This failure to shut down is not a normal process; indeed, it is an abnormal process that lies at the base of comedogenesis. It is most likely triggered by a pathogenic change or chain of events under the influence of an extraneous factor for which evolution has left the follicular duct unprepared. Diet is the key that fits.

7.4 Mediators, cellular and humoral, and neuroimmunology

The number of mediators, the chemicals that effect change and that have been identified in active lesions in the acnes, is vast. This is to be expected, because this is an inflammatory reaction that can be exceptionally "brisk," given the numerous antigens presented to the dermis by the ruptured follicle. They induce all the classic signs of inflammation: *rubor* (redness or erythema), *calor* (heat), *dolor* (pain), *tumor* (swelling), and *functio laesa* (loss of function). The range of activity in each area is wide. In the *pain* category, for example, mild itch occurs at one end of the spectrum [14] (presumably caused by histamine release in response to *Malassezia*), and intense pain is possible at the other end (presumably caused by substance P in response to the deep inflammation and swelling of acne inversa). The search for individual molecules that might be suitable targets for novel medications has led to a whole library of these mediators and effectors.

But one point needs to be made here, and that is that these are, all of them, secondary (and tertiary and quaternary) reactions. They all occur downstream from the main problem. They are all *epiphenomena*, events that follow upon the primary phenomenon, the plugging of the pore. Although neutralizing, counteracting, or even (in the case of inflammation inhibitors) mimicking them may be of assistance, the prime therapy needed in acne is the development of a protocol that will shut down the development of new lesions and allow the old ones to heal up as swiftly as possible.

7.5 Allergy (shared antigens)

Patients have for decades worried about the question of acne being due to an "allergy" to milk. For years I have dismissed the possibility that the adaptive immune system was actively involved in the actual pathogenesis of acne, but now I'm beginning to wonder. There are a few reasons that have made me reconsider. Just as there are those who are adamant that chocolate breaks them out, there are those who have bought into the link to dairy but whose stories are just not what one would expect. In particular, the story I hear over and over is "I was fine until last week when I ate or drank [whatever; dairy of some sort or other] and the next morning I was a mess." Then there is the reverse story (a recurring theme on the Internet sites I monitor): "I stopped all my dairy after listening to you guys (or gals). I'm two weeks into my new diet and my skin is almost clear!"

What is going on here? Could this disorder be partly mediated by a true allergy to milk components? Would acne lesions present and resolve in such a time frame if this is, partially at least, an allergic reaction? I think that the answer in both cases is "Yes." There is at present no proof, and Internet searches are unrevealing, but let's think about this. We know that babies can be allergic to something in cow milk, while allergy to mother's milk is *almost* unheard of. We know these quick-onset lesions are not lactose intolerance and they onset too fast to be due to hormones. Fats are not great allergens, so it is likely that the proteins in milk are to blame. In testing regular cow milk allergy, immunoglobulin E directed at casein (specifically, alpha S1-casein) and directed at whole milk is higher in patients than controls. Alpha-lactalbumin and beta-lactoglobulin both produce skin prick reactivity [15]. At the moment, all the allergenic proteins have not been identified, but it appears that some of these presumptive allergenic proteins survive the digestive process often enough and long enough to make trouble [16]. And that brings us to the question of

what these proteins actually are. The challenge is that proteomics allows us to identify thousands of different proteins in milk. Sorting out the allergens from the innocent bystanders will take a few years.

At this point in the discussion, it is important to note that the proteins in milk are all produced by mammary glands. These proteins are partly specifically formulated as food for the nursing infant, whether human or bovine, but some have a structural source. Remember that the mammary gland is a modified apocrine gland, and that means a very specific event, decapitation secretion, is part of the milk production process. The top of the milk-producing cell actually comes off and is shed into the milk. That in turn means that proteinaceous material that starts out as the cellular wall and roof of every lactiferous cell winds up in the milk as small and quite possibly allergenic fragments. On the list of work that needs to be done, we should attempt to identify these fragments in unprocessed milk and see if they are particularly antigenic. This work must be done on raw milk prior to homogenization. The high-pressure process of homogenization consists of forcing milk through small holes in stainless-steel plates or valves to break up the remaining fat globules either before (for whole homogenized milk) or after separation of most of the cream (for low-fat or skim milk). It may also "homogenize" the bits of lactiferous cell wall that are still present in the milk. We need to know what effect that has on the possible allergenicity (less or more) of the protein or lipoprotein.

In any event, I no longer discount these stories of swift exacerbation and quick resolution. I suspect patients are telling us a story worth listening to, even if we are not certain why. There certainly seems to be, in some patients, a relationship to the local folliculopapular and folliculopustular inflammatory response.

7.6 Inflammation, pigment, and PIH

One of the most difficult parts of acne to treat is the hyperpigmentation (increased color) due to inflammation. Usually abbreviated to PIH (for *post-inflammatory hyperpigmentation*), it is remarkably long lasting for many patients, and the darker the patient's skin color, the more difficult the problem is. This temporary discoloration is referred to as "scarring" in some communities.

The cause of the color is simply the impact of the inflammation on the melanocytes that give the skin color. More inflammation=more melanocytic irritation=more color. The vast cultural mythology in the background, the wish to try "bleaching agents," the cultural *pressure* to try bleaching agents, the lack of safe and effective bleaching agents, the wish to try steroids to calm the inflammation, and the need to avoid excessive sun exposure: all of these are tripwires in a therapeutic minefield. This is especially true when counseling darker patients of color. (See Section 8.5.7.)

7.7 Inflammation and scarring

One of the challenges in managing scars is that what some people *call* scars are not real scars. The dark marks that comprise PIH (Section 7.6) in darker skins are not scars, nor are the reddish marks that are their equivalent in fair skin. They are *healing areas*. They will fade with time, and time is the absolute best healer. The redness that shows through in light skin is an indication that Mother Nature has dilated the local blood vessels and is at work cleaning up the mess. The same thing shows up as temporary darkness in darker skins. Picking, squeezing, rubbing, getting facials, and using irritating bleaching creams—all will make the problem last longer. This is where patients need patience, for weeks or months. It is essential to avoid the cycle of color → color reduction methods → irritation → more color → more color reduction methods → and around we go again. It is a vicious (and expensive) cycle.

Real scars come in several varieties, and the easiest to treat are the fresh ones. Indeed, one of the most important parts of scar therapy is scar prevention, even before the fresh scars are present. That means aggressive acne prevention, aggressive but thoughtful care, and an early start, especially if there is a family or personal history of bad scars. Isotretinoin should be used if at all possible. While its use does not guarantee that *no* scars will form, it helps to get the patient over the inflammatory phase of therapy as quickly as possible. It should be combined with cortisone injections. These can be done every couple of weeks, directly into the thick areas, and can do wonders to smooth things out. These injections do not always yield perfect results either, and they are no fun for the patient, but they are usually worth the discomfort. There is only one way to

see if they work for your patient—try it. The patient is often surprised to find how tolerable they are. They are especially valuable as scar prevention in the early inflammatory nodular phase. Success is marked by the request for more at the next visit. I have seen little else that works as consistently and is so worth the money. On the other hand, remember that treating a simple area of PIH with some of the cosmetic methods may take six months and hundreds of dollars, whereas leaving it to heal by itself may also take half a year but is free.

For thick established scars, it is important to realize that there are two types, hypertrophic scars and real keloids. The word *keloid* comes from the Greek word for *claw*, describing the claw-like extensions out beyond the original location of the damage. They are relatively unusual except following burns. The normal scars that one sees in acne are raised bumps where the acne nodule used to be, and they are contained within the site of the original injury. They have no "claws" but are heaped up vertically. (See Figure 0.18.) They are properly called *hypertrophic scars*. They are not keloids, but are almost as difficult to treat. Most dermatologists use straight intralesional triamcinolone, occasionally working up from 10 to 40 mg/mL in very strictly limited volumes. The injections must be made *into* the scar, not through the scar into the underlying tissue. Some use custom mixtures containing methotrexate or 5-fluorouracil. Another technique is to shave off the scar flush with the skin (under local anesthesia) to flatten it out, and then stop bleeding with ferric chloride or aluminum chloride. After a day or two, imiquimod 5% cream is then applied twice daily in a very thin film for six weeks or so during healing to prevent regrowth.

And then the emphasis goes right back to prevention again. If the patient wants to avoid inflammation, including scarring, he or she must avoid further plugging of the pores. No mystery there. Control those hormones with diet and birth control pills as appropriate, or the FPSUs will be back in trouble again.

References

1 McInturff JE, Kim J. The role of toll-like receptors in the pathophysiology of acne. Semin Cutan Med Surg 2005 Jun;24(2):73–8.

2 Baroni A, Orlando M, Donnarumma G, Farro P, Iovene MR, Tufano MA, *et al.* Toll-like receptor 2 (TLR2) mediates

intracellular signalling in human keratinocytes in response to *Malassezia furfur*. Arch Dermatol Res 2006 Jan;297(7): 280–8.

3 Leyden JJ. Antibiotic resistance in the topical treatment of acne vulgaris. Cutis 2004 Jun;73(6 Suppl):6–10.

4 Williams HC, Dellavalle RP, Garner S. Acne vulgaris. Lancet 2012 Jan 28;379(9813):361–72.

5 Kurokawa I, Danby FW, Ju Q, Wang X, Xiang LF, Xia L, *et al.* New developments in our understanding of acne pathogenesis and treatment. Exp Dermatol 2009 Oct;18(10):821–32.

6 Jeremy AH, Holland DB, Roberts SG, Thomson KF, Cunliffe WJ. Inflammatory events are involved in acne lesion initiation. J Invest Dermatol 2003 Jul;121(1):20–7.

7 Zouboulis CC. Is acne vulgaris a genuine inflammatory disease? Dermatology 2001;203(4):277–9.

8 Watanabe S, Kano R, Sato H, Nakamura Y, Hasegawa A. The effects of *Malassezia* yeasts on cytokine production by human keratinocytes. J Invest Dermatol 2001 May;116(5):769–73.

9 Danby FW. Ductal hypoxia in acne: is it the missing link between comedogenesis and inflammation? J Am Acad Dermatol 2014 May;70(5):948–9.

10 Kim SH, Kim S, Choi HI, Choi YJ, Lee YS, Sohn KC, *et al.* Callus formation is associated with hyperproliferation and incomplete differentiation of keratinocytes, and increased expression of adhesion molecules. Br J Dermatol 2010 Sep;163(3):495–501.

11 Leire E, Olson J, Isaacs H, Nizet V, Hollands A. Role of hypoxia inducible factor-1 in keratinocyte inflammatory response and neutrophil recruitment. J Inflamm (Lond) 2013;10(1):28.

12 Lai Y, Li D, Li C, Muehleisen B, Radek KA, Park HJ, *et al.* The antimicrobial protein REG3A regulates keratinocyte proliferation and differentiation after skin injury. Immunity 2012 Jul 27;37(1):74–84.

13 Roupe KM, Nybo M, Sjobring U, Alberius P, Schmidtchen A, Sorensen OE. Injury is a major inducer of epidermal innate immune responses during wound healing. J Invest Dermatol 2010 Apr;130(4):1167–77.

14 Davidson S, Giesler GJ. The multiple pathways for itch and their interactions with pain. Trends Neurosci 2010 Dec;33(12):550–8.

15 Lam HY, van HE, Michelsen A, Guikers K, van der Tas CH, Bruijnzeel-Koomen CA, *et al.* Cow's milk allergy in adults is rare but severe: both casein and whey proteins are involved. Clin Exp Allergy 2008 Jun;38(6):995–1002.

16 Lonnerdal B. Human milk proteins: key components for the biological activity of human milk. Adv Exp Med Biol 2004;554:11–25.

CHAPTER 8
Management

The vast body of writing on the three acnes has been heavy weighted toward medical and surgical management until the past 15 years. Gradually, the mechanisms of formation of the acnes are becoming understood, and that in turn is allowing us to look toward prevention, in the hope of avoiding the expense and side effects of the traditional lines of attack.

8.1 Prevention

The management of any disorder should start with prevention, and that should look at *all* preventable aspects of *all* the causes of the disease. The classical approach is to discuss primary, secondary, and tertiary prevention. Quaternary prevention has been added, as have universal, selective, and indicated prevention. Even further, *environmental* prevention is worth considering.

Primary	To avoid occurrence of the disease. This can be done on a universal, selective, or indicated population.
Secondary	To diagnose and treat early to prevent significant marking and both physical and psychological scarring.
Tertiary	To treat to reduce existing scarring, post-inflammatory hyperpigmentation, and psychological trauma.
Quaternary	To avoid unnecessary or excessive healthcare interventions.
Universal	This involves the whole population.
Selective	This involves the population at risk, those with a personal or family acne history.
Indicated	This identifies populations at risk, aiming at early identification.
Environmental	Regulated avoidance of an identified cause of the disorder.

Looking at this chart as it applies to acne, it is apparent that accepting diet as the prime cause of acne in the majority of cases means we have a lot of work to do. The evidence that diet is indeed the prime modifiable cause of acne has accumulated steadily over the past decade (Figure 2.16). The recent review by Melnik [1], discussed in this section, illustrates the mechanisms involved with a precision never achieved before (Figure 2.15).

Universal primary prevention would be the ideal way to eliminate acne. That would involve the entire population stopping dairy and high-glycemic-index foods. It is an impossibly impractical undertaking in a free and unregulated society because "regulated avoidance" is not a viable option. Universal voluntary avoidance is also likely a pipe dream—unless the idea and its implementation suddenly "go viral." That means that public education, where possible, and gradual recruitment patient by patient (and physician by physician) will remain the prime methods of prevention for now.

For practical clinical purposes, it is sufficient to discontinue all dairy products that are provided in bulk or used as a major portion of a food. That means no milk or cream of any sort, no butter, cheese, cream cheese, yogurt, ice cream, cottage cheese, sour cream, raw milk, pasteurized milk, goat milk, or indeed anything that comes "from the south end of the cow", or from any other mammal for that matter. Derivatives of dairy products are also eliminated. This particularly includes any of the protein products that contain whey or casein, which have been documented increasingly [2] but noted

Acne: Causes and Practical Management, First Edition. F. William Danby.
© 2015 John Wiley & Sons, Ltd. Published 2015 by John Wiley & Sons, Ltd.

clinically to be a problem around the world. Unfortunately, we are not sure exactly what hormones and growth factors are present in these derivatives, but the whey alone seems to be a sufficient threat. These protein sources are commonly used by bodybuilders and in weight training. The question arises, given the involvement of this hormone-infiltrated industry, whether these supplements are adulterated with steroids. At the moment, there is no published material touching on the hormone content of these materials, so this comment is speculative. There are no publicly available assays; indeed, even the US Food and Drug Administration has not studied the existence and quantities of hormones in dairy products, nor was there any plan to do so as of the FDA response to me July 2012 [3].

Besides diet, there is little one can do as primary prevention to avoid the acnes. Genetics play a well-defined role but choosing new parents is not an option. We note the close relationship between the rise in insulin-like growth factor 1 (IGF-1) during the teens and the incidence of acne [4], but stopping puberty to control one's elevated level of IGF-1 is likewise not an option, because that would mean stopping normal growth and development as well as stopping acne vulgaris.

Total avoidance of the sun to prevent acne rosacea by minimizing the risk of sun damage to blood vessels and the collagenous support tissues of the folliculopilosebaceous unit (FPSU) during one's entire early life is likewise unlikely to happen. Although the concept of *pre-rosacea* has been suggested, rosy cheeks are not generally considered a *pre-disease state*, even though this may actually be the case for patients with actinic telangiectasia and with true acne rosacea. On the other hand, careful sun avoidance and the use of effective sunscreens or sun blocks makes the use of vitamin D3 supplements mandatory to avoid the numerous adverse effects of vitamin D3 deprivation.

Sunscreens and sun blocks are of two basic types, absorptive and reflective. The chemical para-amino benzoic acid (PABA) was used in the earliest absorptive sunscreens that achieved general use in the 1970s. Its disadvantages were several and it is rarely used now, but one major problem with PABA is still with us today. Because PABA's capacity to protect against ultraviolet B's (UVB) burning rays minimized sunburn, the public was led to believe that stopping the burn from the sun would stop the damage from the sun. That misconception has allowed a couple of generations to stay out in the sun longer than unprotected exposure would have allowed. We were robbed of our warning system (the redness and sensation of burning from UVB) and so we were able to remain too long in the sun. That extra exposure allowed us to accumulate far too much of the UVA that slipped right past the UVB blockade. In Europe, as early as the 1970s, broad-spectrum chemical sunscreens were available. The best sun protection products are still available there, while the products in the United States play catch-up. New FDA guidelines insist on documented adequate protection up to 370 nm to earn the *broad-spectrum* label, and that should clear the playing field of the deceptive labels on many sunscreens.

The classic zinc oxide paste used on the 1955 beach lifeguard's nose provided superb reflective protection but was an aesthetic joke. It has been improved upon over the years and now we have zinc oxide, titanium dioxide, and mineral pigments like ferric oxide that have been developed to provide newer physical blocks that are much more socially acceptable. They also provide the broad- to full-spectrum protection the general public thought it had enjoyed for the last 40 years or so. Gradually, over the past decade, these products have shown slow but steady acceptance by the public. Addition of silicone derivatives to several of these products has minimized the irritating features that made many products unacceptable to patients with combined acne rosacea and actinic telangiectasia [5].

Stopping smoking is always wise. The only better idea is to not start in the first place. Smoking's likely influence in adult-onset acne [6], and particularly its influence in acne inversa/hidradenitis suppurativa (AI/HS) [7, 8], emphasizes the need to avoid not only smoking but all sources of nicotine. The challenge of stopping smoking without nicotine substitution is significant, but using nicotine substitutes just prolongs the problem.

The only other general preventive advice that would be worth offering, particularly with regard to universal prevention, would be universal maintenance of ideal weight. Saving $3 billion per year in the United States on acne care would be a drop in the bucket compared to the savings achievable throughout the entire health care industry if maintenance of a normal-range Body Mass Index (BMI) or ideal weight became a national pastime. Certainly this would impact on many cases of AI/HS as well as the incomes of bariatric surgeons.

That leaves us with diet as the single most effective means of preventing acne vulgaris and AI/HS, and sun avoidance as the major means of avoiding acne rosacea. Diet is discussed in Section 8.3 in much greater depth.

8.2 General principles of management

Because almost all of my patients are referred, they and their referring physicians are expecting my best efforts to clear them as quickly as possible. They are not referred by their primary care physicians to serve as experimental subjects. This means that my observations, not being part of a randomized clinical trial (RCT), will never rise to the level of evidence of such formal work, so they cannot be considered EBM (evidence-based medicine). This allows me freedom to customize treatments, learning as I go, and my patient and I can explore therapy "outside the box" to the best of our combined abilities. This flexibility is essential to comprehensive management, but systematically reporting on such nonstandardized treatment courses is problematic. One winds up with broad impressions, a personal practice pattern, and what I call XBM (or *experienced-based medicine*). The advantage of this method of practice is that it is truly patient oriented—and the newest term is *patient driven*. Every patient gets a customized approach. The disadvantage (if it really *is* a disadvantage) is the simple fact that XBM cannot be plugged into a drop-down menu or treatment template. It takes thought, and experience, to guide one's patients through the complexities of acne.

The encumbrances and hurdles set up by restrictive guidelines (even those that claim to be nonrestrictive), "preferred drug" lists (which actually are the opposite of *preferred*), restrictions on use of drugs for non-FDA-approved indications, limited and self-serving formularies, "branded" but still expensive generics, highly inefficient government-level dictates such as iPLEDGE, and the imposition of "step therapy" that disallows the proper treatment until the improper treatment has been proven to fail—all these meddlesome economic barriers tend to produce a counterproductive and anti-intellectual practice environment. It is really quite wonderful to see clinical trials showing up from other countries where the legal system has not developed a pervasive, extensive, and expensive stranglehold on research productivity. Their work is much appreciated.

The other side of the problem with referred patients is that they have usually been previously treated. Not only does this create numerous variables not of my (or my patients') making, but also the patients or their parents have often invested significant money in therapy, often failed therapy. I usually take advantage of that fact to have them continue to use, when reasonable, the therapy from the past. Doing so helps maintain their relationship with their primary care providers (even though some doubts sometimes remain), and helps to retain or even build confidence in that physician, when possible, to encourage the patient to return eventually to primary care. As a former general practitioner, I am sensitive to the need to minimize criticism of prior attempts to treat. Inexplicable failures? Nothing ever works 100%. Unscientific successes? Never argue with success. Why didn't my other doctor (or dermatologist) know (or do) that? We all have different training and experience paths. And so on …

If the patient is having significant symptoms, or they are distressed, I press forward with the most aggressive therapy possible but insist that patients adopt a full zero-dairy and low-glycemic-load diet from the beginning, no matter which of the acnes is present. There are two reasons. The first is that prevention must start as soon as possible, and the first visit is the best time for a full review of causes and consequences. Secondly, prevention of new lesions takes time, so the earlier the start, the earlier the clearing.

When patients are actually in trouble, they tend to remember better what is necessary to prevent the acne from coming back. Nevertheless, constant reminding is wise. It sometimes borders on nagging. I tell them I know that I'm nagging. I tell them I get paid to nag, that it is part of my job, but they can get it for free from their parents if they prefer.

8.3 Diet

There are three reasons to modify diet in managing acne vulgaris. The first is to lower insulin levels, the second is to lower levels of IGF-1, and third is to avoid the steroid and polypeptide hormones and the growth factors that are present in dairy products. High-glycemic-load diets impact on only one of these three factors—they open the androgen receptor by perpetuating chronically high insulin levels.

But dairy impacts on all three promoters of androgen empowerment.

8.3.1 Dairy

Restricting dairy intake has a profound effect on acne vulgaris. This is usually more obvious in teenage boys than teenage girls. The girls have the disadvantage of cyclical menstrual hormones that confuse the picture, and they seem to be more impacted by stress than most boys. This is not to say that simply stopping all dairy clears all acne within a couple weeks. It does not. It takes months. The patient needs to know this right up front. While it is possible to clear acne with nothing but dairy restriction, I have encountered only a few patients over the years who had the patience to follow that course. The most memorable are described elsewhere in this book. The low-glycemic-load (low-carbohydrate-load) diet should be introduced early as well.

This restrictive diet is best maintained for a full six months. During that time, with or without isotretinoin, one can usually clear acne almost 100%. There may be some scarring or post-inflammatory hyperpigmentation (PIH), and perhaps a few residual lesions, but the war is pretty much won by six months. After six months, or after the patient is clear, more liberal dietary choices may be offered. The better choice would be to continue the restricted diet, and generally this is a wise lifelong choice. Alternatively, the patient can begin slowly liberalizing the diet. I generally discourage them from going back to the fluid milk. That includes not using it on breakfast cereal. There are many alternatives: milk substitutes made from soy, rice, almonds, coconut, and hemp. One can find, on the Internet, ways of making one's own "milk" from nuts by using a blender. As far as cheese is concerned, the less the better, and zero is best. But to keep the patient "on side," I permit the occasional nibble of small amounts of whatever dairy they particularly miss. There is a large population of cheese lovers among acne vulgaris patients and hidradenitis suppurativa patients, and they are some of my most recalcitrant patients. They tell me they are "addicted to cheese." I tell them they can have one ounce of cheese per week, or that they may have a taste on occasion, but they must no longer consider cheese to be a food. It is just an occasional "taste treat."

It is interesting that, in the Harvard study, pizza did not show up as a risk factor [9]. On a speculative basis, I suggest to my patients that it may be that the high temperatures in the pizza ovens (750° F average and up to 900° for some cooks) will almost certainly cook and therefore destroy the activity of (denature) the polypeptide hormones and growth factors. Having said that, I have no proof whatsoever that this is true. The reproductive hormones, the steroids, have significant resistance to high temperatures and are likely not destroyed, but this also needs investigation. Unfortunately, this lack of data on hormone content is almost universal.

I have looked into the costs of defining all the different hormones in all different types of dairy products from all the different breeds of cows, on many varied fodders, prepared as raw milk, organic milk, and pasteurized or unpasteurized milk; soft or hard and cream or cottage cheeses; yogurts (Greek or not); and other derivatives. It would take years, and several millions of dollars. The dairy industry does not seem interested; nor, as I have learned, does the US Food and Drug Administration (FDA). For now, a blanket avoidance rule is the safest approach, much like the FDA's approach to contaminated food. The recall is general, and does not require the testing of each sample before excluding it from the diet.

That brings up one of the major objections I hear every day—is it safe to NOT drink milk? The fact is that there are hundreds of millions of individuals who grow up quite healthy in this world without milk. It simply is not part of their diet for reasons of economics, geography, religion, custom, or choice. There are millions who are allergic to it and fully 65% of the entire world population is lactose intolerant and generally avoids the volume of fluid milk consumed here in the United States. Although estimates vary, 85–95% of African-Americans are lactose intolerant, as are almost 100% of Asians. Both groups are quite capable of developing serious acne when exposed to a Westernized diet. AI/HS in particular is a major problem when it occurs in African-Americans.

Then there is the question of "organic milk." Even the definition of *organic milk* leads to confusion. For a specific group of organic-conscious American consumers, this means milk produced without injecting the cow with recombinant bovine growth hormone (rBGH or rbGH), also called bovine somatotropin (BST). In some areas milk from such non-injected cows has been marketed as "hormone-free milk," a concept that advertises ignorance of the facts more than anything else. Monsanto's Posilac® injection, which is illegal in Canada and Europe (and too expensive for most of the rest of the world), is fading away, unmourned by most, thanks in particular to the marketing power of several major grocery retailers who in 2008 refused to sell milk and milk derivatives produced this way. I thank them, and so do the cows.

And, just to be perfectly clear, there is no such thing as hormone-free milk. Actually, milk could be legitimately considered a specialized, highly evolved, and species-specific hormone delivery system that happens also to have the fats, proteins, and carbohydrates needed to do the hormones' bidding [10].

For other consumers, *organic* means a generally more expensive product that has been produced with extra care by cows that are fed healthy, natural diets and are exposed to no unapproved pesticides, herbicides, fungicides, or antibiotics. It also means no exposure to the fodder that had in the past been formulated by recycling pieces of cows that had already gone to market, as ground-up bits of protein. That was the problem with "mad cow disease" (bovine spongiform encephalopathy). While such fodder was in a strict sense "organic," it was a far cry from the sense intended.

To the farmer, *organic* means extra expense, greater care, and adherence in the United States to a list of permissible chemicals published in the Federal Register. In the United States, the National Organic Program sets the standards at http://www.ams.usda.gov/nop. In Europe, extensive Council Regulations are in place. Straying beyond those guidelines means loss of the organic certification for the farm and an expensive few years of waiting to have the farm recertified. Interestingly, organic milk in the United States has been shown to have higher levels of estrogen and progesterone—evidence of healthier animals, we presume [11]. This is not a positive selling point when dealing with a set of disorders like the acnes that are postulated to be made worse by these same hormones.

The next most common concern I hear from parents is that their offspring will not get enough calcium if they don't drink their milk. It is worth pointing out that human beings are the only species who believe they must rely on dairy products for calcium. Cows have huge bones, they never take calcium supplements, they eat mostly grass, and they never drink milk after they are weaned.

There is also a widespread belief that the major source of vitamin D3 should be from milk. The fact of the matter is that milk contains very little natural vitamin D3. Calves get their vitamin D3 from the sun. For generations,

vitamin D3 has been added to milk one way or another during the manufacturing (dairying) process as a public health measure to minimize the risk of rickets. The only reason why humans need to take vitamin D supplements is that they do not spend their days standing in the sun in a pasture without clothing, having their own vitamin D made by the action of sun on the cholesterol in their skin. We dermatologists are forever cautioning patients to avoid excessive sun and to use sunscreens, so we bear some responsibility for the fact that the population in general is low on vitamin D3. The major responsibility for low levels of 25-hydroxy vitamin D3, however, must be borne by our weather, our clothing, and our indoor lifestyle. Just as we use iodized salt to provide an appropriate level of iodine in our diets, we really do need adequate daily supplements of vitamin D3.

Thus, it is entirely responsible and wise to recommend and take vitamin D3 supplements. The question arises "How much?" Although the highly respected US Institute of Medicine (IOM) has placed an upper limit of safety at 2000 international units (IU) of vitamin D daily, the real experts in the field are comfortable with doses well in excess of that number; indeed, an informal 2009 survey of such experts' own consumption came up with "an average of 5,000 IU" daily [12].

Why the discrepancy? The IOM is composed of a broad range of experts chosen from the tops of many fields, but they are *not* experts in vitamin D3 metabolism. That means they relied on a vast number of scientific papers, some reaching back decades to the days when the only known value of vitamin D was to provide the small amount needed to prevent rickets. They were basically looking for data to support their eventual published opinion. Unfortunately, no large population studies have been done, using the higher doses recommended by the real experts, to demonstrate the benefits that active vitamin D researchers are now learning about. For instance, it is standard to recommend both calcium and vitamin D, combined, to treat osteoporosis. This is despite there being no large study, of adequate length, of osteoporosis, whether for prevention or therapy, in which fully adequate doses of Vitamin D have been provided in the range of 2000–5000 IU per day *without* supplemental calcium. Lacking such studies, the IOM experts simply could not recommend the higher doses. Their understandably obsessive "evidence-based medicine" criteria were fulfilled only for what many now consider suboptimal doses.

Their view was crystal clear but it was, of necessity, a look in the rear-view mirror.

Two points on closing. Note that Vitamin D3 is a fat-soluble vitamin and should be taken with food, preferably fatty food, to assist and permit full absorption. And note that vitamin D2 is far less effective than vitamin D3 [13]. The only reason that weekly capsules of 50,000 IU of vitamin D2 are used seems to be that it is the only *prescription* preparation of vitamin D available, so it may be covered by insurance plans and it also offers prescribers a sense of control over the dose. I would be happy to see vitamin D2 disappear, taking with it the confusion it causes.

Calcium supplements are another story, because taking extra calcium at the same time as vitamin D supplementation can cause hypercalcemia (a high level of calcium in the blood), hypercalciuria (excess calcium in the urine), and kidney stones [14]. To look at this from a physiological point of view, vitamin D supplementation restores to normal what would be normally obtained by sun exposure if modern clothing, housing, sun protection, and geographic location did not interfere with this natural process. Calcium supplementation, on the other hand, corrects no such deficiency or physiological process. I can find no evidence that taking calcium supplements alone (without vitamin D supplementation) improves bone mineralization. There is no doubt, however, that ensuring that normal blood and therefore tissue levels of vitamin D are maintained is the most physiological means of enabling the body to absorb the correct amount of calcium from food.

A year's supply of this very inexpensive vitamin costs less than the single blood test needed to determine your personal blood level of 25-hydroxy vitamin D3; it requires no visit to the physician and no needle stick at the lab, and the risk of side effects from hypervitaminosis D at this dose is essentially nil (as long as you stay away from calcium supplements).

8.3.1.1 The deli-planning heiress

Ms. Bleu came to me with extensive nodular acne that involved her lower face, jawline, and upper neck literally from ear to ear.

A few years previously she had inherited some money and after college, she decided that she would like to open a restaurant on the very small Atlantic coast of New Hampshire. She wanted to understand the whole operation and decided to spend her inheritance on

further education. She headed to France and spent 2 years in a famous cooking school. Finishing that, and having seen how restaurants are run in France and elsewhere in Europe, she decided that it would be good to have a delicatessen associated with the restaurant. She travelled all over Europe learning everything she could about the products she planned to sell.

During history taking at her first visit, I was discussing her diet over the past couple of years and of course she had a very broad experience of a wide range of fabulous foods. When I asked about dairy, she almost exploded, "Oh, my God, it's the cheese!" She had specifically concentrated in the previous several months on sampling the "best of the best" cheeses in Holland, Denmark, France, Belgium, Germany, Italy, and Switzerland. She had never had acne as a teen but it was during the cheese-sampling months that her acne developed and blossomed.

She was a certain candidate for Accutane, but for two problems. She was uninsured and didn't have any money left, and she didn't want (or need) to go on birth control pills (BCPs). Her acne had set her social life aside.

Perfect!

I explained that she was exactly the case I was looking for—someone I could treat with diet alone, who was mature enough to adhere to dietary rules, had dairy-induced acne, and would be willing to try management with no medications. As a bonus, she was an accomplished and willing professional chef who could design her own diet with care and taste.

We agreed to meet at three-month intervals. No charge. She was essentially 60–70% improved by three months and 95% clear by six months, with no medications whatsoever.

Patients like Ms. Bleu are hard to find, and even harder to convince to manage their acne with diet alone. But when they follow the rules, the rewards are self-evident.

The purists will of course insist that only by returning to the dairy, and having the acne return and then disappear again on withdrawal, can one "prove" the relationship. I'm a pretty good salesman, but I have been unsuccessful in selling that approach to patients who have just escaped from the grip of years of acne. They don't want to go back and, to my mind, it borders on the unethical to suggest that they should take the risk of further recurrences.

But there is no doubt in my mind, or Ms. Bleu's, that simple withdrawal of all dairy works wonders.

Lesson learned: Freedom from acne as a teen is no guarantee of freedom from acne when exposed to a heavy dairy diet.

8.3.1.2 The pharmaceutical executive

Much of the content of this book has been shared over the years in various venues from Jaipur, India, to Copenhagen, Denmark, and from Cuzco, Peru, to Whistler, Canada. As it has evolved, I've regularly presented the story at Focus sessions at annual meetings of the American Academy of Dermatology.

While most lectures are a concentrated one-way delivery of information to the audience, I sometimes learn fascinating things during the informal question period that follows when the presentation is over.

After one session a few years ago, a pharmaceutical executive volunteered a story that made me just shake my head in amazement. He was never a patient of mine, but I had known him for years, and his career and company has impacted on millions of acne sufferers.

I had been talking about the relationship of milk to acne, and he related the following:

"My brother and I and some friends used to play basketball two or three nights every week for a couple of years during our teens. We played hard and were pretty tired and sweaty after every session, and I remember I would always down almost a quart of milk after the game. Listening to you, I realized that I had really bad acne during those years but when I went to college and the basketball and the milk stopped, my acne cleared up. I never connected the two until now."

This man is a very senior executive, highly respected in the industry, and has built and grown a huge multinational drug company, with his core products being an anti-acne line of topical preparations. My colleagues would likely recognize both his company and his product line.

What would his life have been like if he had made the connection between his milk intake and his acne 50 years ago? We can only wonder.

Lesson learned: You are never too old to make the connection between milk and acne.

8.3.2 Carbohydrates, glycemic load, and hyperinsulinemia

The word *glycemic* simply refers to sugar, specifically glucose, in blood (*heme*). If the level of glucose in blood is high, that is hyperglycemia. A high-glycemic-load diet is one that causes higher elevations in blood glucose than a low-glycemic-load diet. Hyperglycemia leads to a compensating elevation in blood insulin levels, which forces the blood glucose levels back down toward normal. If the levels go too low, that is hypoglycemia, low blood sugar, and you get hungry. The tendency is to eat at that point, to increase the level of sugar in your blood, and then you are no longer hungry. The result is that there is a constant attempt by your body to control the level of sugar in your blood by trying to control the amount and the timing of insulin produced by and then released from your pancreas into your blood.

All diets contain elements from various food groups and types. In general, the foods that cause high-glycemic-index ratings are those that contain highly refined carbohydrates such as the sugar refined from sugarcane and the fine white flour refined from wheat. All will push sugar up in the blood quickly, causing insulin to be released. This elevated insulin level (hyperinsulinemia) is one of the two factors that open the androgen receptor, allowing it to accept androgenic molecules like testosterone (T) and dihydrotestosterone (DHT). They stimulate growth in tissues that are dependent on androgen signaling. This is one of the major links between diet and acne.

Quite unexpectedly, it has been shown that another cause of hyperinsulinemia is the ingestion of milk itself [15, 16]. We knew that the lactose in milk (a mixture of glucose and galactose) raised blood glucose, but the effect on insulin levels in the blood of drinking whole milk is independent of this sugar. It is also about four times as powerful. This hyperinsulinemic reaction is caused by a small polypeptide called *glucose-dependent insulinotropic polypeptide* (GIP) and appears to be "purpose-built." Whey proteins in milk are the most potent inducers of GIP, which is secreted by the baby's entero-endocrine K cells. GIP, working together with essential amino acids from hydrolyzed whey protein, stimulates insulin secretion by the baby's pancreatic beta cells [17].

The reason for this reaction is actually quite simple, and is quite natural at this stage of life. Milk is designed as a hormone-signaling messenger to be consumed in the early stages of life. At that point, it is essential to activate the androgen receptor so that the powerful anabolic (growth-enhancing) effect of milk on infant growth and development can be fully expressed. That is, after all, why babies drink milk. It is designed to make them grow. So the whey portion of milk, acting through GIP, really does open the throttle that controls the growth of babies, by providing part of the stimulus to open the androgen receptor. This, combined with the impact of IGF on the androgen receptor, adds to the overall de-repression (activation) of this important receptor. With the androgen receptor open, ready, and waiting, milk is also ready, loaded with the anabolic androgenic steroids that provide the stimulus to growth.

8.3.3 The paleolithic diet

The attention of the acne research community was drawn to low-glycemic-load diets by Professor Loren Cordain's 2002 paper [18]. The complete absence of acne in the remote populations studied in New Guinea and Paraguay was attributed by the Lindeberg research team to the low-glycemic-load diet consumed by both these tribes of hunter-gatherers.

Cordain has subsequently substantially developed and elucidated the science and the human dietary history behind the low-glycemic-load diet consumed by our distant ancestors. His publications are widely read and explain the basis for promoting a diet consisting of food that was available to our forebears during the millions of years prior to the availability of refined flour and sugar and the development of herding practices that introduced regular dairy intake to our diets. This is generally referred to as the *caveman, Paleolithic,* or *Paleo diet*. It is apparent that the lack of dairy plus the low level of simple-carbohydrate elements combine to provide a very healthy diet. The testimonials are positive, the effort is definitely worth it for most who adhere to the diet, but adherence to any strict diet can be a challenge on an individual basis. It remains to be seen whether such a diet could be the subject of universal and environmental primary prevention measures. Such measures would require a widespread change in attitude toward nutrition, business practices, farming methods, and the products produced.

8.3.4 High-fructose corn syrup (HFCS)

No discussion of sugar and insulin response is complete without an understanding of HFCS. Because it is cheaper to make and sweeter than regular table sugar (sucrose), fructose-containing corn syrup is the preferred sweetener for soda-type drinks. In 2004, the *American Journal of Nutrition* noted that HCFS represented "more than 40 percent of caloric sweeteners added to foods and beverages and (was) the sole caloric sweetener in soft drinks in the United States" [19]. So, that means cheaper

drinks, right? So what's the problem? Well, there are two main problems with fructose.

The first concern is that fructose does not stimulate the release of insulin. This is important because insulin controls leptin, a hormone that tells you when you are full. So you get no "full feeling" from fructose. That means that you are likely to drink or eat more of the fructose-containing drink or food before your body tells you that you are full. This is not good for weight control.

The second problem is that fructose is not handled in the body like other sugars. Instead of being broken down like glucose to produce energy in a process called *glycolysis*, it tends to produce the building blocks of fatty acids, setting us up for fat deposition. In animal studies, but less so in humans, fructose also raises blood pressure, raises triglycerides, impairs glucose tolerance, and promotes insulin resistance. Although a moderate amount of fructose intake in fresh fruit is a natural part of a healthy diet, consuming the excessive amounts available in artificial man-made "foodstuffs" (including sweetened drinks) is neither physiological nor natural.

The impact of HFCS on acne occurs because of a mass effect. Normal sugars raise insulin levels to a normal degree. That triggers leptin and the appetite is satisfied, shutting down your wish to drink or eat more. When fructose is a part of the sugar mix, the signal to cease eating or drinking is diminished. You tend to consume more and that eventually boosts the insulin levels higher (from the other sugars, not the fructose), and that helps to de-repress the androgen receptor. That turns up the throttle on androgen-dependent processes from acne to hair growth to increased muscle and bone mass. This, combined with the tendency of fructose to store as fat, may be a significant player in the obesity epidemic that is driving up health care costs at a frightening rate. Limiting fructose to natural sources, taken in moderation, seems to be the best way to limit its impact on acne or other unwanted metabolic effects.

8.3.5 Metformin

As we have learned over the past few years, anything that can be done to normalize the everyday levels of glucose and insulin in our acne patients' blood will reduce the tendency toward insulin resistance and will also assist in reducing the availability of the androgen receptors to androgens of whatever source. Metformin has recently been recognized to assist in this regard, and positive reports of its effective use in AI/HS have appeared [20]. It has been assigned FDA Pregnancy Category B so is worth consideration in the patient trying to achieve pregnancy (especially if she is overweight or has a diagnosis of polycystic ovarian disorder or metabolic syndrome). There is also reasonable evidence that metformin would be a wise addition to the anti-acne regimen [21]. The most common side effect is nausea and vomiting, so metformin's introduction would be best done prior to achieving pregnancy, given the risk of morning sickness. Start low and go slow.

8.3.6 Synthesis and summary

There is a massive crossover in the influences of dairy and high-glycemic-load foods between acne and several other diseases and disorders of modern man and woman [22–24]. Prevention of the acnes presents lifelong dietary challenges, and these challenges are shared by the entire population exposed to processed foodstuffs, not just those with the genetic predisposition to the acnes.

Acne vulgaris is linked with obesity, obesity is linked with polycystic ovaries (PCO), and PCO is linked with excessive facial hair growth. That is linked with balding in women and is also linked with obesity. Obesity links with AI/HS, acne inversa is linked to smoking, and smoking links to adult acne in women. The links through hyperinsulinemia and diabetes to insulin resistance and the metabolic syndrome are well established, and all appear to be related to dairy and increased glycemic load. There is recent evidence [25] that part of the blame may be shared by meat consumption, but we have (at the moment) no epidemiologic or clinical evidence that meat consumption is part of the problem in acne.

Insulin resistance is a challenging problem, and its story is thoroughly interwoven into the pathogenesis of the acnes. Chronically elevated blood levels of diet-sourced glucose induce chronically elevated levels of insulin. The insulin attempts to lower glucose by storing it as glycogen in the liver and in other peripheral tissues. This chronically elevated insulin is one of the triggers of the de-repression of the androgen receptor, and is therefore a persistent pro-acne influence. The most effective product so far to counter this situation is metformin, a biguanide that decreases intestinal absorption of glucose and stimulates glucose's entry into muscle and liver cells, where it is converted to and stored as glycogen, thus lowering the blood level. It has other useful metabolic effects (plus some side effects) and has proven of value in both acne and AI/HS [21, 26]. It is likely to see greater use in these conditions as we continue to search for alternatives to isotretinoin, and should probably be regularly used hand in hand with the dietary regimen.

Other diseases and health problems that share dairy as a potential cause include prostate and breast cancer, decreased female fertility, overweight neonates, increased risk of Caesarean sections, increased fetal mortality, and increased rates of twinning [27]. Numerous other dairy-related problems that are mediated by allergy, lactose intolerance, and other factors that do not depend on the insulin mechanism, so they are not included here.

The science is not yet complete, but the messages are clear. If you suffer from one or more of the acnes, you should:

Avoid all dairy.

Consume a diet that is low in glycemic load.

Avoid fructose-predominant sugar sources.

Normalize your weight.

8.4 Comedolytics and other topicals

Some patients still show up believing the blackheads are dirt caught in the pores. They need to know that these plugs are made of keratinocytes, the cells that line the duct, and they are "stuck in a traffic jam" at the opening of the duct or just under the skin. The color is due to the same chemical, melanin, that gives our skin color or makes us tan. Each and every comedo in a case of acne needs to be emptied out of the follicular duct. Leaving it behind invites future trouble.

While gentle cleanliness to remove the oil and makeup and other surface material at the end of the day is wise, it is impossible to scrub out comedones below the skin surface. Scrubbing just adds insult to injury and is to be discouraged, whether with wash cloth, loofah, or "complexion brush" (manual or electric). Soap and detergent selection alone will not clear acne, but on general principles I recommend the gentlest products possible, basically because I will be using other irritating chemicals on the face and I want to "reserve the irritation" for the medications the patient really needs. Unscented and pH-balanced synthetic detergent (syndet) cleansing bars are preferred, but gentle liquid facial cleansers or mild "super-fatted" soaps are usually sufficient. They should be applied with bare hands, warm water, and a gentle circular motion with fingertips only, and followed by a gentle rinse in clear warm water. No face cloths or washrags are permitted. Especially oily faces may need a second wash to get "squeaky clean." The face is patted or blotted dry with a clean terrycloth towel, preferably laundered in an enzyme-free detergent and not exposed to dryer sheets or fabric softeners. This is all the preparation needed for the application of the products discussed throughout this section.

Antibacterial soaps have been recommended for mild acne [28], but that recommendation was made before the realization that such products are likely partly responsible for the biotropic effect that shifts the balance of the facial flora toward production of *Malassezia* yeast by killing off the "easy-to-kill" bacteria. I have patients avoid such products unless there is clear evidence of bacterial infection, which is rare.

Comedones (the plural) can be physically forced out by pressure (Section 8.7.1) or dissolved (lysed) by the action of a comedolytic. Some comedolytics do nothing but dissolve or unplug pores. Others have additional roles.

8.4.1 Standard topical comedolytics

These chemicals have long histories as valuable and effective products.

8.4.1.1 Retinoids

The retinoids originated as drugs derived from vitamin A, whose chemical name is *retinol*. The first to be introduced was *vitamin A acid*, technically *all-trans retinoic acid*, which was available originally as a very effective but very irritating liquid, applied topically (Figure 8.1). Patients were warned that there would be redness, irritation, and peeling. It was easy to tell 40 years ago if your patient was using the medicine or not. Because there was little else available at the time, most put up with it, mainly because it *really* worked if used as directed, not only on open comedones (Figure 8.2) but on closed comedones as well (Figure 8.3 and see "Practical Acne Therapy").

With time, gentler formulations were developed with different strengths, different vehicles, different indications (including fine wrinkles), and numerous different names. Dermatologists generally pride themselves on being able to juggle drugs and fine-tune them to match

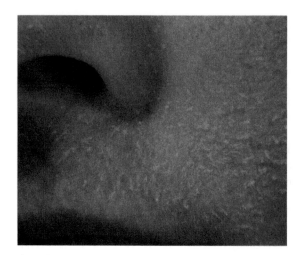

Figure 8.1 The original liquid preparation in the mid-1970s was a challenge to tolerate, but alternatives were few.

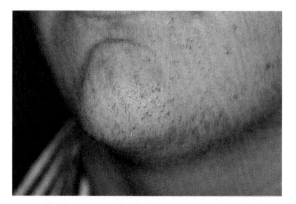

Figure 8.2 These comedones developed in a 16-year-old while he was on a full anti-inflammatory dose of doxycycline as successful treatment for pityriasis lichenoides chronica.

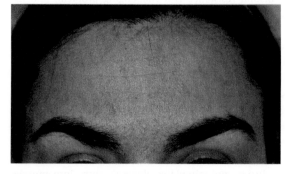

Figure 8.3 This variety of fine closed comedonal acne with hundreds of lesions is a challenge, but proper use of topical retinoids will clear the tiny milia-like folliculopapules.

their patients' skins and needs, so the variety is welcome. As a starting point today, the generic vitamin A acid 0.05% cream is reasonable, perhaps three nights a week to the entire involved area. The frequency of use is increased as tolerated. My pre-printed prescription forms indicate that the applications may vary "from 3 to 14 times per week," and patients are instructed and encouraged to gradually increase (or decrease) the frequency to tolerance. The use of these products *over the entire involved area* is highly important in a population that is used to "spot treatments." Patients must understand that comedolytics work by doing two jobs at the same time:

1 If the pore is plugged, the comedo in each pore will be lifted to the surface, often making the individual spot appear worse, until the entire pore is emptied out. This needs to be continued until every pore is empty.

2 If the pore is NOT plugged, then the comedolytic will get down into the pores in the entire involved area and *prevent* the nonplugged pores from becoming plugged.

These applications are continued until all is clear and then the frequency is reduced to more tolerable maintenance levels, which (with luck and gentle skin care) are often below the level that causes redness and peeling or flaking.

The next retinoid to reach the market, adapalene, is similar in effect to retinoic acid but was not based on the vitamin A molecule, even though it is called a retinoid. Adapalene was originally introduced as Differin® 0.1% cream, and a gel followed shortly. It had the advantage of being somewhat gentler than retinoic acid/vitamin A acid [29] but was just as effective. In addition, it is stable when exposed to sunlight so it can be used in the morning even in sunny locations. As a result of competition from generics and from a stronger product, Differin's strength was boosted to 0.3% in the gel vehicle and it is a stable, reliable, albeit expensive product.

The third retinoid, tazarotene, was introduced as a topical for psoriasis but in the hands of the dermatology community, always experimenting, it found a place as a comedolytic and that is now its preferred use. It is available in a cream and a gel, as both 0.1 and 0.05% Tazorac®. It is photostable and rates above the Differin 0.3% gel both as a comedolytic and as an irritant. I find it particularly useful as a supplemental tool to clean out the most resistant comedones that may be refusing to leave with low-dose isotretinoin (the oral retinoid—see

Section 8.4.3.2). Using any of these to get out the last resistant comedo always requires persistence and tolerance. Persuading patients to remain adherent to a long-term preventive maintenance program is almost as difficult.

8.4.1.2 Benzoyl peroxide

A potent oxidizing agent, benzoyl peroxide (BP), has been in use as a solo ingredient and in various combinations for decades. It works to dry and peel the top layers of the skin, gradually thinning and flaking away the keratin that makes up the comedonal material plugging the pores, qualifying it as one of the earliest true comedolytics. It is also a moderately effective bactericidal (killing bacteria) and bacteriostatic (slowing their reproduction) agent. As such, it has been especially useful in the decades that saw the worldwide spread of antibiotic-resistant *Propionibacterium acnes*. Because its mode of action is not susceptible to induction of bacterial resistance, it has been and still is an ally against the antibiotic-resistant *P. acnes* strains [30]. It penetrates well into sebum, so it is capable of reaching not only the skin surface but also the follicular portions of the FPSU [31].

In the animation available at http://www.acnemilk.com/acne_animation, you can see how the low oxygen content of the follicular structure is produced by pressure from the overgrowth of the lining keratinocytes. The oxygen content is so low that *P. acnes*, which grows best in a low-oxygen (or no-oxygen) location, multiplies happily in these anoxic (no-oxygen) ducts. It is happy to do so as long as there is enough food. Fortunately, the same hormones that turn on the keratinocytes are equally busy producing lots of sebum. It is no accident that sebum is the preferred food of both *P. acnes* and *Malassezia*, so they are quite happy to take up residence in this sebum-saturated niche in the skin, at least until BP is added to the mix.

Consider that BP, just like hydrogen peroxide, releases fresh oxygen as it reacts with other substances. And remember that it is quite soluble in sebum. So if you rub it on your skin, there is a pretty good chance that it will dissolve in the sebum, penetrate the pores, and then travel down into the duct to flood the deeper parts of the follicle with oxygen. This is likely to slow the growth of *P. acnes*, dropping the population of that organism. This has always been thought to be a bactericidal effect but it may be due simply to the inhibitory effect of the fresh input of oxygen flooding the living space of the anaerobic *P. acnes*. Although speculative and unproven, there is reason to wonder if one reason for its effectiveness may be the provision of sufficient oxygen to the depths of the follicle that the formation of hypoxia-inducible factor 1 (HIF-1; see Section 7.3) may be prohibited.

BP has been used in concentrations from 2% to 20%, and both the effectiveness and the amount of irritation experienced by the patient are quite variable. This depends upon the concentration of the drug itself, the vehicle (cream, gel, lotion, wash, shower bar, shower gel, etc.), the length of application time (from a wash on–rinse off 2% shower gel to an overnight 10% spot treatment), and individual patients' sensitivity. The last is somewhat unpredictable. Some patients may become truly allergic to BP; the estimates vary from 1% to 10% of patients exposed. More common is simple primary irritant contact dermatitis, which is dose or frequency related and so can be managed by varying the product used and the frequency and exposure time. There is also a population of extra-sensitive individuals, often atopics (patients with personal or family histories of allergies, eczema, hives, hay fever, etc.), who cannot tolerate using this (or many other topicals) at all. They have the *sensitive skin syndrome* [32], for which the only effective therapy is avoidance of irritants. Basically, they are best treated only with systemic medications unless they are prepared to put up with stinging, burning, itching, and general irritation during a prolonged course of gentle-as-possible topicals.

BP is available both alone and as a combination with other medications. As Sulfoxyl 5 Lotion®, a mixture of 5% precipitated sulfur and 10% BP, it was a mainstay of therapy during the 1970s. The sulfur may have been responsible for the lack of problems with *Malassezia* during those years. Subsequently, BP was added to erythromycin and clindamycin topicals when studies showed that this decreased the incidence of resistant strains of *P. acnes*. The combination was marginally better than the topical antibiotics alone but did have the advantage of concurrent comedolytic therapy while the *P. acnes* was being treated. Like the retinoids, the BP products should be applied to the entire involved area for their preventive effect. Higher strength (10%) products may be used as "spot treatment" to dry up specific lesions. This is especially useful overnight, for example following "acne surgery" (Section 8.7.1).

8.4.1.3 Salicylic acid

This simple relative of acetylsalicylic acid (Aspirin®) has been used for decades in low concentrations and is remarkably safe, cheap, and gently effective as a comedolytic for clearing mild acne. It is a *beta-hydroxy acid*; in fact, it is the only one used in acne care. This "beta" configuration means it is lipid soluble, so it can actually get down into the sebum (oil, lipid) in the follicular duct. It is available as a cream, cleansing bar, shower gel, lotion, body wash, and *spot stick*. As with BP, the effectiveness and tolerance vary from person to person.

If salicylic acid worked for all acne, we dermatologists would never see a case.

If it worked for no cases, we would be overwhelmed by acne.

If a gentle product for maintenance after isotretinoin is needed, salicylic acid is worth a try.

8.4.1.4 Alpha and beta-hydroxy acids

Salicylic acid is the only *beta-hydroxy acid*; all the others are *alpha-hydroxy acids*. The original one, promoted as an effective anti-aging facial peel by van Scott, was glycolic acid [33]. More than with other comedolytics, the variables of concentration, vehicle, pH, exposure time, skin "prep" preoperatively, "neutralization," and aftercare determine the results with glycolic acid. At one extreme, the aggressiveness of the reaction is such that it is best monitored only by a cosmetically trained dermatologist with considerable experience, a well-trained staff, excellent handholding skills, and excellent liability insurance. At the low end of the potency scale, it can be rendered so gentle that it is sold over-the-counter and self-administered, but it is almost as ineffective at low potency as the high potency is risky. It has gradually become an aesthetician's tool, even when dispensed or used by dermatologists or their staff.

8.4.2 Unclassified topicals

Many chemical compounds have been tried over the years. Their method of action is not always well defined. Nevertheless, some of them work for some people, some do not, but most are worthy of mention.

8.4.2.1 Azelaic acid

This rather gentle compound is found naturally in some grains. It is a mild bactericidal against *P. acnes*, and is a gentle comedolytic. It is also a mild anti-inflammatory and a tyrosinase inhibitor, so it finds use in treatment of

PIH, especially in those with darker skin types. The vehicle in which it is used has a significant effect on its potency, and the 15% gel is most often prescribed. While it suffers from the disadvantage of having little effect on *Malassezia* [34], it is FDA category B, so it is safe for use in pregnancy.

8.4.2.2 Sulfur

Sulfur, in its many forms, has been used for centuries in dermatology. It is a mild antibacterial, is quite effective against *Malassezia*, and is a gentle comedolytic. Overuse will cause irritation and peeling, but it is otherwise non-toxic when used topically. It is often combined with salicylic acid or sodium sulfacetamide in various strengths in topical lotions and creams [35].

8.4.2.3 Zinc compounds

Correction of a presumed zinc deficiency has recently been shown, in specimens taken from patients with active lesions of AI/HS, to appear to enhance the expression of all the markers of innate immunity that were depressed [36]. This observation may explain why various forms of zinc have been found useful in managing acne vulgaris, acne rosacea, and acne inversa. When used topically in antibiotic combinations, it has been shown to be as effective as oral tetracycline [37]. Zinc has been associated with a decreased systemic absorption of clindamycin from a topical preparation containing both, a possible protective effect. It has also been found to be sebosuppressive. An oral proprietary mixture of nicotinamide 750 mg, zinc 25 mg, copper 1.5 mg, and folic acid 500 µg [38] produced positive results comparable to the effect of oral antibiotics in patients with acne rosacea or acne vulgaris. In AI/HS, oral zinc has been found to be effective. While it has been suggested that zinc supplementation might be useful only in those who suffer from a zinc deficiency, defining this deficiency is expensive. From a pragmatic point of view it is much more cost-effective to supplement with the dose used in this last study, zinc gluconate 30 mg with each meal [39], administering zinc gluconate or chelate with meals (30 mg twice or three times per day in adults). Zinc may reduce copper absorption by displacing copper, so copper supplementation has been advised [40]. A proprietary capsule containing the recommended proportion of 50 mg zinc and 2 mg copper in an amino acid chelate used once or twice orally daily likely avoids problems.

8.4.2.4 Resorcinol

Resorcinol is a simple benzene ring molecule with two hydroxyl groups at the 1 and 3 positions. It is an antiseptic, disinfectant, analgesic, and hemostatic (stops bleeding). In low concentrations (2% or less), it has been an active ingredient in anti-acne products for decades. Paired with sulfur, it was present in Acnomel® and is still present in certain Clearasil® products. It is useful for both acne vulgaris and acne rosacea.

A recent innovation is its use in a stable proprietary base at a fairly high 15% concentration. It is used to treat early or resistant lesions of HS/AI [41]. As formulated, it decreases the redness and swelling and helps dry up early inflammatory nodules. Even though it is not a classical comedolytic, it dries and peels the surface of such lesions. Note that extemporaneous mixtures at this concentration tend to disintegrate. A proprietary vehicle that allows compounding without subsequent breakdown of the mixture has been developed.

8.4.3 Systemic comedolytics

Topical therapy depends upon the ability of the active molecule to gain access to the targeted areas of the follicle at an effective concentration. Systemic administration has proven more effective than topical for the most important retinoid comedolytics.

8.4.3.1 Vitamin A

The original retinoid, vitamin A (retinol), has been available in such bland and innocuous topical products as Vitamin A&D ointment for generations and is included in all multivitamin oral preparations. Its effect on any of the acnes when applied topically is essentially nil. In high doses (300,000–400,000 IU daily), given orally there is a significant acne-clearing effect, even before obvious toxic effects are approached. Kligman and others [42] worked with such doses prior to the arrival of isotretinoin on the scene. These high doses have been associated with documented teratogenicity, and so must be avoided where there is risk of pregnancy [43].

8.4.3.2 Isotretinoin

Although available in some countries as a topical in a gel base, isotretinoin works far better when introduced to the follicular unit through the bloodstream following oral administration. The same is true of the need for delivery to the sebaceous gland itself, a feat that cannot

BOX 8.1 ISOTRETINOIN, A CHALLENGE TO PRESCRIBE

The risk that isotretinoin presents to developing babies has led to quite reasonable controls implemented to minimize the risk. Unfortunately, many former isotretinoin prescribers were lost to the system as a result of the botched introduction of the iPLEDGE program in the United States, a triumph of constructive obstructionism. Although it initially made a difficult situation worse, it has served to maintain the availability of an exceptionally valuable drug. Isotretinoin remains on the market, and the hurdles thrown up by iPLEDGE serve at least as daily reminders of the need to prescribe this drug with caution. The use of a standard educational package provided by hand plus the signed consent forms retained in the chart certify that the patient (and parent) has read the required information. This not only underlines the importance of the informed consent process but also provides some defense against claims of malpractice based on lack of informed consent. Nevertheless the loss of hundreds of caring prescribers because of the iPLEDGE debacle has been both counterproductive and incompatible with comprehensive and appropriate clinical care.

   A similar patient-unfriendly set of rules evolved in the European Union, the so-called European Directive (Article 29 of Directive 2001/83/EC), with the recommendation that isotretinoin be reserved for those "with severe acne … resistant to adequate courses of standard therapy with systemic antibiotics and topical therapy." An international group of dermatologists noted, "The new recommendations suggest isotretinoin should only be used in severe acne (nodular, conglobata) that has or is not responding to appropriate antibiotics and topical therapy. The inference of this being that it should now not be used at all as first-line therapy" [50]. It is impossible to know how many unnecessary cases of inflammatory bowel disease, candidiasis, and *Malassezia* folliculitis have been caused by the inappropriate oral antibiotics prescribed to follow this rule. Likewise, how much prolonged physical and psychological scarring and inflammatory disease have been added by delaying effective treatment? This unfortunate dictate simply added to the load carried by the EU's acne patients. In fairness, the Directive was formulated before discussions of a risk as yet unproven, the recent question of isotretinoin causing inflammatory bowel disease. It is time to see the Directive revised.

be achieved topically. Following Peck's introductory article in 1979 [44], isotretinoin arrived on the scene in 1982 and the entire picture of acne therapy changed. As Accutane in North America and Roaccutane elsewhere, it was quickly recognized as the most effective therapy available. Despite significant side effects, almost all of which are easily managed with conservative dosing and careful monitoring, it retains pride of place as the most effective of all therapies for acne.

Isotretinoin is a powerful drug and must be treated with respect, consideration being carefully given to the following five areas of concern. See also Box 8.1, "Isoretinoin, a Challenge to Prescribe."

8.4.3.2.1 Teratogenicity

The major concern over the years with the use of isotretinoin has been teratogenicity (physical and mental abnormalities developing in the unborn baby caused by its mother's exposure to the drug in early pregnancy). Programs mandated by government and underwritten by the drugs' manufacturers have been in place for years, the most recent being iPLEDGE [45]. The object is to minimize the risk, and careful adherence to protocols has been shown to stabilize but not eliminate the occurrence of unwanted pregnan-

cies. Although contraceptive failures occur and patient failures are often to blame, prescribers share the blame, occasionally excusing patients from adherence to the protocol or inadvertently trusting the untrust-worthy [46, 47].

Adherence to the birth control regimen is a matter of trust, and it is essentially impossible to enforce. Religious objections and personal commitment need to be discussed openly, a difficult prospect if mother and underage daughter have differing agendas. Frankness and honesty, even though uncomfortable, is the best policy.

8.4.3.2.2 Contraception

It can be very helpful to view the newer progestins as being used for acne control, rather than exclusively as conception control. By presenting acne in all its variations as a disorder triggered by hormones, one can lead the discussion naturally to the use of hormonal control as a medical decision, not open to religious or moral concerns. This is admittedly a "sidelong glance at reality," but it may allow the patient and her parents to see "the Pill" in a different light, as a valuable part of the therapy, and therefore as an acceptable choice.

From the opposite side of the question, the physician always retains the right, indeed the responsibility, to withhold any medication that he or she suspects may be used inappropriately, putting an unborn child at risk. A patient who deceives the prescriber, accepts a prescription for a BCP, then sets it aside for religious or other reasons and takes the isotretinoin that was prescribed by the physician in good faith may create a very difficult situation. If a pregnancy occurs in the face of the physician's misplaced faith in the patient, an innocent life is threatened.

The iPLEDGE program assists in guiding, recording, and documenting the informed consent process, but the ultimate risk is the patient's, or the unborn child's.

8.4.3.2.3 Inflammatory bowel disease

The question that is presently preoccupying and enriching lawyers in North America is whether or not isotretinoin may cause inflammatory bowel disease (IBD). Several cases have reached court. The financial settlements have been monumental. Nevertheless, the science is unsettled. One problem is that most patients who have been treated with isotretinoin have had their acne previously treated with broad-spectrum antibiotics. The incidence of IBD among patients who have taken isotretinoin may actually be lower [48] than that among those treated with broad-spectrum antibiotics [49], but this is insufficient evidence to totally exonerate isotretinoin. The only way to obtain data unconfounded by previous antibiotic therapy (topical or systemic) would be to identify a population with severe acne but no prior experience of broad-spectrum antibiotics and no family or personal history of gastrointestinal symptoms suggestive of (and so predisposing to) IBD. They could be treated with isotretinoin prospectively in a randomized clinical trial, but now that the drug is "off patent" there is no interest from the manufacturers in funding such expensive studies.

That leaves standing the question of whether acne and IBD, both being inflammatory diseases (whether primary or secondarily), occur in individuals who have a genetic or acquired predisposition to inflammatory disease itself. It is possible that some individuals, like atopics, are simply more prone to certain kinds of disease driven by certain types of mediators, such as tumor necrosis factor alpha (TNFα) and others. And, of course, IBD existed long before isotretinoin came on the scene in 1982.

To complicate matters, a pre-authorization policy of some pharmacy benefit managers in the United States insists on a failed trial of broad-spectrum antibiotics prior to the introduction of isotretinoin. A European directive on the use of isotretinoin mandates a similar approach (see Box 8.1, "Isotretinoin, a Challenge to Prescribe").

These "trial of antibiotics first" protocols (financially influenced by insurance companies in the United States) ignore the pathogenesis of the disease, encourage the overgrowth and influence of both *Candida* in the bowels and *Malassezia* in the FPSUs, put patients at further risk from scarring and perhaps even induction of IBD, hinder investigative science, and so are profoundly counterproductive, in my opinion.

8.4.3.2.4 Depression

The fourth problem we need to consider is the question of the induction of depression by isotretinoin. The drug remains under suspicion as a true, if infrequent, idiosyncratic cause of depression. While the studies of depression and isotretinoin therapy generally support the lack of association, it is essential that we recognize the risk and possibility of depression occurring in rare individual patients.

There is no denying that there are cases in which a temporal relationship exists between isotretinoin and depression or isotretinoin and suicide. The question is whether isotretinoin itself is the cause.

Over the past 30 years, I've seen four patients in whom the depression question arose. The first was a young woman who was so severely depressed after 6 weeks on isotretinoin that she required admission to a psychiatric unit. This occurred before the question of depression associated with isotretinoin had been raised. She had, in order to take the isotretinoin safely, been started on a BCP. At the time (the early 1980s), the estrogen level in BCPs was higher and the potential for depression from the BCP far outweighed our concern regarding isotretinoin. Her depression was attributed to the BCP. She remained off both drugs subsequently, and no challenge was performed. The next two cases were patients, one male and one female, who reported depressive symptoms shortly after starting the isotretinoin. Both were interviewed in depth about their diet. Both habitually avoided vitamin A–containing vegetables and took no supplements. Both stopped the isotretinoin for two weeks and were placed on vitamin A supplements (8000–10,000 IU) for 10 to 14 days. Both then returned to isotretinoin and completed the course without incident [51].

I learned about the fourth patient from his parents, who reported his suicide four months after the very successful completion of the course of isotretinoin. There were extenuating personal problems in his case, and the call was to thank me for helping provide the young man with what they called "the best few months of his teens" before his passing.

In the first case, there is no doubt that BCPs cause depression in a fair percentage of women, opening the possibility of simple coincidence.

In the second and third cases, I suspect (but cannot prove) that vitamin A–deficient individuals have numerous vitamin A receptor sites in their bodies that are unoccupied by their natural ligand, vitamin A itself. This may leave these receptors open to accept isotretinoin, an unintended ligand, with unpredictable results, including the possibility of night blindness. There is unfortunately no practical way of proving this theoretical suspicion. Nevertheless, there is little risk of additional vitamin A toxicity if one simply advocates a daily dose of 10,000 IU vitamin A for a week or 10 days prior to starting isotretinoin therapy in any patient with a poor history of vitamin A intake. The admonition in the June 2000 Accutane package insert, "Because of the relationship of Accutane to vitamin A, patients should be advised against taking vitamin supplements containing vitamin A to avoid additive toxic effects," was written without apparent regard to the relative safety of 400,000 IU of vitamin A in Kligman's series [52]. There was no evidence in support of the warning in the product insert, written long before "evidence-based medicine" was invented.

My experience with the two patients who suffered depression, then had vitamin A supplementation followed by successful isotretinoin therapy, suggests that vitamin A deficiency may predispose to isotretinoin toxicity [53, 54]. This is anecdotal, so the idea is probably an insurmountable distance from clinical proof, and it will likely never see the Cochrane stamp of approval of "evidence-based medicine." Nevertheless, I occasionally supplement an isotretinoin candidate whose dietary history suggests inadequate vitamin A intake, and I offer it as a practical and low-cost preventive approach whenever the question of depression is raised.

With regard to the fourth patient, it is becoming apparent with more reports that there is a population of individuals who appear well adjusted, normal, productive, and happy in every way, but who suffer from covert depression. A recent review states,

Psychological disturbances, including depression and other suicidal tendencies, are extremely common during adolescence and are clearly increased by acne, particularly where it is severe. Isotretinoin does not appear to increase this risk. Routine screening should be performed for psychological disturbance in adolescents, particularly among those presenting acne. Prescription of isotretinoin is not contraindicated in subjects presenting depression. [55]

So what is the practical approach to isotretinoin in the face of psychological or psychiatric worries? If the patient is already depressed, under psychiatric care, and taking appropriate medications, I explain the vitamin A deficiency hypothesis, take a dietary history, and recommend two weeks of 10,000 IU of oral vitamin A. Because isotretinoin is a derivative of vitamin A and vitamin A is a fat-soluble vitamin, both are taken daily with fatty food. Here in the United States, I recommend a tablespoon of peanut butter—but not cow or goat butter. Olive oil works well, but is harder to use. A square "pat" of (oleo) margarine spread on toast or a cracker will do, as will a couple of gelatin capsules of fish oil. The vitamin A is recommended irrespective of the food history, to eliminate doubt. If the patient (or parent) wishes, or if my concerns are high, I communicate with the psychiatric therapist. I explain that the use of isotretinoin in patients already under treatment for depression is normal and accepted and that most psychiatrists are well aware of this and welcome the help that isotretinoin provides. Indeed, as I tell my patients and their parents, "I would also likely be depressed if I had to come to work with acne like this. I hope we can get rid of one of the major causes of depression for you." This may sound "promissory," and with any other drug it would be a risk to make such a statement, but isotretinoin has passed the test of time and can deliver superb results when used properly.

When all involved are counseled, consented, and comfortable, I then proceed with a low dose (20–40 mg isotretinoin daily with peanut butter) and the solid (sometimes written) understand that if there appears to be any adverse response, the drug is stopped and I am to be notified immediately—I provide my cell/mobile number for that purpose.

If there is a family history of depression or bipolar disorder, but there is no clinical depression, I explain the situation. The explanation is communicated to the primary care physician. Again, the vitamin A supplementation is highly recommended, despite the iPLEDGE proscription against it. To repeat, there was no evidence provided in support of that warning, which was written long before evidence-based medicine was invented.

If the concern springs from the patient's or the family's reading of the Internet or the iPLEDGE booklet, in the absence of depression, the approach is the same, with the vitamin A offered as an option.

In an obviously depressed patient, or the rare patient with body dysmorphic disorder or obsessive-compulsive disorder (anything from destructive self-manipulation to obsessive use of the magnifying mirror), I recommend professional psychiatric help before we go further. As an aside, from a practical point of view, patients who are obsessive pickers will stop "obsessing" and picking if they run out of targets to pick at—and there is no drug that eliminates those targets better than isotretinoin.

In ALL cases, the question needs to be asked about self-destructive thoughts.

The additional psychological burden added to patients' lives by the iPLEDGE program does have benefits, but we do lose patients who would benefit from a less heavy-handed administrative approach. And that, of course, prolongs the problem. On the other hand, if the negative power of the iPLEDGE program could be used to persuade all parents and professionals who care for acne patients to manage them from the first contact according to the principles set out in this book, aggressive prevention could lead to much less need for isotretinoin.

The iPLEDGE process is uncomfortable for all concerned. This is one reason that in my practice I never prescribe isotretinoin to females, and very rarely in males, to a new patient on the first visit. I insist they take 48 hours, or a weekend or a week, to review the iPLEDGE booklet in detail. If aged less than 18, the review is also done by parents (mandatory when a parent's signature is required), or with a trusted second or third party. This booklet is available online [45] and raises the question of depression and suicide in some detail, preparing patients and parents (assuming they read the whole booklet) for my eyeball-to-eyeball question before I sign off on the iPLEDGE consent form and write the prescription. My script is simple: "You have read the manual, you are aware that there are concerns about depression and suicide, do you have any further questions or concerns?"

To the general public, the iPLEDGE pamphlets and the consent forms that go with them are scary documents. They pull no punches. They are designed to protect. They help to protect the patient against a lack of informed consent, they help to protect the physician against claims of failure to provide informed consent (when used as part of the full informed consent process), and they help to prevent exposure of an unborn child to a known teratogen.

The documents are a "heavy read" for many patients and their parents. Indeed, of those who are sent home with the iPLEDGE documents for review, approximately 15% never come back to the office. Often this is a vote against the need for birth control, judging from the conversation when the question is introduced, rather than a vote against isotretinoin itself. Another 10% or so come back, but wish to avoid the drug for various other reasons. Alternative therapies, initially presented as options at the earlier visit, are then detailed.

8.4.3.2.5 Other side effects

That leaves us with the physical side effects. Prior to its commercial introduction, and during the early years, the dosage of isotretinoin was often as high as 2 mg per kg per day. As a result of experience elsewhere [56], I now rarely go beyond 0.8 mg per kg per day. I explain to patients that we once used a fairly high dose over a short period of time, but that we now use a lower dose over a longer period of time. The total dose (and the effectiveness) of the medication is approximately the same, but the side effects are far less [57]. The long list of cutaneous and mucous membrane side effects that were such a challenge in the early years (see table) have diminished significantly with this lower dose regimen.

acne fulminans	nail dystrophy
alopecia (which may persist)	paronychia
bruising	peeling of palms and soles
cheilitis (dry lips)	photoallergy or photosensitivity
dry mouth	pruritus (itch)
dry nose	pyogenic granuloma
dry skin	rash (including facial erythema,
epistaxis (nose bleeds)	seborrhea, and eczema)
eruptive xanthomas	Stevens–Johnson syndrome
erythema multiforme	sunburn susceptibility
flushing	increased sweating
fragility of skin	toxic epidermal necrolysis
hair abnormalities	urticaria
hirsutism	vasculitis (including Wegener's
hyperpigmentation and	granulomatosis)
hypopigmentation	abnormal wound healing
infections (including disseminated	(delayed healing or exuberant
herpes simplex)	granulation tissue)

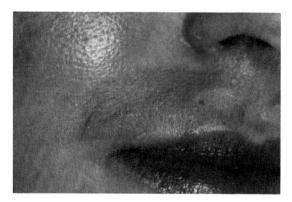

Figure 8.4 One of the earliest cases of a very upset bridesmaid whose waxing while on isotretinoin took off a strip of upper lip epidermis.

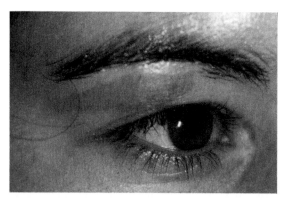

Figure 8.5 Her eyebrows also lost a layer—fortunately, the wedding was over a week away.

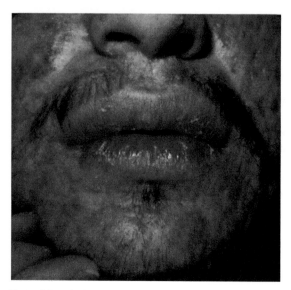

Figure 8.6 High-dose Accutane. Note the (pre-existing) facial scarring as well as the extensive cheilitis (chapped lips).

The chapped lips and dry skin remain, and are very valuable in judging the patients' adherence, but the peeling of upper lip and eyelid from waxing is now seldom seen (Figures 8.4, 8. 5). We still discourage waxing (in any area) for isotretinoin users for at least two months after finishing the drug. There are other side effects, once quite common, such as the pyogenic granuloma-like lesions around toenails that I have not seen for over 10 years. We still hear the occasional complaint about aching backs, we rarely hear about sore muscles at this dose, and the incidence of hypertriglyceridemia is so low on the zero-dairy, low-glycemic-load diet that blood tests are ordered on my patients only when there is a strong positive family history of diabetes or blood lipid anomalies. The exception is a strong parental presence that is insistent upon

testing. In essence, the management of acne with isotretinoin in low doses is a much simpler process than it was in the early years.

The major surprise has been the excellent response achieved over a 120-day course at the low dose. My bias is to attribute this to the zero-dairy, low-glycemic-load diet that I encourage all patients to follow. Certainly, those with significant lesions on the back, neck, and chest often require an additional 30- or 60-day course to achieve full clearance, but that is certainly not an excessive total dose. All are taught to consider isotretinoin as a means to clear their dairy-induced disease faster than avoidance of dairy alone will permit. All know that even the worst acne will clear over time with diet alone—but that it will be a much faster clearance (and with less scarring) with isotretinoin. As always in medicine, opinions and protocols change with time and there is now new evidence that a higher dose produces better long-term results [58], and discussion at a recent symposium pointed out some interesting facts about the guidelines being used. I'm not sure I wish to revisit the high-dose days. The reactions were sometimes quite impressive (Figures 8.6, 8. 7).

There is a problem created when a strict dosing schedule is used in setting up the clinical trial of a new drug. If the drug is successful in reaching the market, it comes with some baggage—the dosing schedule used in the

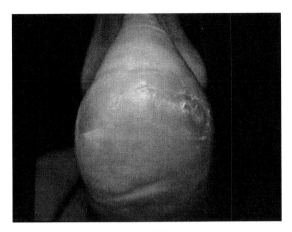

Figure 8.7 Same patient—a peeled heel.

trial usually becomes part of the FDA-regulated package insert. While useful as a guideline, the daily doses, the total doses, and the length and timing of treatment courses are subject to evolution and modification and individual patient sensitivity over years. Patients and physicians are both presented with choices every day, and there is now a background of 30 years of "experience-based" advice as well as "evidence-based" advice to consider on all sides of the discussion [59].

8.4.3.2.6 The convict who looked like Chief

Before isotretinoin was introduced as Accutane® in 1982, it was available on a select basis to some investigators for clinical use. I had several patients on this early program, the most memorable being an inmate in a local penitentiary. This was in the days when inmates could earn "time off for good behavior," and one of the good behaviors was to assist with clinical trials of drugs. This is now considered an unethical practice—times change—but it was mutually beneficial to all concerned in many cases. Even taxpayers benefitted, long before "Win, win, win" was ever invented.

If you've seen the movie *One Flew Over the Cuckoo's Nest*, you will remember Chief, the massive aboriginal basketball player whose declared love of Juicy Fruit® gum was a highlight of the film. My patient was cut from the same cloth; he could have been Chief's twin, but he had horrible bleeding nodular acne that made him a prime candidate for the trial. He was involved from just beneath his ponytail down his back to his belt-line, and his face, neck, shoulders, and upper chest were almost totally submerged in nodular acne.

In isotretinoin's early days, the dose was high and the side effects were a major concern. Because this was a clinical trial, no adjunct therapy was permitted by the protocol, so we saw the full major initial flare; peeling, cracked, and swollen lips; peeling and dry face; and even calluses peeled off feet and particularly off the heels. Special appeals for extra linen, extra issues of clothing, extra shower time, and excuses from manual labor—all were honored by his keepers, but he was still pretty uncomfortable. By six weeks, he could see some improvement and his natural stoicism carried him forward. He steadily improved, and the side effects became tolerable.

By 16 weeks, he was essentially clear of active lesions. He was still putting up with peeling, swollen split lips, and dry skin but could get through the nights with no bleeding, and the nodules had almost all disappeared.

His last appointment was for the four-week post-therapy follow-up. He failed to show. Clinical trial managers really frown on incomplete records, so my staff called the institution to check on him. It seems he was sufficiently happy with the results that he had decided to "take it to the streets." One satisfied customer, he had "gone over the wall," and that was the last I ever heard of him.

8.4.3.3 Acitretin

Another retinoid is available for use in the acnes, but it was actually introduced for the management of conditions in which there is a "disorder of keratinization." This occurred at a time when acne was considered to be due to overproduction of sebum and the role of disordered keratin metabolism took a back seat. Acitretin has the disadvantage of a very long half-life, and because it is teratogenic (like isotretinoin) and because its long half-life can be extended even further if it is taken concurrently with alcohol, it is normally avoided in women, especially those of childbearing capacity.

Acitretin is not approved for use in acne vulgaris, nor is it used in acne rosacea. It is, however, quite useful in managing the abnormal keratinization of the follicular ductal canal that is the cause of the follicular rupture in AI/HS [60]. In managing this disease, all involved must be aware that the time frame is extended because patient and physician are looking for *prevention of new lesions* while the old lesions are managed with antibiotics, anti-inflammatories, and surgical approaches as each case dictates.

8.4.3.4 Summary

If I were asked to design the most cost-effective therapy for acne, even non-inflammatory comedonal acne, it would consist of a zero-dairy, low-glycemic-load diet and an initial course of low-dose isotretinoin, accompanied in women by a non- or low-androgenic progestin-based oral contraceptive, preferably using the "extended" 84/7 regimen and likely supplemented with spironolactone.

This would achieve both effective secondary prevention and effective treatment. It would eliminate the need for aggressive and risky long-term broad-spectrum antibiotics, expensive topicals that now run into the hundreds of dollars per packaged unit in the United States, and would have the added benefit of teaching a dietary lifestyle that could produce a lifetime of healthier choices. While we still do not have any epidemiological evidence that diet is important in true papulopustular acne rosacea, it is not unreasonable to expect that it is developed by the same processes that trigger acne vulgaris, so I make parallel recommendations to my acne rosacea patients regarding both diet and isotretinoin use. Increasing experience in my personal group of HS/AI patients has likewise shown the value of diet, but isotretinoin is of less value here. Acitretin is more effective and deserves broader use.

Until all comedones are prevented, comedolytics are an essential part of acne care.

8.5 Anti-inflammatories and antimicrobials

The first tetracycline, Aureomycin®, was originally brought to bear on acne vulgaris over 60 years ago as a topical ointment in a case of a highly inflammatory acne known then as *acne varioliformis* [61]. The initial intent was to use the tetracycline as an antibiotic, to kill the "acne bacillus," then called *Corynebacterium acnes*, now *P. acnes*. Twenty years later, we learned that tetracycline and other antibiotics, even in doses below the concentration needed for lethal or static antibacterial effect, were fairly potent as suppressors of inflammatory activity, at least as measured by neutrophil chemotactic activity [62]. Subsequently, other antibiotics employed in managing acne have showed varying degrees of anti-inflammatory activity, and varying degrees of success. The problem throughout this discussion over the

years has been deciding to what degree the anti-inflammatory response is purely anti-inflammatory and what response is due to the elimination of the organisms. The problem that has evolved, and has not received adequate discussion, is the fact that reducing or eliminating *P. acnes* does away with one enemy, but tends to enhance the activity of another, or of several others. (See Sections 6.1 and 6.2.)

8.5.1 Antibiotics as anti-inflammatories

The short story here is that every antibiotic that has been used for managing acne vulgaris has anti-inflammatory properties [63, 64]. That said, the choice of antibiotic is based more on overall clinical effect on inflammatory acne lesions and on safety than on a rating of the drug's anti-inflammatory capacity. Topical dapsone, a moderately effective anti-inflammatory when applied topically, is much safer when administered this way than by mouth. Topical clindamycin, on the other hand, has been known to cause its major side effect, pseudomembranous colitis, even when applied topically [65]. Tetracycline applied on the skin surface has never been very effective in acne and is generally not used. Erythromycin ointment, on the other hand, does have some limited topical use, but mainly for its antibacterial capacity rather than its anti-inflammatory properties.

8.5.1.1 In acne vulgaris

In managing acne with tetracycline prior to the arrival of Accutane® in 1982, I regularly used 1–4 g of tetracycline daily. That high dose has not been much used since isotretinoin became available. Now that tetracycline, after disappearing temporarily from the American scene, has reemerged at approximately 100 times its cost of a few years ago, the emphasis will be on the continued use of doxycycline (also subject to a significant price rise) and minocycline. Both are normally used in a dose of 50 to 200 mg daily, in a divided dose, and either **may** be taken with food and water (minocycline) or **must** be taken midmeal with 8 oz. of water (doxycycline) despite the inaccurate instructions provided by pharmacists' computerized handouts in the United States. Because of side effects [66], minocycline has been used less than doxycycline, but the new prices may change these practices.

With the arrival of azithromycin, erythromycin has faded into the background. Numerous regimens have been suggested for azithromycin, one of the 500 mg tablets taken daily for 3 days every 10 days being one of my favorites because of improved compliance, limited side effects, and gentle efficacy.

Amoxicillin and ampicillin have their advocates, as do clindamycin and trimethoprim–sulfisoxazole. In unusual situations such as Gram-negative folliculitis, the antibiotic selection will be determined by culture.

8.5.1.2 In acne rosacea

In managing acne rosacea, almost all the same antibiotics used in acne vulgaris have been tried at various times. Nevertheless, topical metronidazole has held pride of place for a few decades now. In spite of the fact that even the manufacturer denies knowing how it works, it has recognized anti-inflammatory activity. There is little clinical difference between the efficacy of the cream, gel, or lotion. Personal preference of the patient seems to dictate the choice of vehicle. Likewise, there appears to be little difference between the 0.75% and 1% preparations, and between the brands and the generics. I tell patients that 80% of cases respond almost completely to the original 0.75% gel applied topically twice a day for 8 weeks. It works so well that I rarely see an untreated acne rosacea because primary care providers look after that 80%. That leaves 20% that will require a different type of therapy. Interestingly, about 40% of patients (half of the original 80%) who are clear upon discontinuation of the initial 8-week trial will stay that way, sometimes indefinitely. Certainly, topical metronidazole should be the first thing tried. Beyond that, things get complicated. (See Section 1.2.)

8.5.1.3 In acne inversa

Antibiotics have been leaned upon quite heavily in this disease. While many authors freely admit that bacterial cultures may bear little relevance to the pathogenesis of the disease, just about everyone admits that antibiotics are useful [67]. While they may be very effective in getting rid of secondary infection, escalation to more and more powerful combinations seems more likely to rely upon the anti-inflammatory capacity of these antibiotics than their ability to eliminate the organisms.

Certainly, when an inflamed acne inversa nodule or sinus is unroofed and allowed to granulate in from below, there is usually no need for any antibiotic whatsoever. This strongly suggests that the inflammatory component of the disease is driven by something other than the bacterial load. (See 1.3)

If I were convinced that AI/HS is due to a bacterial infection, I likely would be inclined to use antibiotic on a regular basis. In general, however, it is better to address the cause of the problem than it is to expose the patient to the risk of long-term, broad-spectrum antibiotic therapy.

Nevertheless, when there is secondary infection obviously present, antibiotics are warranted. Really hot solitary nodules can also be cooled to a certain extent using the anti-inflammatory capacity of antibiotics, but they clear more quickly and heal faster and with much less pain if unroofed. Grossly infected sinuses are rare but do require antibiotics, and the choice varies from simple full-dose doxycycline to trimethoprim–sulfamethoxazole to rifampicin. They may be used preoperatively to cool the inflammation, making the surgery easier, and then for a short period postoperatively to calm residual inflammation. That said, the healing response without antibiotics, and without the risks of antibiotic resistance and allergic reactions and secondary yeast, is an argument in favor of avoiding them unless cellulitis is apparent.

The risk of secondary yeast infection, especially if the genital areas are involved, is significant. Fluconazole given weekly in a dose of 150–200 mg is normally quite satisfactory to control yeast, and is best used weekly until the signs of infection have disappeared. Once again, unroofing would be preferred, thereby eliminating the need for the antibiotics and for the covering antifungal.

Patients suffering from the extensive sinuses and hypertrophic scarring of Hurley Stage III disease need far more than broad-spectrum antibiotics. They need surgery, and that may be accomplished either by aggressive widespread staged unroofing or by en bloc excision with grafting. See Sections 8.7.3.3 and 8.7.3.4.

8.5.1.4 In dissecting terminal folliculitis (DTF) and acne keloidalis

These recalcitrant disorders require a "full court press," treatment that addresses all potential contributors to the problem. Concurrent anti-*Malassezia*, antibiotic, anti-inflammatory, comedolytic, and intralesional steroid therapy plus diet are used to settle the process. I have not found surgery necessary in DTF if the patient will accept the risk of some residual scarring, but wide excision in acne keloidalis does give remarkably good results.

8.5.2 Antibiotics as antibiotics

When dealing with acne vulgaris, acne rosacea, or AI/HS, there will be times when true hot secondary infection needs aggressive culture-guided antibiotic therapy. The practitioner's experience-based best 'educated guess' as to the offending agent should lead to initial antibiotic therapy while awaiting culture results. The need to switch to a different antibiotic is unusual, but one certainly does not wish to compromise the result by ignoring the availability of culture and sensitivity.

In addition, it is essential to keep in mind that inflammation does not always mean infection. That hot red nodule on the back may be a sterile epidermoid cyst, requiring no antibiotic whatsoever, but simple evacuation instead. The hot red nodule in the middle of the cheek may look the same as the back lesion but may contain no cyst whatsoever, and an attempt to excise or evacuate the lesion may lead to a cosmetic disaster. In the latter situation, intralesional triamcinolone is far better therapy. The same hot red nodule in the inguinal area or under a breast in a patient with other signs of AI/HS may respond to intralesional triamcinolone (a steroid) but more likely needs unroofing as definitive care. Not antibiotics. Not excision. Not "I&D" (incision and drainage). If the lesion is fresh, and especially if solitary, then biopsy punch mini-unroofing is best. (See 8.7.3.1.)

Lastly, remember that the biotropic effect of antibiotics is always there. Antibiotics encourage yeast to grow, whether *Candida* below the navel or *Malassezia* above. Watch for these predictable side effects, and treat with fluconazole or ketoconazole, respectively. Their effective spectra of antifungal activity are reasonably specific with little overlap. Lipophilic ketoconazole for lipophilic Malassezia and hydrophilic fluconazole for hydrophilic Candida.

8.5.3 Ketoconazole, ivermectin, and crotamiton

Ketoconazole, like most of the azoles, is both anti-inflammatory and antimicrobial. It is very useful in acne vulgaris and acne rosacea, but I've not tried it in AI/HS other than dealing with the remote side effects of excessively long courses of broad-spectrum antibiotics.

When it was first introduced, it was dosed on a daily basis, and soon earned the reputation of causing liver problems. Shuster, an early fan, studied its use in seborrheic dermatitis using ketoconazole 200 mg per day for 4 weeks and then 400 mg daily for 4 weeks. He set it aside in 1984 with these words: "ketoconazole may occasionally produce hepatotoxicity … the drug is not suitable for prolonged treatment of seborrheic dermatitis and dandruff, its minor manifestation. It is to be hoped that an equally effective topical preparation or derivative will be developed" [68]. Professor Shuster's hopes for an alternative have not been realized but ketoconazole, despite its reputation, can be used with remarkable safety at one-seventh of its original dose.

One needs to realize that the primary impact of the drug on the liver is its ability to compromise the cytochrome P450 3a4 enzyme system. If this interference occurs on a regular daily basis, at the dosage approved at its introduction, general hepatic metabolic function is severely compromised. On the other hand, given once a week or less, ketoconazole in a dose of 400 mg is remarkably well tolerated. I have used it with patients for almost 20 years. Of course, working in a consulting practice, one does not double blind the treatment. Referred patients expect active treatment, the best available. That is what they are paying for, and that is exactly what they get with this drug. But a challenge has arisen. (See Box 8.2, "Ketoconazole Warning July 2013.")

BOX 8.2 KETOCONAZOLE WARNING JULY 2013

Daily use of 400 mg of ketoconazole (two Nizoral oral 200 mg tablets), as prescribed and approved for several deep life-threatening fungal infections, exposes the patient to sufficient inhibition of the cytochrome P450 3a4 enzymes to risk serious side effects, and this has led to the withdrawal of the drug for first-line use in such conditions in the European Union and the United States.

There has been no limitation on its "off-label" use in the United States for treating *Malassezia*.

The FDA "has not prohibited use of oral ketoconazole for indications that are not FDA-approved; these remain off-label uses for oral ketoconazole" and "agrees that off-label use should be based on firm scientific rationale, sound medical evidence, and a consideration of risk and benefit for the patient" [61].

Using ketoconazole 400 mg weekly is remarkably effective, at a dose that was not expected by the manufacturer to be effective, and so the drug was never subjected to FDA trials at this dose, nor for this organism. What seems to happen is that the remarkably lipophilic yeast *Malassezia furfur* concentrates in the sebum, its food of choice, which includes long-chain fatty acids essential to its metabolism. The drug is itself also remarkably lipophilic [69] and so is selectively absorbed into and retained in sebum. The reason the drug works is that a fungicidal dose is not needed because it is not necessary that the organism be killed. The yeast is instead "disabled" if exposed to an adequate dose of ketoconazole. Changes in the *Malassezia* cell wall render it unable to "hold on" to the walls of the duct, and it is pushed out of the follicular unit onto the skin surface in the natural flow of sebum and is washed away. In addition, presumably due to these changes in the structure of its cell wall, the yeast is unable to resist being phagocytized (eaten up) by the body's white cells and so, in the presence of ketoconazole, it is consumed and digested and disposed of by macrophages [70].

One problem is that it takes weeks for this to happen, so the patient needs to take the ketoconazole ("keto") for an eight-week course. Shuster noted recurrences after discontinuing the 4 weeks of ketoconazole. This is not unexpected because, in Shuster's trials, it had not been given for a long enough timeframe. The low-dose, long-term regimen gets around this limitation quite neatly.

A second problem is that keto, if one takes it *daily*, is stored in the fatty areas of the liver, seriously impairing liver enzymes, making the patient feel unwell, and interfering with the metabolism of other drugs the patient may be taking. This historical information is generally upsetting to the patient, other physicians and pharmacists, and other prescribers unless they are briefed on the safety of keto when used in this weekly, low-dose pulsed fashion. Adjustments may be needed for patients taking the cholesterol-lowering medications generally known as *statins*; the patient simply omits the statin dose the evening before the keto. My patients taking warfarin (Coumadin) are instructed to always take keto on Sunday and get their INR (international normalized ratio) on Wednesday. A weekly INR with a minor downward adjustment of Coumadin dose is usually needed. Patients taking proton pump inhibitors are permitted their morning dose as long as peanut butter is used to enhance absorption.

A third problem is that keto is not easily absorbed, even when taken with food. I usually order it for Sunday mornings, when neither school nor work interferes. It was thought best to take it on an empty stomach with a low-pH (acidic) drink like apple or orange juice. Coca-Cola Classic® provides the same low pH with less gastric upset but with an unhealthy dose of sugar [71]. Three ounces or 100 mL will do. The mixture rested in the otherwise empty stomach with no interference from added food or drink for an hour, and then breakfast was permitted. Patients occasionally felt a little queasy, but breakfast normally settled that. When there was gastric upset, the full dose was given with food or divided into two separate administrations, the second taken an hour before (or with) the evening meal on the same day.

Patients weighing less than 50 kg are prescribed one 200 mg tablet per week; those over 100 kg receive two at each weekly dose. There have been no FDA-sanctioned studies of these dosage schedules. These are considered "off-label" uses [72].

Grapefruit juice was initially recommended because its low pH enhanced absorption. More recent research on grapefruit interactions with many drugs suggests that caution is needed when grapefruit and other fruit juices are used when ketoconazole is given concurrently with several medicines. Grapefruit (the juice or the fruit) can inhibit cytochrome P450 3a4 and increase the absorption of several medications, risking toxic levels of dihydropyridines, terfenadine, saquinavir, cyclosporin, midazolam, triazolam, verapamil and possibly lovastatin, cisapride, and astemizole [73]. It can also lower the oral bioavailability of acebutolol, celiprolol, fexofenadine, talinolol, and L-thyroxine, while orange juice did the same for atenolol, celiprolol, ciprofloxacin, and fexofenadine [74].

For the past year, to minimize the gastrointestinal upset, and to take advantage of the drug's lipophilicity to enhance absorption, I have instructed patients to take the weekly dose with a swallow of water, followed by a tablespoon of peanut butter to enhance absorption. This is the same routine I use for isotretinoin, a derivative of the fat-soluble vitamin A. This works remarkably well, with excellent patient acceptance.

Fourth, it appears that *Malassezia* does not actually cause disease in the ways that other organisms do, by excreting exotoxins like the highly potent strangling diphtheria toxin, or botulinum's famous paralyzing

"Botox" toxin or the epidermolytic toxin of staphylo-coccal scalded skin syndrome. Such toxins directly harm the host. *Malassezia*, however, sits quietly on the skin and in the pores of almost all of us. As is the case with pollen allergies, only if we become allergic to the anti-genic surfaces of these little balls of protein do we trig-ger, and then suffer from, the allergic reaction that is generated. *Malassezia* yeast, at an average of 5 and up to 7 μm in diameter is about one-third the size of ragweed pollen, at a diameter of 16–27 μm. As with 'friendly fire', the reaction to both of these allergens originates in our own defensive weapons but harms us more than it harms the enemy, whether pollen or yeast.

The fifth problem is that recurrences are not at all unusual, as one would expect with an organism that is ubiquitous (lives everywhere). Remind patients that *Malassezia* lives on heads, hats, helmets, headrests, headbands, hairbrushes, hoodies, and housemates. Patients can markedly reduce the risk of reinfection by using selenium sulfide 2.5% shampoo/lotion or 2% ketoconazole shampoo or even selenium sulfide 1% shampoo. It is rubbed into the wet scalp weekly with fingertips, and left on the scalp for 5 minutes. This can be followed by the use of the patient's regular shampoo and conditioner to restore the hair's manageability.

In my undocumented experience, well over 50% of patients who respond to the oral regimen will be back within a year to 18 months with a recurrence. To reduce this 'failure rate' (as patients see it), I prescribe 16 tablets with three refills. Initially, two tablets are taken every week for eight weeks (for clearance), with the second prescription of 16 taken as two tablets every two weeks, the third prescription taken as two tablets every three weeks, and the fourth prescription taken as two tablets taken once a month. This is remarkably simple and remarkably effective, and is another example of early advice lost to time. Faergemann noted 20 years ago that a prophylactic treatment schedule of "a single dose of 400 mg every month" was effective [75].

8.5.3.1 In acne vulgaris

Ketoconazole is becoming more and more valuable to me in managing acne. Most of the patients I see are referred or previously treated, and most have already been on broad-spectrum anti-inflammatory antibiotics. Some of these are topical; some are oral. Almost with-out exception, they are referred because these are "anti-

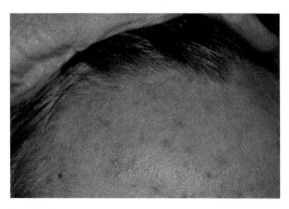

Figure 8.8 There are only two or three active lesions in the hairline, but the little folliculopustules on the forehead are classic.

biotic-resistant acne." In truth, they *are* "antibiotic resistant" but not because the *bacteria* are resistant. It is because the *Malassezia* is not at all inhibited by the anti-biotic; indeed, the reverse is true, and the yeast has sim-ply overgrown. This is generally unrecognized, and it is remarkably easy to turn around. The prescriber (because it is a prescription drug almost everywhere) has the option of simply starting the ketoconazole and continu-ing with the antibiotic or stopping the antibiotic, prov-ing the point with 8 weeks' worth of oral ketoconazole, and then reintroducing the oral or topical antibiotic on an "as-needed" basis.

In deciding whether to use ketoconazole in acne vul-garis, it helps to look for other signs of the *Malassezia* yeast. This includes small folliculopapules and papulo-pustules along the hairline (360° from the central fore-head to nape of the neck and back) and up into the scalp hair itself (Figures 3.10 and 8.8). This is exactly the pres-entation that was described early in the last century as *acne varioliformis* by early dermatologists. T. Colcott Fox in 1909 noted "typical papulonodules … along the bor-der of the scalp on the forehead" [76] that Graham Little later in 1925 called "characteristic of this eruption on the forehead at the junction of the hair and skin, on the temples … on the intermammary portion of the chest" (Figure 8.9) [77].

Itchy scalp is a sign of *Malassezia* at any age, as are the tiny pustules around the back of the neck and the excoriated folliculopustules in the scalp. Watch for the patient to unconsciously scratch his or her scalp during the interview. *Malassezia* is no respecter of social station; I've seen this scratch performed by all ranks

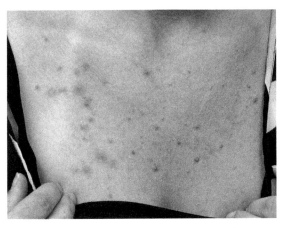

Figure 8.9 Often monomorphic folliculopapules, the lesions can be obvious folliculopustules and the surrounding urticarial erythema hints at the itch.

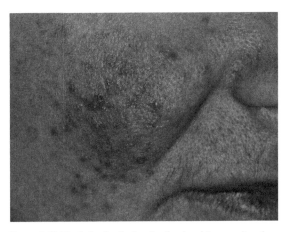

Figure 8.11 The lady also had active forehead "rosacea" and about four pre-sternal folliculopustules.

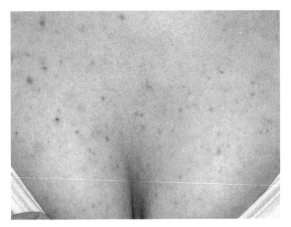

Figure 8.10 It is quite common to find all the diagnostic lesions with their tops scratched off.

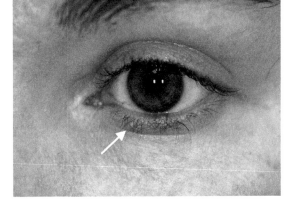

Figure 8.12 First visit April—blepharitis noted but thought to be bacterial (note pustule—white arrow—medial to telangiectatic area) with a history of styes.

from bus drivers to one Crown Princess. Often these patients have been on sufficient oral antibiotic that they have *Malassezia* folliculitis on the upper chest and upper back. Even though there may be only a half dozen little folliculopapules or folliculopustules, they are enough to suspect the diagnosis, and if they have had their tops scratched off, well, the diagnosis is essentially confirmed (Figure 8.10).

8.5.3.2 In acne rosacea

For papulopustular acne rosacea, a similar approach is taken. Again, these patients have often been on long-term antibiotics before they arrive for consultation. Many of them will describe the itchy little pimples, and

the question is whether the itch is due to *Demodex* or *Malassezia*. Simple physical examination may be all that is necessary to differentiate these two (Figure 8.11).

If there are small papules or pustules around the 360° "halo" area of the forehead and scalp, this is more likely *Malassezia*, especially if there is an associated itch. If the patient has been on broad-spectrum antibiotics, again *Malassezia* is more likely. If the patient has a somewhat suffused, marked central facial erythema and tiny superficial pustules over the nose, lower forehead, and cheeks (Figure 8.12), then *Demodex* is more likely. The eyelids should be closely examined for blepharitis, a

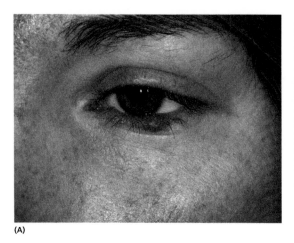
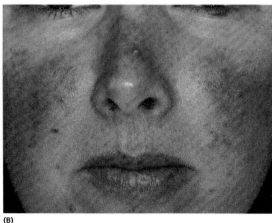

(A) (B)

Figure 8.13 (A) In August, the cheeks were worse despite antibiotics. The forehead is also involved, but the left lower eyelid tells the tale. (B) The bacterial pustules were gone, but the telangiectatic eyelid area had become nodular. KOH from the nose pustule was positive for *Demodex* and was cleared with ivermectin.

finding very suggestive of *Demodex*. A positive KOH coverslip sample of a pustule for *Demodex* (see Section 6.4) will show the way, but the blepharofolliculitis is a better marker (Figure 8.13).

Remember, of course, that every patient is allowed to have more than one disease. If there is confusion, use eight weeks of ketoconazole, assess the results, and decide whether or not it is time to shift to therapy that will deal with *Demodex*. If you wish to cover your bases, you can cautiously give doxycycline or minocycline in standard doses at the same time, reducing slowly as clearance occurs. The problem is that if you introduce two medications at once, you create two problems:

1 If there are side effects, it may be hard to decide which is responsible.

2 When the problem clears, it may be hard to decide which one to credit.

Be prepared for failures and recurrences. Patients with rosacea are sometimes incredibly complex and challenging.

If the problem is complicated by prior ineffective therapy, it is confused by unexplained flares and remissions, or the patient is impatient or demanding, it is wise to explain early that there is likely more than one organism causing trouble and it will take time to discover and eliminate all the causes. The patient may be expecting to see the problem gone quickly. This is an unreasonable expectation given the complexity, but the patient doesn't know that. An explanation is warranted "up

front" so that the patient's expectations can be brought into line with reality.

For Demodex, 0.2 mg/kg ivermectin (Stromectol®)—or one 3 mg tablet for each 30 pounds of weight—in a single dose weekly for three weeks may be given in *addition* to the anti-yeast and antibiotic. If the patient is averse to using the oral ivermectin, then a scabicide such as topical sulfur (2% precipitated sulfur in a cream base), permethrin 5% cream (Elimite®), or crotamiton 10% cream or lotion (Eurax®) is worth considering. These topical medications are best used overnight in order to catch the mites at play. I tell patients these are contraceptives for the mites and they will eventually die out.

If blepharitis unresponsive to antibiotic is present, the options are limited. Stromectol is a "specific" therapy, but I have used oral isotretinoin twice in this situation with success. Both patients had experienced years of trouble and were very grateful. Topical ophthalmic medications containing tea tree oil (TTO) are coming into use, but TTO is somewhat irritating for use around the eyes and the clearance rate is less than optimal. I prefer the safety and efficacy of ivermectin despite the cost.

Start using the topicals two nights a week for a week or two and move up to nightly if tolerated. Four weeks should empty the pores of all live mites. Hot new tiny pimples may break out as the deceased mites are recognized by the innate immune system and expelled in little pustules. The dead *Demodex* are recognizable on

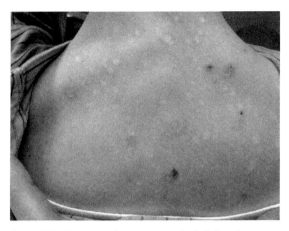

Figure 8.14 The *Malassezia* yeast causes the itch, but the patient does the damage. This is the excoriated shawl syndrome.

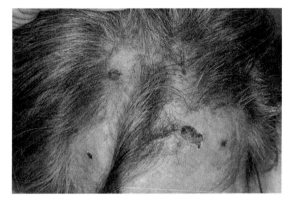

Figure 8.15 Patients are often labeled neurotic or psychotic when the problem reaches this extent. The itch *can* drive them crazy.

KOH examination as deformed and shrunken shadows of their former selves.

8.5.3.3 In acne inversa/hidradenitis suppurativa and dissecting folliculitis and cellulitis

There are no indications for these medications in pure AI/HS, but they must be considered in the event the patient is suffering from concurrent facial involvement with the deep and recalcitrant nodular variant of acne called *acne conglobata*, or the aggressive deep dissecting cellulitis and folliculitis of the scalp called *perifolliculitis capitis abscedens et suffodiens*.

In the scalp, *Malassezia* is a constant threat. It thrives on the sebum from our oil glands, is tremendously antigenic and pruritogenic (causes itch), and can cause patients to dig deeply into their scalp and upper back areas, producing the holes illustrated by Fox (Figures 8.14, 8. 15) [76].

Failure to suppress the pruritus by eliminating the *Malassezia* antigen is a common cause of therapeutic failure in several diseases. The common ill-advised symptomatic use of strong topical steroid scalp lotions, solutions, and shampoos simply worsens and prolongs the problem, especially when combined with broad-spectrum antibiotics. Even the condition known as Morgellons may be related.

8.5.4 Steroids

Corticosteroids, also known as *steroids* or as *cortisone*, or by their numerous proper generic and trade names, are wonderful friends and vicious enemies. They do an excellent job in calming inflammation.

But steroids are double-edged swords:

Steroids slow healing.

Steroids thin the skin.

Steroids encourage infection.

The last is an interesting feature, and is responsible for what we see as "rebound." If cortisone in a cream or ointment or other vehicle is repeatedly applied on an area that has a low-grade background infection, the body's natural control over that infection is reduced by the cortisone. Suppressing the immune response allows the background infection to increase, and sometimes the numbers of bacteria, yeasts, fungi, and even scabies multiply wonderfully. Then, when one stops the topical steroid, a "double whammy" occurs. There is a *sudden recognition* by the body's immune systems of the *increased population* of these uninvited guests. The defensive immunological reaction restarts very quickly and tries to catch up. If one had taken the precaution of either cleaning the skin beforehand with an antiseptic or prescribing antibiotics and/or antifungals to keep the population of multiplying organisms under control, the rebound should not have occurred.

When used with care, steroids are highly effective, and they do have a place from time to time in managing the acnes, but overuse can cause major difficulties. Years ago there was a wonderful preparation called Neo Medrol Acne Lotion®. The combination of neomycin and methylprednisolone in a sulfur-containing topical lotion would not stand up to the FDA requirements of today, but it was remarkably useful in managing both acne vulgaris and acne rosacea. If one considers that acne really is more of an inflammatory reactivity to materials trapped in and then released from within the follicular duct rather than a true infection, it makes reasonable sense to consider using steroids on the face, provided the bacteria and the yeast are under control. This approach has broad acceptance in European countries, particularly France. In the United States, the level of caution (or paranoia) with regard to the use of steroids on the face is very high. This is likely because of our extensive experience with strong topical steroids inducing rosacea-like dermatitis, the variant known as *iatrosacea* (iatrogenic rosacea = rosacea caused by the physician) [78]. In fairness, much of this was actually a variant that I call *reprosacea*, caused by pharmaceutical sales representatives claiming that their product was "safe for use on the face." We dermatologists should have known better than to believe the sales pitch. But I digress.

For acute situations (weddings come to mind), it is sometimes necessary to cool down acne vulgaris on an inflamed face in a short period of time. Several options are available.

If the oral antibiotic and antifungal coverage is already underway, for 3 to 5 days for example, a 3–4-day topical application of medium-strength steroid ointment can be justified to gain immediate control. If not, it would be wise to initiate immediate concurrent ketoconazole, full-dose doxycycline or minocycline, and the topical steroid of choice, perhaps triamcinolone 0.1% ointment nightly for a week. This is not something that should be repeated often, and the patient must be thoroughly cautioned to discontinue it after no more than seven days.

This could also be considered for acne rosacea. The patient must be warned that lack of discipline in stopping this steroid at the end of the prescribed seven nights is an invitation to trouble.

The eruption of hot inflammatory facial nodules likewise could be considered an emergency treatable with steroid, and the appropriate approach is with very small volumes of intralesional triamcinolone acetonide, saline diluted to 2.5–5 mg/mL, administered through a 30-gauge needle, and preferably given under cover of oral antibiotic and anti-yeast. The actual injection is administered through the healthy nearby skin into the center of the active lesion. It bears repeating that only a tiny volume is required, barely enough to be visible as faint blanching on injection; otherwise, visible and palpable pits (usually temporary, fortunately) may be induced as a result of local steroid-induced fat atrophy.

Systemic use of steroids is generally frowned upon, except in special situations. Again, emergency social situations sometimes qualify, but the most frequent use of systemic steroids is in the management of secondary flares due to isotretinoin. This drug induces an initial temporary flare of lesions in many patients, as X-ray therapy did in the distant past. It is sometimes necessary to stop the isotretinoin for a week or two, but usually it is possible to cool things down with oral or intramuscular steroids. The dose is normally 1 mg per kilogram of body weight, when given as intramuscular triamcinolone acetonide, with a maximum dose of 80 mg. This is given very infrequently. Oral prednisone is occasionally used at the same dose for a short 5–7-day pulse in managing such flares, but steroid side effects occur more frequently with the oral medication. Long-term use of either oral or intramuscular steroid is unwise, carries risks to several body systems, and is discouraged.

Acute flares of AI/HS occasionally require similar intralesional or high-dose, short-term systemic steroids, but carry the same risks referred to above.

8.5.4.1 The Marine

He came to see me in 2003, a high school senior. He had the worst acne I had seen since coming to the United States. His face, back, and chest were a mass of draining nodules. He bled as he took off his T-shirt. He regularly woke himself up when he stuck to his sheets. He ripped off crusts when he turned over in bed while sleeping. He had true acne conglobata. He wept in my office. It was pitiful. He had been on just about all the available antibiotics and topicals.

On enquiring into his diet, I found him heavily into dairy and the high-glycemic-load carbohydrates. Milk, macaroni and cheese, cheese, and pizzas were staples in his diet.

We discussed options. One was a zero-dairy diet. Another option was Accutane®. Eventually the family agreed to the Accutane and we got started on 40 mg daily. He flared, and he required pulses of prednisone, erythromycin, and ampicillin; dose reductions in Accutane; and holidays from Accutane. After eight months and a very rocky course, he was clear. Scarred, yes, but clear. No active lesions. I turned him loose, and I didn't hear from him again.

In 2009 I began an informal study looking into the recurrence rates of acne in patients who adhered to the diet versus those who slipped back into the high-carbohydrate and high-dairy world. My staff contacted him by mail with a short questionnaire. He didn't respond because he was out of the country. His mother did, though—she was handling his mail.

It turns out that his skin was so clear that he was able to pass the physical examination for the US Marine Corps (USMC). The Corps is well aware of the risks that hot climates and heavy backpacks and sweaty, stress-filled environments present to acne-prone individuals. Indeed, one of their dermatologists introduced me to a new variant of the disease—they call it *Iraqne*. They take care to screen out recruits with potential problems.

He was accepted into the Marines and is serving with real pride. To see his formal USMC portrait in dress blues and remember how he looked in a bloody T-shirt a few years previously is a lesson in itself. But the kicker was the note I received from his mother.

She wrote:

I have talked to (my son)—and we both agree—it was the dairy products that contributed to his Acne Conglobata.

He has been "Dairy Free" since his first O.V. (office visit) with you.

After (he) left for Boot Camp I found many unopened packets of Accutane under his bed!!

I learned later → he did not want to take such a powerful drug.

He cleared up on Accutane?! NOT

This result was due to him never drinking milk, Mac and Cheese, cheese, pizza, etc --- ever again.

The Marine Corps builds men—but I don't think they need dairy products to do it!

Lessons learned: Even acne conglobata will respond to zero dairy, and once again, "It isn't all it seems … at seventeen."

8.5.5 Nonsteroidal anti-inflammatory drugs (NSAIDs) and biologics

The use of NSAIDs in acne vulgaris and acne rosacea is limited. Ibuprofen was used in combination with tetracycline and with minocycline for acne years ago, but this combination of therapy never really caught on [79]. Oral dapsone has been used (its success led to the use of topical dapsone), and even clofazimine has been tried in a very rare variant called *acne agminata* [80].

In acne inversa, however, the class of drugs called *biologics* is undergoing extensive clinical testing and the results are mixed. When used to calm the widespread inflammatory component of Hurley Stages II and III, the first biologic used, infliximab (Remicade®), continues

to display its superiority over other TNFα inhibitors and the more recent interleukin (IL) antagonists. These agents cool the fires, reduce the swelling, diminish the drainage, and clear the odor. They also prepare a more hospitable field in which to operate surgically, providing less drainage and greater clarity of the margins, and sometimes they are successful in achieving full remission. Regrettably, they can only rarely be discontinued without a recurrence showing up within weeks or months.

So far, none of the biologic treatments have been paired with the full dietary, hormonal, and lifestyle changes that are part of long-term prevention of new lesions, and without them they are doomed to fail. We need clinical trials that combine a strict zero-dairy and low-glycemic-load diet with a pharmaceutical manufacturer's product. This is likely to remain an unmet need for some time, barring sudden enlightenment at the FDA.

8.5.6 Phototherapy

Ultraviolet light has been used in the treatment of acne for years. It has several points of impact on acne, depending on the wavelength used, the intensity, the frequency of use, and the length of the exposure.

UVB is known to cause sunburn, and if it is sufficiently acute the skin will peel in response. This desquamation, traumatic though it is, can provide a temporary improvement in acne by opening some pores and allowing them to empty. Unfortunately, UVB damages the underlying collagen at the same time, weakening the support of the dermal blood vessels and presumably also the support tissues of the FPSUs. UVB is also capable of killing superficial bacteria and yeast, eliminating some of the antigens that are partly responsible for acne vulgaris, acne rosacea, and AI/HS.

UVA penetrates deeper into the dermis, and has a definite effect on inflammatory cell populations. By decreasing the population of inflammatory lymphocytes, there should be a significant improvement achieved as a result of diminished inflammation in the area. Tanning bed users have noticed the improvement in acne offered by such exposure. That real and obvious benefit provides part of the appeal of this dangerous procedure.

More recently, blue and red visible light sources have been introduced as therapies. Some studies looked at blue or red light alone, and some used pretreatment with a photosensitizing drug, a technique called *photodynamic therapy* (PDT). An extensive 2009 review of published work noted that "21 studies reported a reduction in inflammatory lesions and/or a significant improvement in acne. The light sources utilized included blue light, pulsed-dye laser (PDL), intense pulsed light (IPL) and red light. Studies comparing the use of PDT to light therapy alone demonstrated greater improvement in treatment groups pre-treated with a photosensitizer" (the PDT); "All studies reported reduction in inflammatory lesions or significant improvement in acne," and "Adverse reactions including photosensitivity, pustular eruptions, and crusting varied among photosensitizers and light sources" [81].

A PubMed search with the parameters "acne," "phototherapy," "follow-up," and "long-term" produced two relevant papers. One was a small study with "complete clearance" achieved in 100% (14 out of 14) patients with a mean follow-up time of 6.4 months. This PDT-treated group had a short 45-minute incubation of topical 5-aminolevulinic acid (ALA) followed by one minimally overlapping pass with the long-pulse (LP) pulsed dye laser (PDL) (595 nm, 7.0–7.5 J/cm2 fluence, 10-ms pulse duration, 10-mm spot size, and dynamic cooling spray of 30 ms with a 30-ms delay) [82]. The second paper was an update calling for "detailed study of an optimized protocol," a call that has yet to be answered [83].

PDT thus appears to be a useful therapeutic option for acne patients who are recalcitrant to standard treatments and poor candidates for systemic retinoids. Further studies are still needed before a consensus protocol can establish optimal photosensitizers, incubation time, activating light source, and frequency of treatment [84]. Meanwhile "blue light and photodynamic therapy show promise" [85], and "Blue light irradiation was as effective as benzoyl peroxide in acne treatment grades II and III but there were fewer side effects" [86].

A reasoned explanation for the improvement has not appeared. Although Choi showed in vitro that "cultured *P. acnes* were killed with both blue and red LED light illumination" [87] and while it is generally accepted that endogenous porphyrins may play a role as photosensitizers in the death of *P. acnes* under blue light activation, actual decreased counts of *P. acnes* are rare.

Two points need to be made here. The first is that dead *P. acnes* remain antigenic, and so simply killing them is unlikely to effect a swift decrease in inflammatory response. The second is that the arrival on the market

of home units for blue light therapy plus the unpredictability, pain, expense, and lack of an optimized protocol for PDT therapy are likely to lead to a swing toward self-care. Wheeland reports,

> The blue light treatment system offers effective, rapid, convenient and well tolerated treatment of inflammatory and non-inflammatory acne lesions. The majority of subjects consider it much gentler than traditional acne treatments and it facilitates effective treatment without the need for antibiotic exposure. The blue light treatment system and blue light therapy alone are attractive treatment options for acne vulgaris, both as alternatives to traditional acne treatments and as adjunctive treatments to complement existing therapies [88].

It is likely that patients will follow, as they often do, the path of least economic resistance and that may lead them to home therapy.

8.5.7 Post-inflammatory hyperpigmentation

The management of PIH requires understanding on the part of both physician and patient of the mechanism of formation of PIH and its clearance. What follows is my "patter," a straightforward explanation that I hope will be as acceptable to the reader as it seems to be for most (I cannot claim "all") of my patients of color.

First, I have the patient hold his or her hand out so we can both see that the pigmentation on the back of the hands and fingers is rarely uniform. There is hyperpigmentation over the knuckles and finger joints and usually in the creases of the palms as well. I point this out and tell them that this color is a product of one form of irritation, the repeated injury to the skin caused by simply flexing hands and fingers. It is the same over elbows and knees. It is due to minor injury to the melanocytes, the cells that make the brown color. Those cells have only a few ways to protect themselves from injury, and making color is one of them. It is the same process that causes tanning in lighter patients, where the color is caused by sun damage because the melanin that induces that color is designed to act as a protection against injury caused by the sun.

The problem in the acnes is that when an acne blemish is "hot," it injures the melanocytes in the area and the melanocytes do what they can do best—they make color. The problem is that this color stays there for several months. Many acne patients are more worried about the color (the "scarring") than they are about the acne, so that priority needs to be addressed. They need to understand that the real number one priority has to be to eliminate the actual cause of the acne and at the same time cool the acne as aggressively and as quickly (and as non-traumatically) as possible so that no new lesions are formed to make more dark marks. This means that if they want to get better fast, they should look at the most aggressive therapy I can arrange. I tell female patients that "I will not twist their arms to go on birth control pills [BCPs] but if they want to get better fast and want to twist MY arm to get the BCP, I am willing to help, with or without their GP, primary care provider or gynecologist."

If they smoke cigarettes or use other sources of nicotine, this means they must stop or I will refuse to prescribe the BCP. They also need to know that nicotine is a factor in worsening acne all by itself [89]. Although quitting presents another challenge, that lifestyle choice can be modified so that instead of "quitting smoking" being seen as a hurdle, "getting acne better" becomes a strong motivator to quit.

Next, I suggest isotretinoin as the fastest way to go. This is becoming a bigger challenge every year as the lawyers pull the noose tighter, but *nothing* works faster and settles the cause of PIH more efficiently. But that means insisting on absolutely no smoking; careful counseling looking for adverse family histories of clotting, strokes, and heart attacks before using BCPs; arranging for providing a restricted diet, plus obsessive pregnancy tests, attendance of appointments without fail, filling in monitoring forms online, and counseling, cajoling, explaining, and educating parents, siblings, referring and other physicians, significant others, and providers of alternative visions and versions of health care.

If isotretinoin is not an option, I try for BCP alone, with or without spironolactone. Failing the BCP, I push hard with spironolactone alone with appropriate advice regarding pregnancy risk.

The next challenge is getting rid of the *Malassezia*, which is now a routine in my practice. I use ketoconazole in the four weeks prior to starting and during the first four weeks on the isotretinoin. If my hand is forced to use systemic antibiotics, I use the ketoconazole on the same timetable for the first eight weeks of the antibiotics. If antibiotics are the choice, I stay away from minocycline in patients of color—nobody needs blue added to brown or black, even though it is reversible. Now that

tetracycline has reappeared in the United States at great expense, and in the absence of lymecycline, full-dose doxycycline is the best choice here but customs will vary globally. I tend to start doxycycline aggressively and taper as quickly as possible, but am sure to *get rid of the* Malassezia *first*; otherwise, it will trigger more inflammation and that will lead us right back up the road to hyperpigmentation.

Topical care is a real challenge because irritation must be kept to a minimum. My preferred comedolytic is adapalene 0.3% gel, basically because it seems to irritate less for the effect generated than anything else [90]. Once anti-yeast and antibiotic and comedolytic therapy is established, I will sometimes follow the path of our colleagues in France, who have much greater comfort using topical steroids on the face than we North Americans. It works, but I still hold my breath. Ointments are best, especially in our northern winters. The risk of "plugging pores" is inconsequential in the face of isotretinoin and very slight with concurrent topical retinoids. Then it is a matter of waiting until things smooth down.

In parallel with active management of the inflammatory component of acne is "the hard part"—the bleach/no bleach story. Patients of color, and even those Fitzpatrick Type IIs of "Caucasian" heritage and "olive" hue with melasma induced by BCPs, need to understand up front that the usual "bleach creams," even in prescription strength, DO NOT really BLEACH the PIH, the so-called scars, at all well. Period. *What they can do is block the enzyme that makes NEW color.* The old color has to fade slowly away, with Mother Nature's help, and with our assistance and cooperation.

The most important point to make is that the hydroquinone-based so-called bleach or fade or lightening creams are not very good at removing the color that is already there. While there may be a small portion of the melanin color that is broken up by hydroquinone [91], the original work was done on guinea pigs. There may be a problem in translating these studies from the guinea pig to our human patients because melanosomes show significant variations in their size, their tendency (or not) to form membrane-bound clusters, and their distribution both within the epidermal cells and ultimately in the epidermis. These variations are found in comparing Caucasian versus Asian versus African-American (A/A) skin, but I've been unable to find comparisons of guinea pig versus human melanosomes' diameter. The fact that melanosomes are found well up in the epidermis in A/A (but not at all in Caucasian epidermis) suggests the possibility that topical agents would have less need for penetrating capacity to achieve clinical lightening in A/A skin.

There is evidence that bleaching compounds are fairly ineffective on dermal accumulation of melanin, and that has prompted investigations on the effectiveness of physical therapies, such as lasers [92]. That is why it is so important to stop new "spots," because every new spot is a new site of irritation and damage. If the damage allows melanosomes to drop through the basement membrane into the dermis, a process called *pigmentary incontinence*, then that pigment cannot be simply desquamated (peeled off) because it is too deep for that. Aggressive attempts at removal will cause irritation that starts the color all over again, and the new color will again last for months. That is also why the topical steroid is used, to calm the inflammation as quickly as possible to cool the fires that brew up new color.

And all of that is why I encourage the most aggressive anti-acne therapy possible, as soon as possible, so the color can be allowed to start fading as soon and as quickly as possible.

Yes, I do permit *gentle* use of hydroquinone, and there seems to be no reason to use anything stronger than 2%. It can be applied after getting home from work or school, after the evening meal, or after the adapalene is applied at night and it can go on again in the morning, preferably under a true broad-spectrum sunblock. Patients must remember that it is going to allow the light areas to fade at the same rate as (or even faster than) the dark areas, and getting a perfect match is a challenge. There are many other creams and procedures that are offered to lighten the color, from ascorbic acid to kojic acid and from grapefruit extract to lasers and glycolic acid peels, but many of these are irritating, and *avoiding* irritation is highly important. Otherwise, a vicious cycle sets up: irritation → color → "fade cream" → irritation → color, and around again.

Two new products show promise. A new tyrosinase inhibitor, 4-n-butylresorcinol, is much more active than hydroquinone and others. It awaits commercial introduction [93]. There is another new product under development that is also hydroquinone-free and it will be watched with considerable interest [94]. Meanwhile, if you are a patient, choose your products and your advisors with care.

The popular belief in the effectiveness of "bleaching" or "lightening" preparations is deeply held worldwide. While ill-informed fair-skinned individuals seek darker pigment in tanning beds, and the wiser ones use spray-on color, they are hugely outnumbered by those with darker skins seeking a lighter skin tone. Wherever this market exists, it is exploited, and this leads to exposure to hydroquinone concentrations that approach or exceed toxic levels [95]. Counsel your patients to avoid especially the stronger ones available in the "gray market" behind the counter in beauty shops. The only cream that really bleaches melanin effectively and predictably is compounded with monobenzylether of hydroquinone, the chemical that Michael Jackson used to remove the residual color left behind by his vitiligo. I tell my patients that is not an option.

This raises still another problem, because one of the side effects of high levels of topical hydroquinone is the production of a darker color that is created on top of the melanin pigmentation. It is due to the action of homogentisic acid. Hydroquinone blocks tyrosinase, the enzyme that governs the change of tyrosine into melanin, and a parallel inhibitory action of hydroquinone on homogentisic acid oxidase is thought to produce the homogentisic acid responsible for the color [96]. Although it is diagnostic of exogenous ochronosis, this color can mislead the patient into thinking the melanin pigmentation is getting darker, encouraging her (or him) to use the hydroquinone with added enthusiasm, inducing even further pigmentation.

Now, there are two other major concerns with PIH.

First is to be certain there is *no new trauma*. That means absolutely no picking, squeezing, or scrubbing, and absolutely no facials, waxing, stringing, or laser hair removal. *Any* injury or irritation (remember the knuckles) will cause more color. If in doubt about what might or might not cause more color, call your dermatologist's office—not your best friend or your cosmetician or aesthetician or beauty consultant—talk to a *real* dermatologist.

Second, and this is a tough one, something most of my patients of color have never had to think about. *Patients with PIH* MUST *stay out of the sun*. They must pretend for the first time in their lives that they are freckled Irish redheads. Really. They need a big broad-brimmed hat. Find some big "Jackie O" or wraparound sunglasses. Perhaps a change in hairstyle will be needed to cover as much of the face as possible. Yes, use a tinted broad-spectrum physical/mineral sunscreen, or a cosmetic "foundation" that will do the same job. They must keep the sun, especially the deeply penetrating ultraviolet A (UVA) rays, off their dark spots. They should consider getting a clear (not dark-tinted) 99.9% UVA-blocking plastic film like Llumar® fitted to the inside surface of the door windows of their car or truck. UVA comes right through ordinary window glass and through most auto glass (unless you are driving a "high-end" Mercedes).

Has somebody in your world suggested a few tanning sessions to "even out" the color? We are not going there, either. Don't even think about it.

Dr Pearl Grimes, the African-American dermatologist with the highest credibility in this area, in a 2009 review of this subject, stated, "In addition, ultraviolet protective measures such as broad-spectrum sunscreens are fundamental to the successful management of these conditions " [97]. Since then, numerous "studies demonstrating skin lightening effects in soy, niacinamide, n-acetylglucosamine, licorice extract, arbutin, vitamin c, kojic acid, emblica extract, lignin peroxidase, and glutathione have led to the development of a growing list of non-prescription skin care products that can be incorporated (mostly as adjuncts) in the management of hyperpigmentation" [98]. The bottom lines? First, if hydroquinone really worked, who would bother developing an alternative? Second, if you want to fade those spots, you need to give the project ample time. Mother Nature's a slow old gal, but she will get the job done if you let her.

One final thing. Stop the steroids on the face as soon as possible. I cannot prove that this is important because finding experimental subjects who would volunteer to have repeated face biopsies would likely be impossible, but we know that healing in general is slower with steroid applied to the skin (that is why steroids make stretch marks). Once the redness has faded, the overall healing should be better *without* the steroid at this point in the process. You *must* allow the *healing* part of the inflammatory reaction to get back to work. Timing is a challenge, but the longer you wait to stop the steroid, the greater the risk of causing side effects from the treatment.

Yes, this is a tall order. It is a very difficult problem and every single aspect of care needs careful attention. You cannot pull that treatment wagon without all four wheels running smoothly. Together, we must clear the pores, cool the flames, calm the irritation, and contain the color. If one of those wheels falls off, progress will drag.

8.5.7.1 Prognosis

That leaves only two pieces missing from the story, the route to the cure and the route followed for maintenance and prevention. They both lead down the same road once again, to the need for adequate control of both hormones and diet. It is very common to see failure to control these twin problems. Unless this control is achieved, the acne problem will almost certainly recur, and so will the scars, marks, and PIH.

8.6 Hormone manipulations and therapy

Hormones drive acne. No hormones; no acne. But it is impossible to lead a normal life without hormones, so removing them completely is out of the question. That means we must look at a number of ways to minimize their impact. We can avoid ingesting them, and avoid ingesting foods that increase their potency. (See Section 4.2.4.) We can also find substitutes for the ones that cause trouble by using different ones that cause less trouble. We can block their effects directly, or alter their metabolic pathways.

8.6.1 Birth control pill selection

It didn't take long to learn that BCPs helped control acne almost as well as they control pregnancy. Most BCPs combine two different families of hormones, estrogens and progestins (also called *progestogens, progestagens,* and *gestagens*). There was so much estrogen (one called *mestranol*) in the first versions of "the Pill" that the impact on acne was obvious. How did it work? Well, the BCPs were taken by mouth and this oral administration led the absorbed estrogens right into the portal system of large veins that go from the stomach and intestines to the liver. There the estrogen increased the production of a protein in the blood called *sex hormone–binding globulin* (SHBG). As its name suggests, SHBG acts like a sponge. It binds the free testosterone floating in the blood and lowers the amount of circulating free testosterone so there is less "free T" available to turn on the acne.

It didn't take long to realize that these original high-estrogen BCPs produced significant bad side effects (like moodiness, depression, weight gain, and swollen breasts) as well as the good side effect (acne control). With time, the amount of estrogen in BCPs was gradually reduced. This slowly lowered the incidence of the bad side effects, but it also reduced the good side effects as well, so BCPs were not very effective in managing acne for a while. For about a decade or more, there was no clear advantage of one BCP preparation over another in treating acne. The estrogen dose gradually dropped to one-seventh of the original daily dose. At the same time, a number of different progestins became available. Eventually, a few were developed to be less androgenic (male-like), and therefore less acnegenic than earlier versions. The first really effective progestin that was truly non-androgenic was cyproterone acetate, marketed in almost every country in the world (except the United States) as Diane® and later in a lower estrogen variant called Diane 35®. Then along came drospirenone, a progestin related to spironolactone that not only was non-androgenic but also acted as an androgen blocker, effectively doubling its effectiveness in reducing acnegenicity. Drospirenone is the progestin in the present "fourth-generation" BCPs, which also contain low (30 µg) and very low (20 µg) doses of the standard estrogen, ethinyl estradiol. Sometimes written as *mcg* instead of µg, each microgram (µg) is 1/1000th of a milligram (mg). Concerns about the capacity of drospirenone to increase the risk of blood clots have focused interest on the progestin norgestimate, a reasonable alternative to drospirenone. Although it is slightly less effective against acne, it carries less risk of venous thrombosis. At least that is the world view at the time of writing.

8.6.1.1 Estrogens

The estrogen family rules femininity. Estrogens are female fuel; they energize women and enable them to fulfil the phenotypic potential that their female genotype maps out. From the time that a preteen or early teen's ovaries get to work until 40 or so years later when they start to fade, the three estrogens that run the show are estr**one** (E1), estra**diol** (E2), and estr**iol** (E3). Estradiol is the major actor, and a variant of this molecule, called *ethinyl estradiol* (EE2), is the estrogen most commonly used in BCPs.

The original estrogen used in the first commercial BCP was mestranol. It was initially found as a contaminant in the first BCP, which was intended to be progestin-only. When the mestranol content was found to control breakthrough bleeding, it was decided to include a specific amount in the formulation of the pioneering Enovid® 10 mg tablets. The 0.15 mg (150 µg) dose of mestranol added to each 9.85 mg norethynodrel tablet

was a much more estrogenic dose than the 20 to 30 µg of EE2 used in today's BCPs. The lower dose of estrogen used now makes BCPs much safer than they were in the past but also contributes less to the direct anti-acne effect of the BCPs.

While the progestins have taken over the anti-acne job, the estrogen component still has an indirect effect. Ethinyl estradiol, besides stimulating SHBG, influences the pituitary gland. It decreases the release of follicle-stimulating hormone (FSH). Giving estrogen early in the menstrual cycle lowers FSH. That inhibits follicular development and so prevents ovulation. By so doing, it also prevents development of the corpus luteum. That stops the output of progesterone and other related acnegenic compounds that normally follow ovulation.

8.6.1.1.1 Warnings

While this all sounds very positive, it is important to consider the downside of estrogens. The biggest problem is the difficulty with increased frequency of blood clotting. Clots in the legs are one thing, painful but survivable, but if the clot reaches the lungs, this is a life-threatening situation called *pulmonary embolism*. Patients past the age of childbearing, the population at risk for acne climacterica or rosacea and taking Premarin (an oral estrogen supplementation or estrogen replacement as used in the Women's Health Initiative study), are exposed to the added risks of clotting that may lead to either stroke or heart attack, especially in predisposed individuals. A recent study using *early* postmenopausal administration of different estrogens and progestins demonstrated much greater safety and more positive results [99].

At any age, the problem appears to be caused by changes in the clotting characteristics of the blood as a result of modification, when exposed to estrogen, of the clotting proteins that are made in the liver. Changing the route of administration seems to help, but it doesn't reduce the incidence to zero. There is some evidence that estrogen administered by patch [100] or by topical cream application is less likely to cause trouble, and the same was hoped for the intravaginal NuvaRing®, but there are already worrisome lawsuits. Reducing the dose of estrogen over the years has helped, but it is down about as low as it can get. While there is a theoretical advantage to avoiding the oral route and first pass of the estrogen through the liver, some of the non-oral techniques still cause higher levels of circulating estrogen. Whether the elevated blood levels of estrogen are themselves a risk, separate from the liver pass-through risk, needs definition.

In fact, nothing reduces the incidence to zero, even *stopping* all estrogens. Women (and men) taking no exogenous estrogen still get blood clots (see Figure 4.6). The risk is higher in pregnancy, in smokers, and even higher in patients who have hereditary abnormalities in their blood-clotting systems. One of these is the factor V Leiden anomaly, in which blood-clotting factor V is dysfunctional, increasing the risk of clotting. The other is the prothrombin II anomaly. Factor V Leiden is present in 4.4% of Caucasians, 0.87% of AA patients and absent in Asians and North American aborigines. A simple blood test can tell patients whether they are at risk. More recently, the relationship of increased clotting risks (both venous clots and heart attacks) has surprisingly and inexplicably been linked to non-O (A, B, and AB) blood type [101].

It is my personal belief that any woman contemplating taking estrogen should be tested for these anomalies. It would be a "once-in-a-lifetime" test and if done on a mass-testing basis would qualify as a public health measure, in my opinion. While I am fully aware that testing would not eliminate the risk entirely, it would certainly allow those with the most common varieties of clotting anomaly to reconsider adding estrogen-containing BCPs to the risk that their genes have already created. Unfortunately, the world experts disagree. They do not consider it to be "cost-effective" at present [102], but with the availability of newer technology [103], it is my hope that routine testing will become universally available soon. As the cost of genomic testing comes down, this is one part of the panel that may prove of value to millions.

8.6.1.2 Progestins

There is an important distinction that needs to be made between progestins and progesterone. The terms are often used interchangeably, an error and a source of confusion, even in the medical press. While there is no single "estrogen"—the word describes a member of a group of similar molecules—progesterone *is* a single well-defined molecule, like testosterone. Estrogens are one family of female hormones; progestins are the other. Progesterone is the prime member of its group and is one of many progestins. The word *progestin* (or *progestagen/progestogen* in the United Kingdom) is the group descriptor for the family of similar hormones that *pro*mote *gest*ation (pregnancy). In actual use, the

---

BOX 8.3 ESTROGENS AND PROGESTINS

*Estrone**	E1	*Progesterone**	P
*Estradiol**	E2	Drospirenone	DSP
*Estriol**	E3	Norgestimate	NGT
Ethinyl estradiol	EE2	Levonorgestrel	LNG
Conjugated equine		Medroxyprogesterone	
estrogens	CEE	acetate	MPA

***Natural human hormones are in bold.**

---

progestins in BCPs, in combination with the estrogens, deceive the ovaries into thinking that there is already a pregnancy present and that they are not needed. That has the effect of preventing follicular development and ovulation, thus ensuring no real pregnancy occurs.

Progestins, like all steroids, have a wide range of activities. They can support pregnancy to a variable degree, they can have variable effects on water and salt retention, and they can raise or lower blood pressure to quite a markedly different degree. They are also quite varied in the degree to which they are androgenic (or, indeed, acnegenic). They have been rated as to their various capabilities, as illustrated in Section 4.2.2.2. The more androgenic, the more impact they have on androgen receptors, and so more acne is generated.

Fortunately, there is one progestin that has an androgenicity rating of zero. Drospirenone not only is non-androgenic but also has the additional beneficial characteristic of being able to block androgens at the androgen receptor. Drospirenone also can retain potassium and thereby allow sodium to pass out of the body instead of accumulating to cause fluid retention. This has the generally highly desirable effect, for those who use it, of not causing weight gain. Its effect on the endometrial lining of the uterus seems to be less progestational, leading to a thinner, less thick, or less "plush" lining of the uterus, and so there is a diminished menstrual flow. This combination of positives has made the fourth-generation BCPs highly successful in the market. There are, of course, some side effects for some women. More appears in Section 8.6.2.4.

8.6.2 Androgen receptor blockade

The androgen receptor represents the location of last opportunity to block an androgenic molecule from turning on acne. There are several ways to do this. One way is to keep the receptor closed (natural repression), as discussed on page 50 in Section 2.9. Another way is to provide a molecule (key) to the receptor (keyhole) that will fit the keyhole but that will not "turn on" the receptor. Several are available to provide this type of blockade, which is called *competitive inhibition*.

8.6.2.1 Spironolactone

Spironolactone was the first androgen blocker to be used in acne. It was originally developed to block aldosterone, an entirely different steroid hormone that is not at all involved with reproduction. Aldosterone is made by the adrenal glands and is responsible for conserving the sodium and water that would normally be lost through the kidneys. Because it is a corticosteroid whose job is to regulate the mineral salt sodium, it is called a *mineralocorticoid*. Retaining sodium retains water as well, so this keeps blood pressure up. Spironolactone was developed to treat patients with high blood pressure by doing the opposite, increasing outflow of sodium and water, conserving potassium, and lowering blood pressure. Early in its development, a side effect was noted—an overdevelopment of breast tissue in men, called *gynecomastia*. This is due to a change in the ratio of androgen and estrogen, and, as it happens, the spironolactone impacts both. The androgen effect is reduced through spironolactone's blockade of the androgen receptor. Estrogens are increased two ways, by increasing the conversion of testosterone to estradiol (actually, a *double* effect because the concentration of *both* is affected) and by displacing estradiol from SHBG, thus increasing the amount of free estradiol available.

This just happens to be exactly what is needed to help manage acne, and spironolactone has earned a permanent place in the care of acne vulgaris. It is also useful as one of the several medications that reduce the activity of the FPSUs in AI/HS, and I expect that its use will increase as a result of a recent paper that associates its use with a decrease in incidence of acne rosacea [104]. It is useful alone, for example in women who cannot or do not wish to take the BCP. It can also be used as a supplement to increase the anti-acne effect of drospirenone-containing and other BCPs. Increasingly, it is being used to achieve the needed hormonal shifts by combining it with the third-generation BCPs containing progestin such as norgestimate. These have a better safety profile than the drospirenone-containing products, but are not

as effective against acne and need the extra anti-acne power of added spironolactone.

The dose varies depending upon the situation, but spironolactone can be effective in a dose as low as 25 mg daily. Most of my patients do well on 50–75 mg daily, and very rarely I have treated acne combined with hirsutism (unwanted hair on the face especially) with 150 and even 200 mg in women weighing over 100 kg. I prefer to "start low and go slow" with spironolactone, using one or two 25 mg tablets daily for the first month in women under 60 kg, and 50–75 mg over 60 kg. The dose is moved up stepwise to a dose just over 1 mg/kg, taken once daily. Cautions include avoiding use if kidney or liver function is impaired, in the face of potassium-conserving diuretics, if diabetes or low sodium or high potassium levels are present, or in the elderly. Postural hypotension (feeling faint on standing because of low blood pressure) can occur especially if fluid intake is less than needed. More importantly, watch for diarrhea (a side effect of high potassium) and for gastrointestinal bleeding (from ages 55 through 74 years, the risk is 13 times the natural age-related risk) [105]. There is a long list of uncommon side effects (See Table 8.1). Medication interactions may occur with lithium and potassium supplements. A host of other medication interactions are listed in Table 8.2.

Table 8.1 Spironolactone side effects.

Signs of high potassium levels (hyperkalemia), including:
    Abnormal sensations, such as burning, tingling, or pricking
    Muscle weakness
    Low heart rate (bradycardia)
Yellowing of the skin or the whites of the eyes (jaundice)
Breast enlargement in men (known medically as *gynecomastia*)
Breast lumps
Signs of an allergic reaction, including:
    Unexplained rash
    Hives
    Itching
    Unexplained swelling
    Wheezing
    Difficulty breathing or swallowing
Diarrhea
Nausea and vomiting
Impotence (in males)
Menstrual problems, including irregular or absent periods
Fever
Confusion
Headache
Drowsiness or lethargy

Table 8.2 Spironolactone interactions.

angiotensin-converting enzyme (ACE) inhibitor–thiazide combos
ACE inhibitors
acetaminophen–aspirin
acetaminophen–aspirin–caffeine
acetaminophen–magnesium salicylate–pamabrom
aliskiren
aliskiren–amlodipine
aliskiren–amlodipine–hydrochlorothiazide
aliskiren–hydrochlorothiazide
aliskiren–valsartan
amifostine
amlodipine–angiotensin receptor blocker (ARB) combos
amlodipine–ARB–thiazide combos
amlodipine–benazepril
antipsychotics
angiotensin receptor blockers (ARBs)
ARB–thiazide combos
aspirin–caffeine
aspirin–chlorpheniramine–dextromethorphan
aspirin–chlorpheniramine–dextromethorphan–phenylephrine
aspirin–chlorpheniramine–phenylephrine
aspirin–diphenhydramine
aspirin–doxylamine–dextromethorphan–phenylephrine
aspirin–phenylephrine
bismuth subsalicylate
bismuth subsalicylate–metronidazole–tetracycline
central nervous system (CNS) depressant–aspirin–caffeine combos
cyclosporine
desvenlafaxine
dexlansoprazole
diclofenac topical
digoxin
drospirenone
duloxetine
esomeprazole
heparin
hydrocodone–ibuprofen
ibuprofen–famotidine
lansoprazole
milnacipran
naproxen–esomeprazole
NSAIDs (Non-Steroidal Anti-Inflammatory Drugs)
NSAID–chlorpheniramine–pseudoephedrine combos
NSAID–diphenhydramine combos
NSAID–phenylephrine combos
NSAID–pseudoephedrine combos
octreotide
omeprazole
oprelvekin
oxycodone–ibuprofen
pantoprazole
polyethylene glycol–electrolytes
rabeprazole

Table 8.2 Cont'd

salicylates
sodium phosphates
sodium sulfate–potassium sulfate–magnesium sulfate
selective serotonin reuptake inhibitors (SSRIs): all
sumatriptan–naproxen sodium
tacrolimus
tizanidine
tolvaptan
trandolapril–verapamil
trazodone
trimethoprim–sulfamethoxazole
venlafaxine
warfarin

Caution Advised

aldesleukin
apomorphine
bile acid–binding resins
COX 2 inhibitors
iloprost inhaled
monoamine oxidase inhibitors, nonselective
maraviroc
mitotane
nitrites–sodium thiosulfate
sildenafil
tadalafil
treprostinil

Where there is a question of potassium levels being affected, intermittent testing is suggested. Fortunately, the population being treated for acne is usually younger and so is less likely to be taking such medications, but caution is advised. Monitoring for possible drug interaction is wise, but routine blood testing in unmedicated healthy women is unnecessary.

The product insert contains the warning "The use of spironolactone in pregnant women requires that the anticipated benefit be weighed against the possible hazards to the fetus." Studies showing adverse effects in rats, mice, and rabbits are generally at doses up to 100 mg/kg per day, far exceeding human use (1–2 mg/kg per day). There is also a warning that spironolactone "has been shown to be a tumorigen in rats." This worry has been set aside by two recent studies: one provided no evidence of an increased incidence of breast cancer in 28,032 patients exposed to spironolactone (hazard ratio 0.99) [106], while the other reviewed 28.5 million woman-years of spironolactone exposure and concluded "there is no evidence of increased risk with spironolactone" [107].

8.6.2.2 Cyproterone acetate

Cyproterone acetate (CypA), the acetylated and more active form of cyproterone, has a number of effects on the enzymes that affect steroid hormone metabolism, but its most important property in acne management is its ability to block the androgen receptor. It is also an effective progestin so CypA can be used for birth control and, at a dose of 2 mg combined with 50 mcg of ethinyl estradiol, it was originally introduced as Diane®. A reduction in the ethinyl estradiol dose to 35 mcg led to labeling as Dianette® in the United Kingdom and Diane-35® in Canada, where it carries the indication for severe acne. Like the other estrogen-containing BCPs, it also carries an increased risk of venous thrombosis (blood clots) and has recently attracted the attention of regulators in France and now Canada [108]. In the much higher doses of CypA regularly used in management of prostate cancer (50–300 mg/day), there is a risk of serious hepatic toxicity and on this basis the drug has never been approved for use as a contraceptive (or for prostate cancer) in the United States, although it is marketed in more than 116 countries [109].

Having prescribed Diane® and later Diane-35® for 134 patients from 1984 through 1997, my personal impression was that it was very valuable as a treatment for acne, but it suffered from significant "nuisance" side effects, the one most complained about being weight gain [110]. When drospirenone became available and it became apparent that it did not promote weight gain and actually helped control bloating and blood pressure, I was delighted (and so were my patients) to switch away from the cyproterone acetate–based Diane-35®.

8.6.2.3 Flutamide

Flutamide was developed specifically as an androgen receptor blocker and has had extensive use in prostate cancer. Unlike other androgen receptor blockers, it is not a steroid so it has no estrogenic, anti-estrogenic, progestational, anti-progestational, anti-gonadotropic, or adrenocortical activity, so theoretically it should be excellent for managing acne. It has been used in a few trials, originally in a dose that was high enough to risk liver toxicity. Although it seems to be relatively safe in lower doses, it has not been approved for use in women or the pediatric population, may cause fetal damage, and requires laboratory monitoring. Its use is sporadic and generally not considered for acne management unless there are special circumstances. A recent review

reports acute liver failure in five young women being treated for acne and hirsutism, all of them requiring urgent liver transplantation. The authors (and I) "believe that flutamide treatment should be preferentially avoided in young female patients with benign pathologies, or if it is used, patients should be warned of its potential severe complications. Also, serial liver tests should be closely monitored and, in case of elevations, the drug should be immediately withdrawn" [111].

8.6.2.4 Drospirenone

Drospirenone is at present the most effective progestin on the market for managing the androgens that cause acne. Its non-androgenicity, coupled with its ability to block androgens at the androgen receptor in the nucleus, is exactly what we and our patients need. The beneficial side effects that include no weight gain, reduced and less painful menstrual flow, and blood pressure control all add positives. In the United States, its ability to provide psychological support is recognized and it is FDA approved for management of premenstrual dysphoric disorder. As a prescriber, my first choice progestin is drospirenone but with that said, it is essential to be flexible. There are negatives, and some are serious. First, it is important for all prescribers and patients to realize that, as stated before, "Every woman is different and every woman is unique." Among the hundreds of patients I've treated with drospirenone, I've had a few who felt "awful" on the drospirenone-containing BCP, and a few whose mood changed dramatically for the worse. The positives? The vast majority of patients "love it," and they love the results. Of the side effects, the most concerning is the increased incidence of clotting disorders. These are basically due to the fact that the estrogen in BCPs goes directly from the stomach to the liver, where changes occur in the proteins that control clotting in the blood. All oral BCPs containing estrogens carry this risk, which seems to be mediated by a drop in free protein S and free tissue factor pathway inhibitor (TPFI) antigen levels. This drop in clotting inhibitors increases the risk of clotting. Although the mechanism is so far unexplained, this drop is associated with an increased resistance to activated protein C (APC), an established risk factor for thrombosis [112]. The real questions are why the addition of drospirenone as the progestin increases the risk compared to levonorgestrel, and whether shifting to a different progestin is warranted. A switch to the more acnegenic levonorgestrel-based BCP reduced the risk in some studies, but is counterproductive. Norgestimate is a reasonable alternative progestin, as it is less likely than drospirenone to cause clotting disorders and less acnegenic than levonorgestrel. This decreased anti-acnegenic effect can be bolstered by adding spironolactone.

8.6.2.5 Topical androgen blockers

The search for a topical androgen blocker has been frustrating. Initial attempts to achieve blockade with topical spironolactone in a cream base did not work out [113]. More recent work with a gel vehicle has shown promise both in reducing sebum output [114] and in reducing lesion counts [115]. Larger clinical trials are anticipated.

A new molecule, cortexolone 17α-propionate, has also been developed that shows some promise. Tested as a 1% cream formulation in a small series [116], it was well tolerated and showed a definite improvement in the acne as assessed using the Investigator's Global Assessment scale. Although absorbed through the skin to reach the androgen receptors, it is reportedly inactivated as it reaches the dermis, limiting systemic toxicity. We await FDA-sanctioned Phase 1 trial results.

8.6.3 Dihydrotestosterone minimization

Because DHT is the most potent natural androgen known, it is assumed that reducing the amount of DHT reaching the androgen receptor will decrease the overall acnegenic effect. To do this, several approaches are worth considering. The most obvious is the need to reduce the conversion of T to DHT, a process that is mediated by the enzyme called 5α-reductase. The second approach is to reduce the availability of 5α-reduced compounds that can be turned into DHT by the intracrine system. That is reviewed in Sections 4.1.1 and 4.2.4.1. Blocking 5α-reductase is a great idea but life is not that simple, because there are actually two 5α-reductase enzymes and they are distributed differently in the hormone responsive tissues of the body. The FPSU-bearing skin harbors predominantly 5α-reductase Type 1. The prostate and hair-bearing skin is host mainly to 5α-reductase Type 2, and this, we have been told, limits the use in acne treatment of the enzyme-inhibiting drugs that are available [117]. Nevertheless, there is some room for modulation of DHT in managing the acnes.

8.6.3.1 Finasteride

Finasteride is an inhibitor of the 5α-reductase Type 2 enzyme, and it has been proven useful at a dose of 5 mg daily for inhibiting prostatic hyperplasia and at a dose of 1 mg daily for slowing male pattern baldness. It is generally believed that the FPSU is populated by 5α-reductase Type 1, so finasteride should not be effective in managing the acnes. Though oft repeated, this may be an inaccurate and outdated concept. Following an initial positive report by Farrell *et al.*, in which finasteride was quite effective, in one man and one woman, at suppressing new lesions of AI/HS [118], Joseph reported significant and prolonged success in a small series of men and women [119]. More recently, it has been used in pediatric patients with AI/HS [120]. Although more work needs to be done, these reports suggest one of three things: 5α-reductase Type 2 is more widely distributed than presently believed, or the FPSUs involved in AI/HS have *both* 5α-reductase Type 2 and 5α-reductase Type 1, or finasteride may not be Type 2-specific.

The problem is that very little study has been put into the question of finasteride and acne by dermatologists and the drug industry, likely because of the teratogenic risk in women. Fortunately, there are always some disbelievers somewhere and a group of gynecological endocrinologists achieved a significant decrease in symptoms of acne in nine of 12 women in a brief clinical trial of 5 mg finasteride [121]. That adds further weight to the likelihood that the Type 1–Type 2 distribution may not be as neatly divided as we have been led to believe, opening the door to use of this drug more frequently in the acnes, particularly in HS/AI.

8.6.3.2 Dutasteride

Dutasteride irreversibly inhibits *both* Type 1 and Type 2 5α-reductase isozymes. If any available 5α-reductase inhibitor should be effective in the acnes, it should be this drug. In benign prostatic hyperplasia tissue, type 2 predominates but *both* isozymes are overexpressed. Data suggest that the same mix of Types 1 and 2 is present in the acnes, seeming to indicate that there is a much lower Type 1–to–Type 2 ratio in sebocytes than the reverse (Type 2–to–Type 1) ratio in prostate tissue [122]. Nevertheless, personal patients with acne and/or AI/HS have done very well indeed with dutasteride and diet. A single male with acne cleared impressively (Figure 8.16), initially slowly without strict dairy and carbohydrate restriction, and much more completely

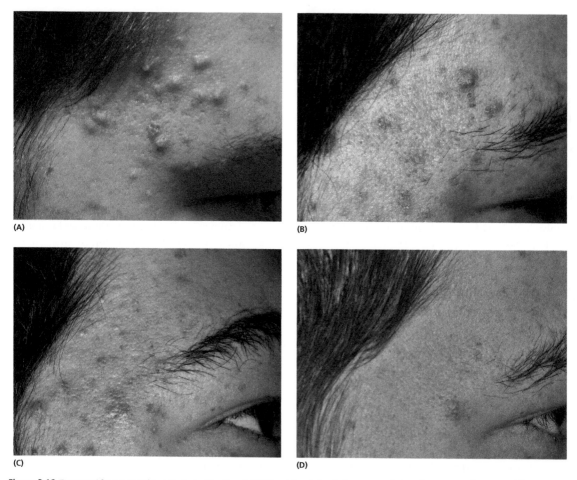

(A)   (B)   (C)   (D)

Figure 8.16 Dutasteride 0.5 mg/day (A) started in March 2007, with minimal dietary restriction due to compliance problems; (B) at seven months, October 2007; (C) at 19 months, October 2008, with dietary compliance improving; and (D) at 22 months, January 2009.

with full restriction. The prolonged course required to achieve success is illustrated in Figure 8.17. This man had a peri-anal sinus that took over two years to heal. There was a relapse midcourse when the patient returned to his dairy, thinking he was clear and could rely on the dutasteride. His symptom relief was almost complete, but it took another year to heal completely, using both dutasteride and dairy restriction.

Experience with the 5α-reductase inhibitors in andro-genetic alopecia reveals little of the impact one might expect on libido, but the very mention of such a possi-bility cools enthusiasm for the drug in a percentage of male patients. Males with severe AI/HS tell me that their sex lives are so compromised by the disease that "there is nothing left to lose." For women in the United

States, use is limited, except in exceptional cases, because of the risk of teratogenic effects and the aggres-sive warning label ("Women who are or who may become pregnant must not handle crushed or broken finasteride tablets, because the medication could be absorbed through the skin.")

8.6.3.3 Diet

As discussed in detail elsewhere, there are other sources of 5α-reduced steroids that are generally unrecog-nized. One of these is the cyclical appearance of 5α-pregnanedione, a product of the ovarian corpus luteum, after ovulation [123]. This molecule and several other 5α-reduced steroids have been found in cow milk (Section 4.2.4) and are present in all mammary secretions.

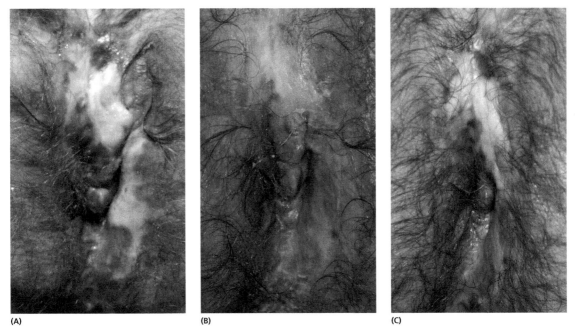

(A)   (B)   (C)

Figure 8.17 Dutasteride 0.5 mg/day (A) started February 2007 with full dairy restriction. From the "tag," the anus is at 11 o'clock and the sinus is at 1–3 o'clock. Note the firm oval swollen nodule at 1 o'clock in the whole complex. (B) At 17 months (July 2008), the nodule has resolved, and the sinus is more obvious at 3 o'clock as the swelling decreases. (C) At 29 months (July 2009), the original nodule has settled, the central tag has shrunk, the sinus has healed from below, and the patient is asymptomatic.

They are products of both the nonpregnant cow ovary and the placenta [124, 125], once that complex but temporary organ takes over from the ovary as a producer of pregnancy-supporting progesterone and its metabolites. Furthermore, it appears likely (although it is unproven) that these molecules find their way to the basal layer of the follicular portion of the FPSU, the basilar sebocytes, and the papillae of the hair roots where they encounter the enzymes of the intracrine system. That system can easily convert these 5α-reduced steroid molecules to DHT, even in the presence of a full blockade of 5α-reductase by dutasteride. These molecules are *already* 5α-reduced, so 5α-reductase is not needed, and the conversion to DHT is accomplished in only a few steps.

To produce the total drop in DHT required for successful prevention of acnegenicity requires a combined approach (Figure 8.18):

- Dutasteride blockade of 5α-reductase blocks *endogenous* DHT.
- Elimination of dietary 5α-reduced precursors stops *exogenous* dairy DHT sources.

A low-glycemic diet adds the finishing touches by repressing and so minimizing the receptivity of the

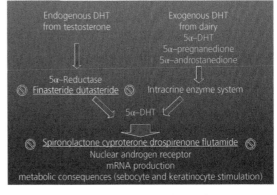

Figure 8.18 Total blockade requires both 5α-reductase inhibitors and avoidance of all dairy.

androgen receptor. This diet will not by itself allow the acnes to quickly heal unaided, but reducing the general levels of the acnegens is expected to help.

8.6.4 Phototherapy–hormone interactions

We have known for years that UVB light, as sunlight, tends to improve acne clinically. We also know that vitamin D is formed when UV light opens the B ring of the

7-dehydrocholesterol (7-DHC or provitamin D3) steroid molecule by a process called *photolysis*. An active pre–vitamin D3 molecule is formed and it isomerizes in the skin to vitamin D3. Thus was the original "phototherapy" born in 1919 [126] as a means of producing vitamin D in the skin of rachitic children (children with the bone disease rickets) in the days before oral vitamin D was available.

Photolysis of the steroid molecule is not limited to 7-dehydrocholesterol. Many steroids can be easily photolysed by radiation at wavelengths shorter than 320 nm [127]. In the early days of the oral contraceptives, it was reported by Ortho Pharmaceutical, Canada, that "the active steroid in Modicon tablets (contraceptive pills), ethinyl estradiol, could be photo-inactivated by light." It occurred to me that photolysis of the steroid B ring of the ethinyl estradiol or the progestin was likely at fault. Another 40 years later, UV light is now being used to degrade endocrine-disrupting chemicals in water, including testosterone and estrogens [128–130]. In addition, it was demonstrated years ago that photoinactivation of the estrogen-binding sites was possible [131].

With this as background, it was no surprise when the first reports arrived describing the effective use of various colored lights and lasers in the management of acne. Photolysis of the B ring of the T and DHT molecule has not been demonstrated in vitro or in vivo, but inactivation of hormone receptor sites, degradation of the testosterone molecule at sites other than the B ring, or photomodulation of other hormones and their derivatives in the skin would certainly seem to be potential ways of limiting or eliminating biological hormonal activity, presenting yet another area for investigative research.

8.7 Surgery

Acne surgery originally meant little more than emptying out plugged pores and pustules. The arrival of isotretinoin and the topical retinoids replaced much of the need for its daily use in the office, but it remains a valuable technique. It is both rarely and poorly taught; indeed, many recently trained dermatologists have never learned how to perform "acne surgery," and in some offices this is delegated to other staff. What follows is a primer of personal techniques.

8.7.1 Acne vulgaris

The idea behind all acne surgery is the removal of foreign material. The principle is very simple and applies equally to the mass of material trapped under the skin in acne inversa as to the comedonal contents of acne vulgaris. Because the innate immune system responds to such material, removal of the material will stop the response. Everyone who has ever had a "pimple" and squeezed out its contents to find that it quickly resolves is aware of this. Although there are standard warnings against "picking pimples," this procedure, glorified by the name *acne surgery*, is a reasonable approach to certain lesions. Indeed, sometimes it is the only effective approach, even in the face of isotretinoin.

8.7.1.1 Acne surgery for patients

The contents of a pustule that is near the surface can often be expressed, eliminating the keratinous core that is stimulating the innate immune system. Care, however, must be taken. Only lesions that are "ready" should be emptied and these should be only shallow pustules, not deep sore nodules that look like boils. It is customary to use an alcohol swab to sterilize the skin surface prior to nicking the top of the lesion. The alcohol swab can also be used to sterilize the end of a simple safety pin, and the top of the lesion can be nicked open with the pin. Pressure on the lesion must be directed carefully to be applied from below the lesion. We want the material squeezed upwards out of the pore, not deeper downwards into the subcutaneous tissue. With the top "opened," the delivery of the contents to the surface should be easy, with only a moderate amount of pressure. If this does not occur, further efforts should be stopped. The open area should be swabbed with alcohol again, and then a dab of 10% benzoyl peroxide lotion or cream applied and left on overnight.

So what happens when we "pop" that "pimple"? If we succeed in getting out just the pus from the top of the pimple, we get short-term cosmetic relief, but then the pus reforms, usually in less than 24 hours and often overnight. If we are successful in popping out the "core," which is the almost pure keratin plug from the ruptured central comedo, the follicle usually heals overnight. Sure, I know you've been told not to do that. That is because it is hard to "squeeze your own zits" safely and effectively. It hurts, and that will often make you stop the pressure before the "core" pops out. But Grandma was right; if you get the "core" out, then everything settles down. Even the ancient Romans knew that, and gave us the instructions "Ubi pus, ibi evacua"—Latin for "where there is pus, evacuate it." If that needs to be done, it is best done by someone with training, but sometimes only the patient is willing and available.

Blackheads (open comedones) may also respond to physical pressure, but likewise must be approached with due care. If they are truly wide open, they may be removed with ease. This is best accomplished after a simple soap and water wash, the main reason being to soften the lesion so that it can be expressed easily. Keratin loves to soak up water (that is why you get wrinkles from staying in the tub too long) but full "rehydration" takes time, usually about five minutes of soaking. The surface of the area is patted dry, and pressure is applied from both sides of the pore using fingertips only, no fingernails. It is best to avoid using any instruments. That should be left to your dermatologist.

Problem pores over the nose can be treated in this way, but instead of using an individual squeeze to each one, the involved area can be "rolled" between two index fingers or the finger and the thumb. This is actually a great way to make sure that topical medications get down into the pores. The routine is fairly simple. During or after the five-minute soak, you lather your face with bare hands, using either a gentle soap or a soapless cleanser to get rid of superficial oil, then rinse with warm water until "squeaky clean" and pat the area dry. Then use the rolled squeezing technique, rewash to remove all the oil that you squeezed out, pat the area dry, and then apply benzoyl peroxide, a retinoid, or other topical. This ensures that the medication gets as far as possible down into the follicle, where it will do the most good.

By the way, warm water does not open pores, nor does cold water close them. And while we are on the subject, pores do not "breathe."

8.7.1.2 Acne surgery for physicians

The use of true "acne surgery" should be restricted to physicians. Although some aestheticians do this work, the quality of the work varies. To be honest, the same is true of physicians, many of whom were never trained in this technique, so to describe this technique as *operator dependent* would be accurate. The main problem I have found with using this technique is that the instrumentation is limited and sometimes inappropriate. Some operators limit themselves to the use of the Unna type of comedo extractor, which is basically a small, bowl-shaped instrument with a hole in the center. The idea is that pressing this over an open comedo will deliver the comedonal contents up through the hole to the surface. This sometimes works, especially in widely open comedones, but there are a couple of tricks, especially for use where the opening is narrow and the comedonal mass is of a substantially greater diameter than the pore. First, lesions should be softened with a five-minute application of plain warm water. Second, for reasons I don't understand, it works better if the hole in the center of the extractor is applied just slightly "off center" of the opening of the pore.

Difficult lesions come in two types. Most difficult is the *closed comedo*, which needs to have an exit to the surface created. This was the reason for the invention of the Saalfield extractor, which has a short sharp lance on one end. This lance is invariably too dull, is often damaged by mishandling, and is a threat to both patient and operator. A handheld disposable 20- to 30-gauge needle is the most cost-effective sterile instrument I have found. The side of the bevel of the needle is used as a tiny knife to enlarge the orifice of a blackhead or incise the top of a closed comedo prior to expression.

For closed comedones, the tiny incision should be made along the skin's natural relaxation lines, basically in the same direction as local wrinkles, either the obvious ones or the ones that can be seen by squeezing the skin gently in various directions. The incision should be about the diameter of the underlying comedonal plug so that the contents can be popped out without excessive (bruising) pressure. For open comedones, again respecting the natural relaxation lines, the needle is inserted about 2 mm directly into the blackhead and is used to flick open a tiny relaxing incision in the sidewall of the follicular orifice (Figures 8.19, 8.20).

The comedo extractor can then be applied, and there are two techniques to be considered. The first is the classic application of the bowl with the hole (the Unna comedo extractor) (Figure 8.21), and the second is a technique using side pressure. This requires the use of the edge of the bowl of the extractor. Using a finger to apply counter pressure, or holding the lesion folded between thumb and index finger, the edge of the bowl is pushed laterally toward the opposing finger, pushing out the contents of the comedo between the two. Because the operator will have already created an easy exit to the surface, the comedo's content is expressed

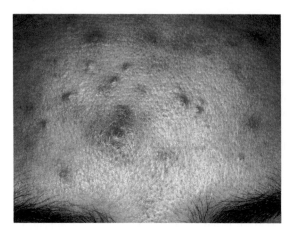

Figure 8.19 These comedones are "pouting" at the end of a third month on isotretinoin. The patient was distressed by the acuteness of the inflammation as each erupted and then left behind the brown post-inflammatory hyperpigmantation "scars."

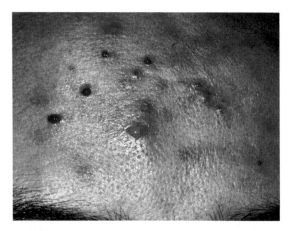

Figure 8.20 After 48 hours, these lesions will be almost imperceptible. All the tiny incisions were made transversely with a 30-gauge needle with no anesthesia, then gentle side pressure was used to pop out the contents using the smooth polished edge of an Unna comedo extractor. Bleeding is stopped with gentle pressure after hydrogen peroxide cleansing and a gentle alcohol wipe. Petroleum jelly or benzoyl peroxide gel is applied about an hour before bed.

with much less pressure than using the bowl technique unaided by this tiny "relaxing incision." One other tip: all surfaces of the comedo extractor must be mirror smooth, blunt, and rounded to minimize shearing trauma. This is especially important if one is doing acne surgery on a patient who is taking isotretinoin, because of the fragility of the skin caused by that medication.

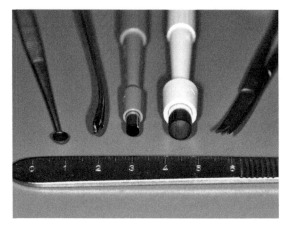

Figure 8.21 Left to right: a semi-sharp spoon curette, a polished and rounded Unna-type perforated spoon comedo extractor, a 4-mm and a 7-mm disposable biopsy punch, and blunt-tipped scissors, SuperCut® curved 5.5-in. Mayo (Miltex, York, PA) or 02.11.10 curved blunt 10.5-cm (Medicon, Germany).

Aftercare consists of a gentle hydrogen peroxide wash to remove blood, an alcohol wipe, and a thin application of simple petrolatum or soft paraffin. It is best to do this at the end of the school day so that the patient's face can recover overnight.

Warning! It is essential that this technique be avoided in managing inflammatory nodules, in draining sinuses, and in wounds that are actually infected as opposed to inflamed.

One other modality has recently arrived that may be worth considering, the combination vacuum suction–phototherapy machine. There are now two of these on the market [132, 133] and the initial trials show results that, from my review of the papers, surpass those using phototherapy alone. This is really not a great surprise, given the fact that eliminating the antigens in the pores by vacuuming them to the surface and cooling the inflammatory reaction down in the dermis with blue light address two drivers of the disease process. Aestheticians and some dermatologists have used less sophisticated vacuum devices for many years, and it will be interesting to see where these devices fit into the marketplace, whether in a dermatology practice or a beauty salon.

8.7.2 Acne rosacea

The phymatous material that is generated by the overgrowth of sebaceous and fibrous tissue can be reduced with several techniques, each with its adherents.

Amazing improvements in the physical appearance and the patients' quality of life can be achieved. Under local anesthetic, with epinephrine for control of bleeding, a simple scalpel blade, a CO_2 laser, cautery with a hot wire, or aggressive electrofulguration can work wonders. A full course of isotretinoin and the full hormonal and dietary regimen should be considered prior to surgery. Photographs illustrating the size and shape of the original nose assist the surgeon in avoiding the removal of excessive volumes of tissue with resulting deep scarring. The healing is usually remarkably efficient, aided by the ready availability of the sebaceous epithelium left at the base of the wound. Re-epithelialization is swift. An artist's eye and a sculptor's hand are valuable assets to the surgeon.

8.7.3 Acne inversa/hidradenitis suppurativa

As dermatologists acquired greater expertise in the surgical side of the specialty, their ability to manage the challenges of hidradenitis suppurativa increased to the point that there is now an overlap between surgical responsibilities and capabilities. Dermatologists, general and plastic surgeons, and urologists and gynecologists now share the responsibility for this area, each contributing areas of expertise. Thus the major surgery of "the acnes" is concentrated on the deepest acne, acne inversa, and its invasive advances into surrounding tissues.

In this disorder, what the patient needs is the physical removal of the epithelialialized sinuses, the proliferative mass, and accompanying inflammatory material. This invasive proliferative gelatinous mass (IPGM) is apparently produced by the combined action of stem cells, inflammatory cells, vascular granulation tissue, and the body's attempt to wall off this pathological proliferative activity in order to permit healing. It needs characterization.

In physically removing this offending material, there must be as little destruction of normal skin as possible, followed by unimpeded healing, with the best cosmetic result possible, and the lowest risk of recurrence possible. The techniques vary, depending upon the age, location, size, and extent of the inflammatory reaction.

No matter what the assigned Hurley stage or Sartorius score, there are only six or seven types of lesions in AI/HS. The earliest is the *solitary inflammatory nodule* involving a single FPSU. Left unattended, it may suppurate and a *fluctuant nodule* or *abscess* will result; and it may drain to the surface, creating a *draining nodule*. Failure to

fully drain and debride the inflammatory material leads to its spread beneath the dermis with further pain and swelling. If a *proliferative mass* is established, presumably by stem cells left behind in the subcutaneous tissue (Figures 1.20–1.26), the invasive gelatinous material spreads along tissue planes, taking the path of least resistance. As the mass spreads, the stem cells (the most likely candidates) attempt to re-create the type of tissue they were programmed to produce, namely hollow duct-like structures lined with squamous epithelium. These structures coalesce and become the *sinus tracts* that grow beneath the skin, forming the complex matrix upon which the hallmark *hypertrophic scars* then grow, thicken, and mature. The top portion of the exploded follicle, having lost its lower portion, its sebaceous gland, and its hair in the initial explosion, seals off its deep end with a scar. It then continues to respond to the acnegenic hormonal environment by producing keratinocytes in the residual acroinfundibulum, forming the sometimes multiheaded *tombstone comedones*. These structures are well named because each marks the site of a deceased FPSU, and represents a battle lost. These comedones are not a sign of early AI/HS; the comedonal plugs that actually start the disease are not generally visible, their deep and inverse presence generally announced only when that first *solitary inflammatory nodule* appears.

Each of these lesion types presents an opportunity to stop the progress of the disease surgically. The technique is chosen to fit the circumstance.

8.7.3.1 Mini-unroofing by punch biopsy

As I write this, I am accumulating experience with a simple technique for dealing with solitary (or multiple) *early* lesions of AI/HS. This is a technique that every dermatologist and many primary care physicians can handle with ease. It is suggested for use instead of the classic stab wound I&D, an overused and overrated technique yielding a high recurrence rate in these lesions. There are two problems with I&D. First, the wound closes and seals over, even if a drain is left in for a few days. Second, the cells that form the proliferative mass that causes recurrences are usually left behind. Both are avoided with early accurate punch biopsy debridement.

This technique is really quite simple and, because local anesthetic is used, it is possible to aggressively squeeze out the residual pus, keratin, and residual follicular wall. Curettage may be used to augment the

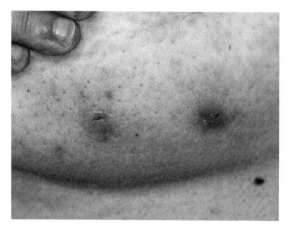

Figure 8.22 The patient was unable to make a timely appointment and took herself to the local emergency room, where the standard of care is incision and drainage (I&D). The healing stab wounds are closed over, and the underlying indurated tissue is palpably indurated and very tender.

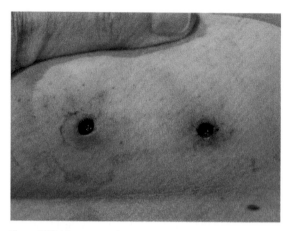

Figure 8.23 These 6 mm biopsy punch excisions yielded pieces of residual follicular material. The ferric chloride and petrolatum are all that are needed postoperatively. Simple adhesive bandage over the petrolatum is all that is required until healing.

clearance of this material but is not needed in a truly early lesion. This works only on fairly small *early* lesions of acne inversa, up to about 2 cm diameter, and this recognizes that the 2 cm is mainly inflamed tissue and edema surrounding an *individual* ruptured FPSU. For painful spots in the areas under breasts, under bra straps, along pantylines, and on buttocks, the pain relief is a joy. The amazing thing to me is the amount of excruciating pain, erythema, and swelling that a *single* ruptured FPSU can cause—and the incredibly fast and effective relief that can be provided with something as simple as a biopsy punch.

Punch biopsy debridement starts with infiltrative lidocaine and epinephrine anesthesia administered well beyond the margins of the wound, so as not to watch the loss of anesthetic solution as it pours out through the wound. This also avoids causing the patient more pain by distending the wound if it is not yet open to the surface. A 10–15-minute wait is allowed for blanching to indicate that both anesthesia and hemostasis are achieved, then is followed by a simple but deep as possible biopsy punch excision using an aggressive rotational twist. This removes the overlying disk of inflamed skin and includes as much of the damaged follicle and surrounding leaked material as possible. A 5 to 7 mm biopsy punch (see Figure 8.21) can be used to take out the whole plugged and leaking inflamed FPSU (Figures 8.22, 8.23). Underlying vessels and nerves can normally be avoided by pinching the involved skin and

subcutaneous tissue into a mound and "punching" the top of the mound. Every attempt should be made to center the cut over the offending follicular orifice so that the punched-out material contains the entire FPSU and surrounding debris. The wound is then aggressively debrided using digital and manual pressure to force any remaining FPSU material to the surface. The prime objective is to remove any of the proliferative mass material that may have started growing in the wound. I suspect suction would be of value, but I have not needed it for success. A spoon or bone curette (Figure 8.21) may be useful on some later lesions, but is not usually needed on early ones. Finally, a cotton-tipped applicator stick covered in coarse cotton gauze is used to forcefully dislodge and remove any residual debris. The wound defect is then sealed with a chemical cauterant or bleeding stopper. Ferric chloride 3.8 molal (37.5% in water) is preferred. The wound is left open with nothing but a simple thick dab of petrolatum, often with no dressing, but a simple adhesive dressing may be applied. Antibiotics are rarely used. Pain relief is almost complete with little or no further analgesia required. Healing leaves behind a small scar.

8.7.3.2 Unroofing

The same principles can be applied in larger, multiloculated, nodular, and abscessed areas and in sinus tract lesions. This is called *unroofing* in the United States and *deroofing* in Europe. It is simply a matter of removing the roof from the inflamed area or sinus, then cleaning out the purulent debris (if infected or seriously inflamed) and the proliferative mass (if present). The edges are beveled with scissors to improve healing cosmesis and to reduce the chances of overgrowth and premature closure. The base of the open wound is then sealed, using ferric chloride as a hemostatic, chemical cauterant, and aggressive biocide. The wound is covered with a thick layer of petrolatum as the only dressing [134]. No wick or packing is used. Such materials are not needed because the wound is not likely to close, nor do we wish it to. That is why we widened it in the first place. Stents, wicks, and drains act as foreign bodies in the wound, causing further irritation, pain, and pressure. They also abrade (rub off) the new epidermis that is trying to move in from the periphery to cover the healing wound after it fills in from below. We do not use them. See the procedure in Figure 8.24A–F.

I prefer to use sturdy scissors with rounded tips for this procedure, so that I can "feel my way." Sharp tips may create false passages while probing so I avoid them. It is faster and more convenient to use the scissors for probing instead of switching back and forth between scissors and probe. Some use a scalpel [135]; others rely on laser [136]. Neither blade nor laser gives me the "feel" of the wound that I rely upon, nor the ability to probe and follow sinuses. Ultrasound has been used to define the extent of the involvement [137], but I prefer direct visualization.

Whether the AI/HS patient is classified as Hurley Stage I, II, or III, it is the individual lesion type rather than the stage that dictates the choice of approach. Hurley III patients are classified according to their worst lesions and are often treated with very aggressive surgery for those difficult lesions (see Section 8.7.3.3). The amount of tissue destruction can be minimized in Hurley Stage III patients by utilizing unroofing where appropriate. This much less destructive technique, used on several of the lesions first, will reduce both the volume of involved tissue and the number of active lesions. Sometimes the anticipated major surgery can actually be entirely avoided by serial unroofing. Final scar revision can smooth out the residual with simple shaving techniques (Figures 3.5, 3.6, 3.7, and 3.8).

The original papers describing this procedure go back many years in the surgical literature [138], but despite a nudge by Henry Ford's Clarence S. Livingood [139], the technique never really took off. It sometimes means a staged approach in the outpatient or office setting, but this approach can keep the patient at work and out of the hospital, as was the case for "The Trucker" in Section 8.7.3.2.1 (and see Figure 8.25).

Preparing to unroof lesions in patients with deep inflamed and intercommunicating epithelialized sinus tracts presents the optimal situation in which to employ "the biologics" (see Section 8.5.5). These expensive intravenous and injectable blockers of various elements of the inflammatory cascade are the best temporary nonsteroidal anti-inflammatories available [140]. The object is to cool the surrounding inflammation and so improve the tissue condition around the active sinus and the invasive proliferative mass (Figure 8.26). This will, one hopes, wall off and localize the inflamed area. This will minimize the extent of the wound and improve the quality of the wound margins. If a flap or rotational graft is planned, the biologics generally make the work of the surgeon less onerous and the quality of the result less tenuous.

It should be noted that there is no evidence that these very selective inflammatory blockers slow the progress of the presumably stem cell–derived invasive proliferative mass. The patient in Figures 1.29, 1.30, 1.31, 1.32, 1.33, and 1.34, whose unroofing yielded classic photos of the cloudy pink and adherent variant of the proliferative mass, had been on adalimumab for six months prior to her unroofing procedure, with steady progression of her lesions.

This conservative tissue-sparing approach goes against the training of some surgeons, but those with the most experience dealing with extensive Hurley Stage III disease are well aware that these patients bring with them special problems, including a tendency to dehiscence (wounds that pull apart despite the best designed flaps and careful suture technique). When unroofing, the smaller the surgical wound, the better. Unfortunately, however, some patients' AI/HS has progressed beyond the stage where unroofing will succeed and these will need to have *ablative, extensive, definitive,* or *curative* surgery through wide surgical excision.

8.7.3.2.1 The Trucker

He was gruff, annoyed, and in pain. He had been to the emergency department three times and said they had "stabbed me and drained out some pus" and put him on broad-spectrum antibiotics. He was a long-distance trucker, on the road days at a time, from coast to coast,

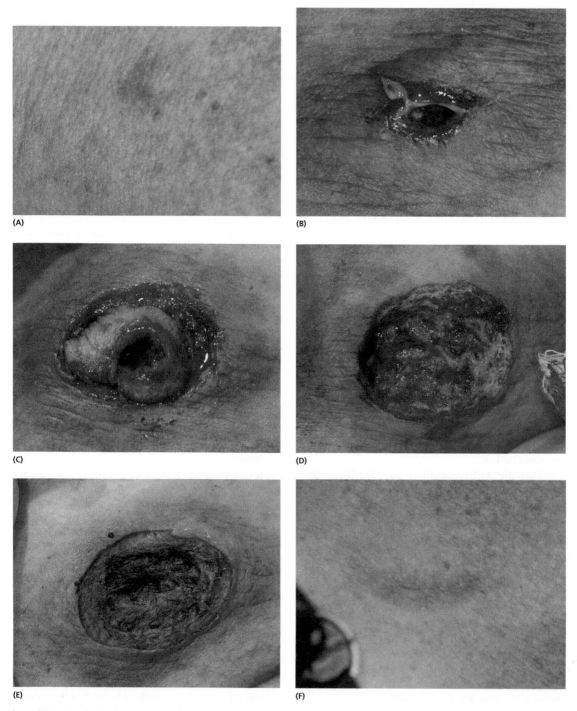

Figure 8.24 (A) Initial lesion thought to be innocent despite patient's warning, (B) three weeks later, (C) scissors excision out to margins, (D) debridement complete using gauze grattage, (E) ferric chloride hemostasis, and (F) result at six months.

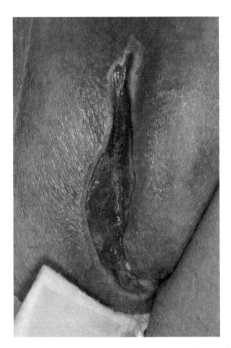

Figure 8.25 This sinus that ran from the 4 cm mid-buttock abscess to the anal verge was unroofed three weeks prior to the photo. The patient had used nothing on it but petrolatum while he continued his work as a coast-to-coast truck driver. When it healed, a second sinus from a second buttock lesion to the perineum and a third from the perineum to the scrotum were likewise unroofed without incident.

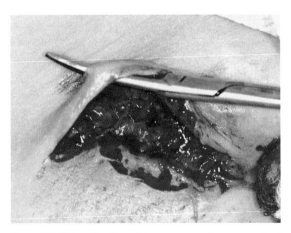

Figure 8.26 This is the closest I have seen to a "pure" sample of IPGM. Whether clear or cloudy, sterile or contaminated with bacteria, avascular or showing a pinkish glow, soft and easily removed with grattage or requiring a curette to separate from the base of the wound, the IPGM is the closest thing to a hallmark of acne inversa that has been described. It is unique in dermal pathology and warrants extensive investigation to delineate its source and functional capacities.

and the inflamed area was right where he sat. It was a 4 cm purplish red nodule in the mid-medial left buttock. He had had it for months.

What was worse, it had tracked, driven by the physical pressure of his sedentary (sitting) occupation. There was a sinus tract that headed downward and inward, toward the anus, where it then turned direction and headed "forward." It ended up in a fluctuant (soft and gel-filled) 5 cm mass on the back of the left side of his scrotum.

Medical therapy was started with doxycycline for the inflammation and dutasteride to block the hormones driving the problem. He went on the full zero-dairy low-glycemic-load diet, no easy chore on the road. I widely unroofed the buttock lesion and the track down toward the anus. I enlisted the aid of a local urologist to unroof the scrotal lesion. Postoperative dressings were with simple petrolatum (soft paraffin). No gauze and no packing were used. He just wore cotton undershorts under his work pants. He took no pain pills. He stopped the antibiotics after the first week, but stayed on the diet and the dutasteride. He sat on the well-greased wound from coast-to-coast until it healed.

And, aside from the surgical days off, *he did not miss a day of work.*

*Lessons lear*ned: Unroofing is the sovereign remedy for the undermining lesions of acne inversa, and the sovereign dressing is petrolatum (petroleum jelly).

8.7.3.3 Wide surgical excision

No matter which technique is chosen for AI/HS surgery, the surgeon needs to define the involved area, remove diseased tissue, leave behind as much normal and viable tissue as possible, and deal with the wound created. As described in this chapter, the involved area can be totally exposed by unroofing, and then there is no need to sacrifice truly healthy tissue. Unroofing takes the operator to the active edges of the disease process, both laterally and at depth, under direct vision. This technique allows the surgeon to minimize the overall size of the excisional area even where there are large involved areas of disease. Reference to the illustrations in Mullins' and Barron's papers is instructive, but the quality is inadequate for inclusion here [138, 139]. Unroofing of some of the more active sites on an outpatient basis during the weeks or months prior to considering definitive excisional surgery reduces overall activity of the disease process and can limit the morbidity caused by the eventual major surgical procedure.

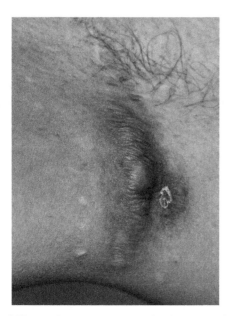

Figure 8.27a (A) The recurrence occurred within six months of the original surgery, despite intralesional steroids and antibiotics. It was unroofed successfully (B) The patient sought surgical care only when her perineal and peri-anal involvement became intolerable. There were only a few Dowling–Degos disease lesions in the axillae, and they were thought to be simple freckles until gluteal cleft biopsy confirmed the diagnosis.

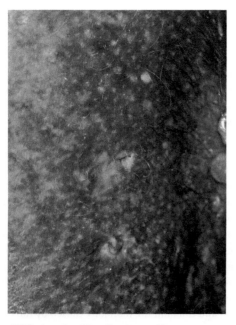

Figure 8.27b Associated Dowling–Degos disease.

As with unroofing, the inflammation in the area can be cooled substantially prior to "ablative" surgery by using one of the biologic medications, whether TNFα inhibitors or the newer anti-IL products. The newer "small-molecule" group of anti-inflammatories will doubtless be tried by the always innovative dermatology community.

To limit damage to normal tissue during wide surgical excision, ultrasound has been used to identify the extent of the subcutaneous sinuses [137], and laser has been used instead of scalpel and/or scissors for these excisions [136].

Total elimination of residual material capable of causing recurrence is the ideal. This is especially true if a primary closure is planned. A blind excision and closure can leave behind unexplored tunnels, unseen stem cells, and their progeny. That leads to the type of result seen in Figure 8.27a. One positive: the need to tidy up the problem with a thorough unroofing led to an unexpected and unsuspected diagnosis (Figure 8.27b).

Once the surgeon has removed the proliferative mass and the scarred tissue, and has explored all the edges for evidence of residual activity, provision must be made for the best healing environment possible. Depending upon the location of the wound, its size, the presence or absence of secondary infection or inflammation, the risk of contamination, and the patient's general health and healing capacity, smoking history, nutritional status, hormonal status, and presence of diabetes or other chronic or recurrent disease (always consider the possibility of Crohn's disease), the surgeon has several options to heal the surgical wound.

8.7.3.4 Healing options
8.7.3.4.1 Primary closure
Some lesions can be closed "primarily." That is simply a matter of cutting out the diseased area as accurately as possible, visually and physically checking to see that there are no residual extensions of the disease, and then suturing the wound closed.

Another way of covering the defect is to loosen up some nearby healthy skin and underlying tissue (called a *flap*) and then move it to cover the area. Flaps vary in size and composition, sometimes including muscle and a blood supply of arteries and veins. This turns what appears to be an "impossible to close" wound into a reasonable possibility and sometimes leads to heroic undertakings [141]. If and when successful, this can provide

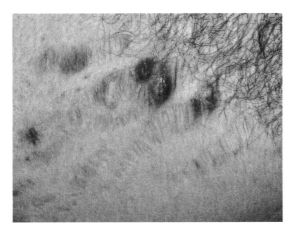

Figure 8.28 This association is not uncommon, suggesting that the tissue defect in follicular support may be responsible for more than just the weakness around the sebofollicular junction.

excellent results in patients whose prayers for true "closure" are finally answered. The vast range of flaps and graft types available is beyond this discussion.

Impressive when it is successful, this type of surgery is not without its problems. Some are specific to this population, one being the generally lax quality of the skin in these patients. Another is suggested by the high frequency of stretch marks, indicating less-than-optimum strength of subcutaneous support (Figure 8.28). I suspect that all AI/HS patients suffer from a defect in collagen metabolism that involves tissues well beyond those required for support of the structure of the FPSU. Indeed, I wonder if AI/HS patients suffer from a familial collagenopathy of sorts. Perhaps it is an elastin deficiency, or a reticulin anomaly, but the unflattering term *poor protoplasm* comes to mind.

Despite fine surgical technique by capable surgeons, the edges of primarily closed (stitched-up) wounds may separate and fall apart. This has a lovely name— *dehiscence*—that basically means losing adherence, either partial or full. Informed consent must include this possibility. Dehiscence leaves open an unpleasant and sometimes unanticipated wound with exposed subcutaneous stitches left to form a focus of infection; can lead to a disappointed, annoyed, or litigious patient; and can leave an unexpected and sometimes really ugly scar.

New lesions may be triggered by the trauma of surgery. Tension at the surgical closure area may generate a whole new set of lesions along the suture line.

Another problem with excisional surgery is the risk of leaving behind some of the proliferative mass. In cases of inadequate debridement, regrowth can occur right under the healing wound. This may possibly occur because surgeons are taught to handle tissue with care and may not be sufficiently aggressive in performing the dermal and subdermal grattage and often curettage needed to remove the somewhat adherent gelatinous proliferative mass (see Figure 8.26).

Infection in the sutured wound is another risk. The location in the armpits, groin, buttocks, or genital areas, where hygiene can be a challenge, can lead to difficulties with infection avoidance and infection control, especially in overweight and diabetic patients.

There is also the risk that a surgeon inexperienced in managing this disease may misguidedly attack the involved area as if it were an infiltrating cancer, removing all the subcutaneous tissue and fat, right down to fascia. The lesions, despite their apparent depth, do not normally grow very deeply. The normal pad of fat beneath the subcutaneous tissue (and beneath the disease) should be left intact to provide a base either for healing by secondary intention or for grafting with a split-thickness mesh (see Section 8.7.3.4.3). In either case, the padding provided by the fat should be spared for reasons of aesthetics and comfort. It is best not to have the healthy epidermis left behind sitting atop a cliff, looking over the edge, wondering how it will ever cover the crater. AI/HS is a disease of the epidermal appendages, so deep ablative surgery is not generally necessary. While there may be incursions of the proliferative mass into fat, it is far safer to leave such areas open, after the best gauze grattage and curettage debridement possible, to allow healing from below, without doing a closure. It is often best to simply leave that part of the wound to heal by secondary intention, even if it is tempting to primarily close or cover cleaner areas of the wound nearby with a flap or graft.

8.7.3.4.2 Secondary intention

For several of the reasons given above, and especially for large areas of involvement, the cumulative risks of primary closure are substantial. The preferred choice may be to perform the surgery without attempting to close the wound. If traditional excisional surgery is planned, this involves very carefully defining the margins by estimating the extensions of the subcutaneous sinus tracts, and then planning the surgical excision to get far enough beyond the apparent disease process to avoid leaving any behind. If laser, simple scissors or scalpel blade are used for unroofing, it is possible to minimize the volume of tissue removed simply by stopping when the edges of the active disease are reached. There is no need to cut beyond the visible disease, and the smaller the wound, the less time and discomfort will be spent on healing. In addition, because the disorder is triggered by trauma to susceptible FPSUs in the first place, putting the margins of the surgical wound under tension, particularly in pressure-sensitive beltline or weight-bearing or bra strap areas, is likely to be counterproductive.

While these wounds are fairly shallow because the disease itself is shallow, most of the time, there can occasionally be problems with true sinuses created by the IPGM burrowing deep into the tissue. This is usually driven to depth by the pressure of sitting, or by tight clothing, along the path of least resistance, usually along tissue planes, the areas where two tissues meet. An example would be an area like the groin crease where abdominal wall fat and the deeper material called *fascia* run side by side but are only loosely connected. The proliferative mass can extend along and between them, as it did in "The Trucker" (Section 8.7.3.2.1).

In this situation, excellent results can be obtained by simply allowing the wound to *heal by secondary intention*. This basically means allowing the fat and subcutaneous tissue and dermis to heal in from below. New granulation tissue grows in from below to fill in the gaps, and then the epidermis grows in from the edges to heal the surface. This allows an opportunity for any trapped areas of residual disease or undiscovered sinuses to "heal up from below," a process that is hampered when the inflammation and the proliferative mass are sutured in, under overlying dermis and epidermis.

The development of true fistula formation, with perforation of a hollow structure such as the vagina or the rectum, is very rare. Detection of such a structure must lead to suspicion that another diagnosis is responsible. Crohn disease or invasive squamous cell carcinomas are the major risks here.

In areas that tend to close themselves naturally, such as armpits and groin areas, secondary-intention healing works well. Mobility must be maintained to prevent the formation of adhesions and unwanted contractures (premature webbed scarring) across the wound. The fill-

ing in of the wound, the close approximation and restoration of the natural contour of the area, and its eventual coverage with new epidermis are wonders to behold. Every location needs to be considered independently. The results of such healing are often better than the surgical scars, because the process of natural contraction of the healing wound seems to automatically adjust to the movements and shapes of the area. Nevertheless, regular visits in the postoperative period are wise in order to detect and forestall unwanted healing and contractures, such as might occur with the adherence of the lateral wall of a labium majus to the medial aspect of a thigh. Such a bridging scar would produce a gaping vulva, a result best avoided with careful monitoring of the healing process.

8.7.3.4.3 Split-thickness mesh grafting

A mixed or hybrid approach is often used in large wounds. Primary closure may be undesirable or perhaps impossible because of the size of the area involved. The large surface area of the wound means that open secondary-intention healing time will be prolonged. Fortunately, special grafts can be used to speed up the process of secondary-intention healing. These grafts cover the wound only partially but they provide a bonus—a source of fresh new epidermal and upper dermal cells that do not need to migrate all the way from the wound edges. Normal skin wounds, like superficial burns or abrasions, heal using skin cells that come to the surface from the deeper undamaged sebaceous and sweat glands and the hair follicles that are left behind during most superficial injuries. They spread out on the surface to make new skin. That is how the donor site will heal.

The problem in AI/HS surgery is that the unroofing technique (and the classic surgical excision) has just been used to remove all the troublesome appendages and has taken all the healthy appendages as well, so a new source of epidermal cells is needed. The meshed skin graft provides this source of new skin cells, so surface healing can begin immediately instead of waiting for the epidermis to migrate in from the edges. This mesh graft technique not only speeds the healing of the wound but also allows any hidden buried residual disease both the time and the path needed to make its way to the surface (Figures 8.29A and 8.29B).

The grafted tissue is the patient's own skin, but the graft is *split thickness*. This means the graft is carefully

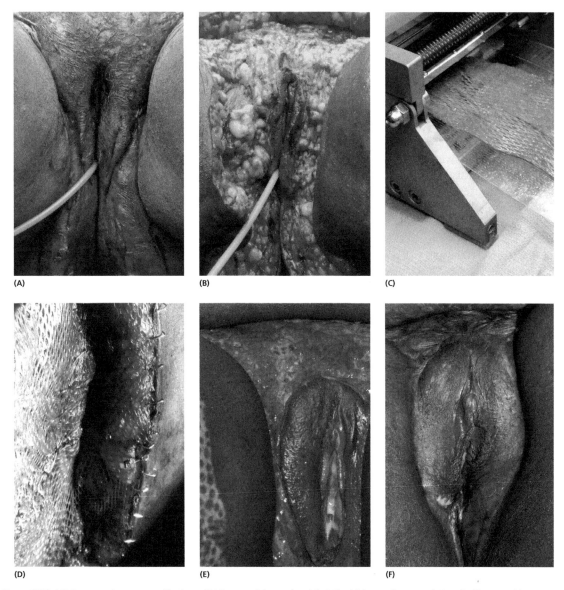

(A)   (B)   (C)

(D)   (E)   (F)

Figure 8.29 (A) Preoperative extent of lesions. (B) Post-excision to fat. (C) Split-thickness donor graft "meshed" to provide drainage, fresh cells, and coverage. (D) Mesh graft applied to wound and secured with staples. (E) Healing wounds showing partial "take" of grafts over pubis and repigmentation of healing donor site on thigh. (F) Final result at 1 year after healing of wounds and repigmentation of donor site. (Images courtesy of Dr. Hope Haefner, University of Michigan)

removed in a thin sheet from the surface of the patient's "donor site," often the front of the thigh or other flat area. A thin "shave" of skin is removed instead of cutting out a full-thickness piece of skin to apply as a patch over the area. Think of the difference between a thick slice of ham or salami (a full-thickness graft) and a sheet of waxed paper (the split-thickness graft).

The thin sheet of donor graft tissue is transferred to a machine that cuts numerous short linear parallel but offset slits into it (Figure 8.29C). The slits are alternated so that the sheet of tissue can be spread in a net-like pattern like the expanded metal lath used in drywall repairs or the open metal gratings used on some outdoor stairs to prevent feet from slipping. This thin mesh of skin (sometimes cut into several pieces) will cover an area three or more times the size of the donor area. It is carefully applied to the surface of the wound and is held in place with staples (Figure 8.29D), pressure dressings, special garments, or a special vacuum dressing that is used to remove excess moisture during the early healing process. Then a simple dressing with petrolatum alone allows final healing (Figure 8.29E and 8.29F) to occur. This process does have a downside—it creates another wound, the donor site, which is left to heal by secondary intention, and it takes time [142].

This is an expensive, labor-intensive, and usually hospital-based approach. Depending upon the size of the defect, it may require hospital admission. It certainly requires a highly skilled team, but it really is the optimal therapy. It represents the only real hope of clearing disease if the AI/HS has been ignored, misdiagnosed, and mistreated to the point that it has gotten beyond the care that can be provided in the office or clinic.

I hope that, some day, medical education and public education will be extensive enough, prevention will be promoted enough, and access to early treatment will be easy enough that all patients with this disorder will be treated while it is in its early stages, rendering this surgical approach unnecessary and obsolete. We are beginning to see this happen in our own patients and will publish on it when we have a large enough series with long enough follow-up.

From a solitary inspissated comedo to Hurley Stage III AI/HS, acne is a disorder driven by trapped foreign material that must be liberated by surgical means when prevention is ignored and the natural and medication-based processes of elimination fail.

8.8 Lights and lasers

8.8.1 Light and other radiation in acne

The beneficial effect of light on acne is not news. Every summer, almost all acne patients with outside summer jobs show significant improvement, even clinical clearing. Then comes autumn, a return to life indoors, and that includes school for most. That brings the stresses of education and, for many, a change in diet from mother's cooking to cafeteria or dormitory food. The stress and the diet share the blame for autumn's eruptions, but much of the responsibility for the flare may be due simply to the lack of sunshine.

So, what role does light have in acne? First, we need to look at the fact that "light" is not a single ray with a single set of physical characteristics. We can start at the infrared part of the spectrum, which produces warmth and even quite concentrated heat. Importantly, by increasing the temperature of the chemical processes in the FPSU, the rate of production of oil and the speed of production of the lining ductal keratinocytes may be increased, explaining the worsening of acne in warm environments. Heat also causes perspiration, and the mixture of sweat and oil on the skin increases the oily "feel" of the skin.

Next is the red end of the visual spectrum. Concentrated red light therapy has been shown to help acne, even when sourced from handheld devices, but the mechanism is not well defined [143]. Red light combined with blue light also provides benefit [144], and the red light used today for acne [145] was used years ago as the original wavelength to activate the porphyrin chemical applied topically in photodynamic therapy (PDT—see Section 8.8.1.2).

At the other end of the visible spectrum is blue light, also used for acne therapy in light sources openly available to consumers, and on prescription by physicians for another variant of PDT [146]. Beyond blue and violet visible light is ultraviolet light, the rays of the tanning–burning–wrinkling–aging–cancer spectrum, responsible for the damage to blood vessels that shows as actinic telangiectasia, the source of much of the rosy complexion behind acne rosacea.

Most light we experience is *spectral*. This means it contains many different wavelengths, seen as the classic rainbow "colors of the spectrum" in refracted visible light. There are also invisible rainbows, such as the UV spectrum that covers numerous wavelengths from UVA (400–320 nm) through UVB (320–280 nm) and into UVC (below 280 nm).

Ultraviolet A (UVA) is closest to the visible spectrum, then UVB and UVC. UVA is further subdivided into UVA-1 and UVA-2, and together they are termed *near UV*. UVA penetrates deeper than UVB, and it is absorbed (and so causes damage) deeper in the skin, and in the skin appendages, than UVB. This is the wavelength that damages collagen and causes wrinkles.

UVB penetrates less and so is absorbed closer to the surface, mostly in the top layer, the epidermis, where its major impact is also superficial, producing sunburn, superficial peeling, and skin cancers.

UVC penetrates so poorly that it doesn't even get through the atmosphere and rarely reaches earth, but it is used as artificial light to provide superficial antibacterial sterilization in food handling, health care, and other "clean" areas.

Even further beyond the UV spectrum are X-rays and then gamma (γ) rays. Although gamma rays have never been used in acne (they go too deep), X-ray therapy was used frequently prior to the arrival of tetracycline in the 1950s. The improvement in acne was thought to be due to the anti-inflammatory effect, but classic work by Strauss and Kligman showed otherwise. They stated, "X-rays have no primary anti-inflammatory effect in acne" [147]. X-ray therapy actually produced an effect very similar to isotretinoin, with a significant increase in inflammation and a marked miniaturization of the sebaceous glands. Clinical improvement occurred *despite* further inflammation caused by the radiation. Just as with isotretinoin, the "value of x-rays is prophylactic: *new lesions are prevented from forming*" [147] Side effects included induction of thyroid tumors in patients who were not provided with proper lead shielding, but it was the arrival of antibiotics that really closed out the X-ray era in acne. Some lessons were left behind (as discussed further in this section).

8.8.1.1 Radiation's targets

There are several targets that can be reached with these various forms of electromagnetic radiation, and the overall impact of any one modality is likely to be diffuse.

Remember first that the original acne lesion is basically caused by androgens. And remember the summer improvement, and that vitamin D is produced by the sun's action in the superficial layers of the skin? The initial step in vitamin D3 formation is caused by UV disruption of the B ring of the steroid molecule at carbon 9. The lysis (splitting) of this bond by packets of light called *photons* is called *photolysis* and is the mechanism by which provitamin D3 (7-dehydrocholesterol) is converted to previtamin D3 through the action of UVB radiation. Cholesterol itself is susceptible to photolysis by UV [148, 149].

We know that a summer in the sun will produce an abundance of vitamin D. One could speculate that the same photolytic mechanism might remove excessive androgens from the FPSU. (See Section 8.6.4.) Unfortunately, the photolysis reaction impacts only the unsaturated B ring of the steroid molecule, so photolysis cannot destructively rearrange T and DHT molecules at that site [150].

Another possibility involves the androgen receptor itself. The estrogen receptor is known to be susceptible to damage by UV light [151], and it is tempting to speculate that this may occur with the androgen receptor, a question that warrants investigation. One might wonder whether Cordain's jungle populations of Kitivan and Aché tribes had the additional advantage (besides their diet) of year-round photodamage limiting the activity of their androgen receptors, helping them to avoid the acne phenotype.

What other structures involved in acne production might be influenced by UV? Consider the wrinkling damage done to the collagen in the upper dermis by long-term sun exposure. Then consider the possible effect of this prolonged UV radiation exposure on the collagen that forms the *glassy membrane*, the basement membrane equivalent that provides support to the follicular part of the FPSU. Is it possible that chronic UV at summer doses weakens the constrictive support of the fibrous material that is wrapped around the follicular tube? Such weakness might allow the tube some flexibility in expansion, diminishing the pressure of actively reproducing keratinocytes so that they would not become anoxic, would not be inhibited in their terminal differentiation, and so would not plug up the duct in the summertime. And during the winter, the absence of light would allow the repair of the basement membrane and its equivalent, a process that perhaps could be measured using a more powerful confocal microscope than is presently available.

Then consider the impact of UV on the support structures of the dilated blood vessels that coexist with acne rosacea as actinic telangiectasia. Perhaps it is no accident that patients "with rosacea have relatively high vitamin D levels compared to control groups "[152]. Vitamin D and actinic photodamage come from the same source.

What of the impact of light on the resident organisms in acne? *Malassezia* growth is inhibited by UV in vitro [153]. UVB at 300 nm is most effective. *P. acnes* colony counts in vivo will drop from 100,000 to 3096 bacteria/mL with only 110 mJ/cm², not even a starting dose for UVB phototherapy for psoriasis [154]. A dose of 900 mJ/cm² totally inhibited in vitro growth of *Malassezia*, *Candida albicans*, and *Staphylococcus epidermidis* while reducing by 50 times the number of *Staphylococcus aureus* colonies [155]. This dose is easily achieved on the skin surface in the narrow-band UVB phototherapy units used in psoriasis. Although not suggesting that they were using tanning beds as treatment, Boldeman reported, "Adolescents with acne/seborrhoea, eczema or psoriasis used sun beds more than others without skin diseases" [156]. It is likely that they perceived or achieved real therapeutic or prophylactic value by lowering their microbial skin load, despite the incremental danger. Importantly, a much lower dose than is normal in a tanning bed would probably have provided the desired medical benefit, although not the same social effect.

And what is the impact of UVA, UVB, and visible light on the various components of the immune systems and the mediators of the inflammatory epiphenomena? In a word, it is *suppressive*. It inhibits antigen presentation, stimulates the release of immunosuppressive cytokines, induces the generation of lymphocytes of the suppressor subtype, and causes apoptosis (death) of leukocytes [157]. In addition to these general effects, the immune system is compromised by UV in an antigen-specific fashion via induction of immune tolerance. This effect is mostly mediated via specific UV-induced regulatory T cells. Upon activation, they release the immunosuppressive cytokine IL-10. This suppresses immune responses in a general fashion, a phenomenon called *bystander suppression* [158]. These suppressive reactions occur at moderate doses of UV.

Taking the same view of this mechanism as it applies to AI/HS would suggest that the *lack* of sun in the areas involved might be contributing to the pathogenesis of AI/HS by allowing the inflammatory cells free rein to destroy the follicular wall at will, basically the opposite of the protective effect that the increased sun contributes to the improvement in acne by damaging and neutralizing the inflammatory cells in skin, an effect we actively encourage (by using phototherapy units) in psoriasis patients whose papillary dermis is filled with the characteristic inflammatory cellular component of that disease. Perhaps we should be using phototherapy in all the intertriginous areas of our AI/HS patients?

At the other end of the exposure range, overdosing with UV creates increased inflammation. Sunburn is the obvious model, and anecdotal stories of improvement in acne induced by inadvertent sunburns are still heard from older patients who had access to "sunlamps" during their teens.

8.8.1.2 Light as a practical acne therapy

Because the thrust of this book is to emphasize preventive therapy first, it would be wonderful to report that regular daily home use of non-damaging blue or red light is all that is needed to destroy DHT or T precursor androgens in the skin, or to damage the androgen receptors, stopping the overproduction of ductal keratinocytes in the follicular unit of the FPSU. Sure enough, as therapy, "infra-red diode lasers used with a low-fluence, multiple-pass approach have … been shown to be effective with few complications" [159]. It must be noted that the mechanism is unknown. We will look forward to studies directed at prevention. The theory, and the references on red light cited in this chapter, support the wisdom of such practical trials, but attention to the long-term side effects of chronic exposure will be needed.

Meanwhile, light as active therapy is under much more aggressive investigation, particularly in the field of PDT. This technique relies upon the ability of a chemical, usually from the photosensitizing porphyrin family, to penetrate selectively (one hopes) to a target area. A dose of light of the specific appropriate wavelength is directed at the target molecules using bright (usually red or blue) incandescent light, IPL, or laser. This excites the chemical and causes the local creation of small but very active particles called *reactive oxygen species* (ROS) that cause almost instant oxidation (essentially burning) of the target tissue. Singlet molecular oxygen, hydrogen peroxide, superoxide anion radicals, and hydroxyl radicals all appear in an instant, react with local tissue, and produce the semi-selective damage that is desired. Numerous protocols have investigated various combinations of sensitizer molecule, concentration, vehicle, time of application, preparation of the target area, type of light source, exposure time and wavelength of light, and frequency of use for therapy and for prophylaxis.

So far, there is no simple, effective, convenient, painless, non-inflammatory, reproducible, inexpensive, insurance-covered PDT available for acne [160]. The home use of a blue light (Section 8.5.6) may come close—if it is safe for long-term use. If it could be guaranteed to eliminate only the exogenous hormones from diet and other sources, leaving innate human hormones alone, it would earn my blessing.

In the meantime, prevention still requires avoidance of dairy, at least in this book.

8.8.2 Lasers

Powerful light of a *single* wavelength can now be delivered using laser. Different lasers are designed to deliver different wavelengths, each wavelength shows a single specific color, and the other characteristics of light delivery vary widely depending upon the light that needs to be delivered. The red light of a HeNe laser pointer, for instance, is generated by activation of a mixture of helium and neon and has a wavelength of 633 nm. One of the variables that can be adjusted in a laser is the intensity of the light in the short burst of single-wavelength light produced; another is the length of time the light is switched on, and there are therapeutic differences between continuous-wave, short-pulse, long-pulse, and fractionated delivery.

A different technique allows spectral light (containing a specific wide range of wavelengths) to be released in a short pulse at high intensity, rather like a super-powered photographic flash. This is called *intense pulsed light* (IPL) and has several useful applications in the acnes. Whether delivered by laser or IPL, the wavelengths are the same as those found in visible light in nature; it is just that they are much more intense and display a highly selected wavelength or spectrum. Because of the intensity of these light sources, they can produce effects that are impossible to achieve with natural light, such as vaporization of tissue, destruction of superficial blood vessels, permanent hair reduction, and coagulation of bleeding blood vessels. In acne vulgaris, laser light can be used to activate porphyrin molecules in PDT (discussed in this chapter). In "rosacea," the accompanying background erythema of acne rosacea and the dilated vessels of actinic telangiectasia can be destroyed by multiple laser pulses or by IPL. In acne inversa, the cutting and destructive ability of the carbon dioxide laser is used by some surgeons to debride and unroof the lesions of hidradenitis suppurativa.

Lasers and other forms of electromagnetic radiation are truly versatile tools in management of the acnes, but they presently lack standardization, proof of superior efficacy, long-term safety, and broad availability.

References

1 Melnik BC, Zouboulis CC. Potential role of FoxO1 and mTORC1 in the pathogenesis of Western diet-induced acne. Exp Dermatol 2013 May;22(5):311–5.

2 Silverberg NB. Whey protein precipitating moderate to severe acne flares in 5 teenaged athletes. Cutis 2012 Aug;90(2):70–2.

3 Yeung A, Sheehan J. FDA measurement of hormone concentrations in milk and milk products [personal communication]. Communication to F.W. Danby, 2012 Jul 2.

4 Ben-Amitai D, Laron Z. Effect of insulin-like growth factor-1 deficiency or administration on the occurrence of acne. J Eur Acad Dermatol Venereol 2011 Aug;25(8):950–4.

5 Nichols K, Desai N, Lebwohl MG. Effective sunscreen ingredients and cutaneous irritation in patients with rosacea. Cutis 1998 Jun;61(6):344–6.

6 Capitanio B, Sinagra JL, Ottaviani M, Bordignon V, Amantea A, Picardo M. Acne and smoking. Dermatoendocrinol 2009 May;1(3):129–35.

7 Schmitt JV, Bombonatto G, Martin M, Miot HA. Risk factors for hidradenitis suppurativa: a pilot study. An Bras Dermatol 2012 Nov;87(6):936–8.

8 Vazquez BG, Alikhan A, Weaver AL, Wetter DA, Davis MD. Incidence of hidradenitis suppurativa and associated factors: a population-based study of Olmsted County, Minnesota. J Invest Dermatol 2013 Jan;133(1):97–103.

9 Adebamowo CA, Spiegelman D, Danby FW, Frazier AL, Willett WC, Holmes MD. High school dietary dairy intake and teenage acne. J Am Acad Dermatol 2005 Feb;52(2):207–14.

10 Melnik B. Dietary intervention in acne: Attenuation of increased mTORC1 signaling promoted by Western diet. Dermatoendocrinol 2012 Jan 1;4(1):20–32.

11 Vicini J, Etherton T, Kris-Etherton P, Ballam J, Denham S, Staub R, *et al.* Survey of retail milk composition as affected by label claims regarding farm-management practices. J Am Diet Assoc 2008 Jul;108(7):1198–203.

12 Martin Mittelstaedt. Scientists taking vitamin D in droves. Globe and Mail 2010 Jul 22.

13 Logan VF, Gray AR, Peddie MC, Harper MJ, Houghton LA. Long-term vitamin D3 supplementation is more effective than vitamin D2 in maintaining serum 25-hydroxyvitamin D status over the winter months. Br J Nutr 2012 Jul 11;1–7.

14 Miller PD. Vitamin D, calcium, and cardiovascular mortality: a perspective from a plenary lecture given at the annual meeting of the American Association of Clinical Endocrinologists. Endocr Pract 2011 Sep;17(5):798–806.

15 Hoppe C, Molgaard C, Vaag A, Barkholt V, Michaelsen KF. High intakes of milk, but not meat, increase s-insulin and insulin resistance in 8-year-old boy. Eur J Clin Nutr 2005 Mar;59(3):393–8.

16 Hoyt G, Hickey MS, Cordain L. Dissociation of the glycaemic and insulinaemic responses to whole and skimmed milk. Br J Nutr 2005 Feb;93(2):175–7.

17 Melnik BC. Evidence for acne-promoting effects of milk and other insulinotropic dairy products. Nestle Nutr Workshop Ser Pediatr Program 2011;67:131–45.

18 Cordain L, Lindeberg S, Hurtado M, Hill K, Eaton SB, Brand-Miller J. Acne vulgaris: a disease of Western civilization. Arch Dermatol 2002 Dec;138(12):1584–90.

19 Bray GA, Nielsen SJ, Popkin BM. Consumption of high-fructose corn syrup in beverages may play a role in the epidemic of obesity. Am J Clin Nutr 2004 Apr;79(4):537–43.

20 Verdolini R, Clayton N, Smith A, Alwash N, Mannello B. Metformin for the treatment of hidradenitis suppurativa: a little help along the way. J Eur Acad Dermatol Venereol 2013 Sep;27(9):1101–8.

21 Badr D, Kurban M, Abbas O. Metformin in dermatology: an overview. J Eur Acad Dermatol Venereol 2013 Nov;27(11):1329–35.

22 Melnik BC. Permanent impairment of insulin resistance from pregnancy to adulthood: the primary basic risk factor of chronic Western diseases. Med Hypotheses 2009 Nov;73(5):670–81.

23 Melnik BC. Milk—the promoter of chronic Western diseases. Med Hypotheses 2009 Jun;72(6):631–9.

24 Melnik BC, John SM, Schmitz G. Over-stimulation of insulin/IGF-1 signaling by western diet may promote diseases of civilization: lessons learnt from Laron syndrome. Nutr Metab (Lond) 2011;8:41.

25 Melnik BC. Leucine signaling in the pathogenesis of type 2 diabetes and obesity. World J Diabetes 2012 Mar 15;3(3):38–53.

26 Arun B, Loffeld A. Long-standing hidradenitis suppurativa treated effectively with metformin. Clin Exp Dermatol 2009 Dec;34(8):920–1.

27 Harvard School of Public Health, McGill University. Milk, hormones and human health [Internet]. 2008 [cited 2006 Oct 23]. Available from: http://milksymposium.mcgill.ca/summary/

28 Collier AP, Freeman SR, Dellvalle RP. Acne vulgaris. In: Williams H, Naldi, editors. Evidence-based dermatology. 2nd ed. Blackwell; 2008. p. 87.

29 Cunliffe WJ, Danby FW, Dunlap F, Gold MH, Gratton D, Greenspan A. Randomised, controlled trial of the efficacy and safety of adapalene gel 0.1% and tretinoin cream 0.05% in patients with acne vulgaris. Eur J Dermatol 2002 Jul;12(4):350–4.

30 Leyden JJ, Wortzman M, Baldwin EK. Antibiotic-resistant *Propionibacterium acnes* suppressed by a benzoyl peroxide cleanser 6%. Cutis 2008 Dec;82(6):417–21.

31 Kircik L, Friedman A. Optimizing acne therapy with unique vehicles. J Drugs Dermatol 2010 May;9(5 Suppl ODAC Conf Pt 1):s53–7.

32 Lev-Tov H, Maibach HI. The sensitive skin syndrome. Indian J Dermatol 2012 Nov;57(6):419–23.

33 Van Scott EJ, Yu RJ. Alpha hydroxy acids: procedures for use in clinical practice. Cutis 1989 Mar;43(3):222–8.

34 Leeming JP, Holland KT, Bojar RA. The in vitro antimicrobial effect of azelaic acid. Br J Dermatol 1986 Nov;115(5):551–6.

35 Gupta AK, Nicol K. The use of sulfur in dermatology. J Drugs Dermatol 2004 Jul;3(4):427–31.

36 Dreno B, Khammari A, Brocard A, Moyse D, Blouin E, Guillet G, et al. Hidradenitis suppurativa: the role of deficient cutaneous innate immunity. Arch Dermatol 2012 Feb;148(2):182–6.

37 Feucht CL, Allen BS, Chalker DK, Smith JG, Jr. Topical erythromycin with zinc in acne. A double-blind controlled study. J Am Acad Dermatol 1980 Nov;3(5):483–91.

38 Niren NM, Torok HM. The Nicomide Improvement in Clinical Outcomes Study (NICOS): results of an 8-week trial. Cutis 2006 Jan;77(1 Suppl):17–28.

39 Brocard A, Knol AC, Khammari A, Dreno B. Hidradenitis suppurativa and zinc: a new therapeutic approach. A pilot study. Dermatology 2007;214(4):325–7.

40 Formigari A, Gregianin E, Irato P. The effect of zinc and the role of p53 in copper-induced cellular stress responses. J Appl Toxicol 2013 Jul;33(7):527–36.

41 Boer J, Jemec GB. Resorcinol peels as a possible self-treatment of painful nodules in hidradenitis suppurativa. Clin Exp Dermatol 2010 Jan;35(1):36–40.

42 Kligman AM, Mills OH, Jr., Leyden JJ, Gross PR, Allen HB, Rudolph RI. Oral vitamin A in acne vulgaris. Preliminary report. Int J Dermatol 1981a May;20(4):278–85.

43 Rosa FW, Wilk AL, Kelsey FO. Teratogen update: vitamin A congeners. Teratology 1986 Jun;33(3):355–64.

44 Peck GL, Olsen TG, Butkus D, Pandya M, Arnaud-Battandier J, Gross EG, et al. Isotretinoin versus placebo in the treatment of cystic acne. A randomized double-blind study. J Am Acad Dermatol 1982 Apr;6(4 Pt 2 Suppl):735–45.

45 The Guide to Best Practices for the iPLEDGE Program [Internet]. 2007 Dec 2. Available from: https://www.ipledgeprogram.com/Documents/Guide%20to%20Best%20Practices%20-%20iPLEDGE%20Program.pdf

46 Werner CA, Papic MJ, Ferris LK, Lee JK, Borrero S, Prevost N, et al. Women's experiences with isotretinoin risk reduction counseling. JAMA Dermatol 2014 Apr;150(4):366–71.

47 Collins MK, Moreau JF, Opel D, Swan J, Prevost N, Hastings M, et al. Compliance with pregnancy prevention measures during isotretinoin therapy. J Am Acad Dermatol 2014 Jan;70(1):55–9.

48 Bernstein CN, Nugent Z, Longobardi T, Blanchard JF. Isotretinoin is not associated with inflammatory bowel disease: a population-based case-control study. Am J Gastroenterol 2009 Nov;104(11):2774–8.

49 Margolis DJ, Fanelli M, Hoffstad O, Lewis JD. Potential association between the oral tetracycline class of antimicrobials used to treat acne and inflammatory bowel disease. Am J Gastroenterol 2010 Dec;105(12):2610–6.

50 Layton AM, Dreno B, Gollnick HP, Zouboulis CC. A review of the European Directive for prescribing systemic isotretinoin for acne vulgaris. J Eur Acad Dermatol Venereol 2006 Aug;20(7):773–6.

51 Danby FW. Night blindness, vitamin A deficiency, and isotretinoin psychotoxicity. Dermatol Online J 2003 Dec;9(5):30.

52 Kligman AM, Mills OH, Jr., Leyden JJ, Gross PR, Allen HB, Rudolph RI. Oral vitamin A in acne vulgaris. Preliminary report. Int J Dermatol 1981b May;20(4):278–85.

53 Danby FW. Night blindness, vitamin A deficiency, and isotretinoin psychotoxicity. Dermatol Online J 2003 Dec;9(5):30.

54 Danby FW. Oral isotretinoin, neuropathy and hypovitaminosis A. Clin Exp Dermatol 2009 Oct;34(7):e260.

55 Misery L, Feton-Danou N, Consoli A, Chastaing M, Consoli S, Schollhammer M. [Isotretinoin and adolescent depression]. Ann Dermatol Venereol 2012 Feb;139(2):118–23.

56 Amichai B, Shemer A, Grunwald MH. Low-dose isotretinoin in the treatment of acne vulgaris. J Am Acad Dermatol 2006 Apr;54(4):644–6.

57 Mandekou-Lefaki I, Delli F, Teknetzis A, Euthimiadou R, Karakatsanis G. Low-dose schema of isotretinoin in acne vulgaris. Int J Clin Pharmacol Res 2003;23(2–3):41–6.

58 Cyrulnik AA, Viola KV, Gewirtzman AJ, Cohen SR. High-dose isotretinoin in acne vulgaris: improved treatment outcomes and quality of life. Int J Dermatol 2012 Sep;51(9):1123–30.

59 Agarwal US, Besarwal RK, Bhola K. Oral isotretinoin in different dose regimens for acne vulgaris: a randomized comparative trial. Indian J Dermatol Venereol Leprol 2011 Nov;77(6):688–94.

60 Boer J, Nazary M. Long-term results of acitretin therapy for hidradenitis suppurativa. Is acne inversa also a misnomer? Br J Dermatol 2011 Jan;164(1):170–5.

61 Howell JB. Aureomycin ointment in acne varioliformis. AMA Arch Derm Syphilol 1950 Nov;62(5):705–6.

62 Webster GF, Leyden JJ, McGinley KJ, McArthur WP. Suppression of polymorphonuclear leukocyte chemotactic factor production in Propionibacterium acnes by subminimal inhibitory concentrations of tetracycline, ampicillin, minocycline, and erythromycin. Antimicrob Agents Chemother 1982 May;21(5):770–2.

63 Labro MT, Abdelghaffar H. Immunomodulation by macrolide antibiotics. J Chemother 2001 Feb;13(1):3–8.

64 Webster G, Del Rosso JQ. Anti-inflammatory activity of tetracyclines. Dermatol Clin 2007 Apr;25(2):133–5, v.

65 Parry MF, Rha CK. Pseudomembranous colitis caused by topical clindamycin phosphate. Arch Dermatol 1986 May;122(5):583–4.

66 Walsh S, Creamer D. Minocycline in the management of acne vulgaris: the challenge of conveying pharmacovigilance data to primary care. Br J Dermatol 2012 Jun;166(6):1158–9.

67 Brook I, Frazier EH. Aerobic and anaerobic microbiology of axillary hidradenitis suppurativa. J Med Microbiol 1999 Jan;48(1):103–5.

68 Ford GP, Farr PM, Ive FA, Shuster S. The response of seborrhoeic dermatitis to ketoconazole. Br J Dermatol 1984 Nov;111(5):603–7.

69 Pyka A, Babuska M, Zachariasz M. A comparison of theoretical methods of calculation of partition coefficients for selected drugs. Acta Pol Pharm 2006 May;63(3):159–67.

70 Ashbee HR, Evans EG. Immunology of diseases associated with Malassezia species. Clin Microbiol Rev 2002 Jan;15(1):21–57.

71 Chin TW, Loeb M, Fong IW. Effects of an acidic beverage (Coca-Cola) on absorption of ketoconazole. Antimicrob Agents Chemother 1995 Aug;39(8):1671–5.

72 Davison L. FDA—Center for Drug Evaluation and Research [personal communication]. Communication to F.W. Danby, 2013 Aug 13.

73 Bailey DG, Malcolm J, Arnold O, Spence JD. Grapefruit juice–drug interactions. 1998. Br J Clin Pharmacol 2004 Dec;58(7):S831–40.

74 Bailey DG. Grapefruit-medication interactions. CMAJ 2013 Apr 2;185(6):507–8.

75 Faergemann J. Pityriasis versicolor. Semin Dermatol 1993 Dec;12(4):276–9.

76 Fox TC. Acne varioliformis in a man aged 37. Proc R Soc Med 1909;2(Dermatol Sect):94.

77 Little EG. Case of acne varioliformis. Proc R Soc Med 1925;18(Dermatol Sect):54.

78 Litt JZ. Steroid-induced rosacea. Am Fam Physician 1993 Jul;48(1):67–71.

79 Wong RC, Kang S, Heezen JL, Voorhees JJ, Ellis CN. Oral ibuprofen and tetracycline for the treatment of acne vulgaris. J Am Acad Dermatol 1984 Dec;11(6):1076–81.

80 Seukeran DC, Stables GI, Cunliffe WJ, Sheehan-Dare RA. The treatment of acne agminata with clofazimine. Br J Dermatol 1999 Sep;141(3):596–7.

81 Riddle CC, Terrell SN, Menser MB, Aires DJ, Schweiger ES. A review of photodynamic therapy (PDT) for the treatment of acne vulgaris. J Drugs Dermatol 2009 Nov;8(11):1010–9.

82 Alexiades-Armenakas M. Long-pulsed dye laser-mediated photodynamic therapy combined with topical therapy for mild to severe comedonal, inflammatory, or cystic acne. J Drugs Dermatol 2006 Jan;5(1):45–55.

83 Morton CA, McKenna KE, Rhodes LE. Guidelines for topical photodynamic therapy: update. Br J Dermatol 2008 Dec;159(6):1245–66.

84 Riddle CC, Terrell SN, Menser MB, Aires DJ, Schweiger ES. A review of photodynamic therapy (PDT) for the treatment of acne vulgaris. J Drugs Dermatol 2009 Nov;8(11):1010–9.

85 Kim RH, Armstrong AW. Current state of acne treatment: highlighting lasers, photodynamic therapy, and chemical peels. Dermatol Online J 2011a;17(3):2.

86 de Arruda LH, Kodani V, Bastos FA, Mazzaro CB. [A prospective, randomized, open and comparative study to evaluate the safety and efficacy of blue light treatment versus a topical benzoyl peroxide 5% formulation in patients with acne grade II and III]. An Bras Dermatol 2009 Oct;84(5):463–8.

87 Choi MS, Yun SJ, Beom HJ, Park HR, Lee JB. Comparative study of the bactericidal effects of 5-aminolevulinic acid with blue and red light on *Propionibacterium acnes*. J Dermatol 2011 Jul;38(7):661–6.

88 Wheeland RG, Dhawan S. Evaluation of self-treatment of mild-to-moderate facial acne with a blue light treatment system. J Drugs Dermatol 2011 Jun;10(6):596–602.

89 Capitanio B, Sinagra JL, Ottaviani M, Bordignon V, Amantea A, Picardo M. Acne and smoking. Dermatoendocrinol 2009 May;1(3):129–35.

90 Cunliffe WJ, Danby FW, Dunlap F, Gold MH, Gratton D, Greenspan A. Randomised, controlled trial of the efficacy and safety of adapalene gel 0.1% and tretinoin cream 0.05% in patients with acne vulgaris. Eur J Dermatol 2002 Jul; 12(4):350–4.

91 Jimbow K, Obata H, Pathak MA, Fitzpatrick TB. Mechanism of depigmentation by hydroquinone. J Invest Dermatol 1974 Apr;62(4):436–49.

92 Briganti S, Camera E, Picardo M. Chemical and instrumental approaches to treat hyperpigmentation. Pigment Cell Res 2003 Apr;16(2):101–10.

93 Kolbe L, Mann T, Gerwat W, Batzer J, Ahlheit S, Scherner C, et al. 4-n-butylresorcinol, a highly effective tyrosinase inhibitor for the topical treatment of hyperpigmentation. J Eur Acad Dermatol Venereol 2013 Jan;27 Suppl 1:19–23.

94 Makino ET, Mehta RC, Banga A, Jain P, Sigler ML, Sonti S. Evaluation of a hydroquinone-free skin brightening product using in vitro inhibition of melanogenesis and clinical reduction of ultraviolet-induced hyperpigmentation. J Drugs Dermatol 2013;12(3):s16.

95 Palm MD, Toombs EL. Hydroquinone and the FDA—the debate? J Drugs Dermatol 2007 Feb;6(2):122.

96 Levin CY, Maibach H. Exogenous ochronosis. An update on clinical features, causative agents and treatment options. Am J Clin Dermatol 2001;2(4):213–7.

97 Grimes PE. Management of hyperpigmentation in darker racial ethnic groups. Semin Cutan Med Surg 2009 Jun; 28(2):77–85.

98 Alexis AF, Blackcloud P. Natural ingredients for darker skin types: growing options for hyperpigmentation. J Drugs Dermatol 2013 Sep;12(9 Suppl):s123–7.

99 Schierbeck LL, Rejnmark L, Tofteng CL, Stilgren L, Eiken P, Mosekilde L, et al. Effect of hormone replacement therapy on cardiovascular events in recently postmenopausal women: randomised trial. BMJ 2012;345:e6409.

100 Olie V, Canonico M, Scarabin PY. Risk of venous thrombosis with oral versus transdermal estrogen therapy among postmenopausal women. Curr Opin Hematol 2010 Sep;17(5):457–63.

101 Sode BF, Allin KH, Dahl M, Gyntelberg F, Nordestgaard BG. Risk of venous thromboembolism and myocardial infarction associated with factor V Leiden and prothrombin mutations and blood type. CMAJ 2013 Mar 19;185(5):E229–37.

102 de Haan HG, Bezemer ID, Doggen CJ, Le CS, Reitsma PH, Arellano AR, et al. Multiple SNP testing improves risk prediction of first venous thrombosis. Blood 2012 Jul 19;120(3):656–63.

103 Svensson AM, Chou LS, Meadows C, Miller CE, Palais R, Sumner K, et al. Implementation of a cost-effective unlabeled probe high-resolution melt assay for genotyping of Factor V Leiden. Genet Test Mol Biomarkers 2011 Apr;15(4):207–13.

104 Spoendlin J, Voegel JJ, Jick SS, Meier CR. Spironolactone may reduce the risk of incident rosacea. J Invest Dermatol 2013 Oct;133(10):2480–3.

105 Gulmez SE, Lassen AT, Aalykke C, Dall M, Andries A, Andersen BS, et al. Spironolactone use and the risk of upper gastrointestinal bleeding: a population-based case-control study. Br J Clin Pharmacol 2008 Aug;66(2): 294–9.

106 Mackenzie IS, Macdonald TM, Thompson A, Morant S, Wei L. Spironolactone and risk of incident breast cancer in women older than 55 years: retrospective, matched cohort study. BMJ 2012;345:e4447.

107 Biggar RJ, Andersen EW, Wohlfahrt J, Melbye M. Spironolactone use and the risk of breast and gynecologic cancers. Cancer Epidemiol 2013 Dec;37(6):870–5.

108 Wu CQ, Grandi SM, Filion KB, Abenhaim HA, Joseph L, Eisenberg MJ. Drospirenone-containing oral contraceptive pills and the risk of venous and arterial thrombosis: a systematic review. BJOG 2013 Jun;120(7):801–10.

109 Collier R. Scrutiny of Diane-35 due to potential dangers of off-label prescribing. CMAJ 2013 Mar 19;185 (5):E217–18.

110 Vrbikova J, Dvorakova K, Hill M, Starka L. Weight change and androgen levels during contraceptive treatment of women affected by polycystic ovary. Endocr Regul 2006 Dec;40(4):119–23.

111 Brahm J, Brahm M, Segovia R, Latorre R, Zapata R, Poniachik J, et al. Acute and fulminant hepatitis induced by flutamide: case series report and review of the literature. Ann Hepatol 2011 Jan;10(1):93–8.

112 van Vliet HA, Bertina RM, Dahm AE, Rosendaal FR, Rosing J, Sandset PM, et al. Different effects of oral contraceptives containing different progestogens on protein S and tissue factor pathway inhibitor. J Thromb Haemost 2008 Feb;6(2):346–51.

113 Walton S, Cunliffe WJ, Lookingbill P, Keczkes K. Lack of effect of topical spironolactone on sebum excretion. Br J Dermatol 1986 Feb;114(2):261–4.

114 Yamamoto A, Ito M. Topical spironolactone reduces sebum secretion rates in young adults. J Dermatol 1996 Apr;23(4):243–6.

115 Afzali BM, Yaghoobi E, Yaghoobi R, Bagherani N, Dabbagh MA. Comparison of the efficacy of 5% topical spironolactone gel and placebo in the treatment of mild and moderate acne vulgaris: a randomized controlled trial. J Dermatolog Treat 2012 Feb;23(1):21–5.

116 Trifu V, Tiplica GS, Naumescu E, Zalupca L, Moro L, Celasco G. Cortexolone 17alpha-propionate 1% cream, a new potent antiandrogen for topical treatment of acne vulgaris. A pilot randomized, double-blind comparative study vs. placebo and tretinoin 0.05% cream. Br J Dermatol 2011 Jul;165(1):177–83.

117 Cilotti A, Danza G, Serio M. Clinical application of 5alpha-reductase inhibitors. J Endocrinol Invest 2001 Mar; 24(3):199–203.

118 Farrell AM, Randall VA, Vafaee T, Dawber RP. Finasteride as a therapy for hidradenitis suppurativa. Br J Dermatol 1999 Dec;141(6):1138–9.

119 Joseph MA, Jayaseelan E, Ganapathi B, Stephen J. Hidradenitis suppurativa treated with finasteride. J Dermatolog Treat 2005 Apr;16(2):75–8.

120 Randhawa HK, Hamilton J, Pope E. Finasteride for the treatment of hidradenitis suppurativa in children and adolescents. JAMA Dermatol 2013 Mar 20;1–4.

121 Kohler C, Tschumi K, Bodmer C, Schneiter M, Birkhaeuser M. Effect of finasteride 5 mg (Proscar) on acne and alopecia in female patients with normal serum levels of free testosterone. Gynecol Endocrinol 2007 Mar;23(3):142–5.

122 Seiffert K, Seltmann H, Fritsch M, Zouboulis CC. Inhibition of 5alpha-reductase activity in SZ95 sebocytes and HaCaT keratinocytes in vitro. Horm Metab Res 2007 Feb;39(2):141–8.

123 Backstrom T, Andersson A, Baird DT, Selstam G. The human corpus luteum secretes 5 alpha-pregnane-3,20-dione. Acta Endocrinol (Copenh) 1986 Jan;111(1):116–21.

124 Belvedere P, Gabai G, Dalla VL, Accorsi P, Trivoletti M, Colombo L, et al. Occurrence of steroidogenic enzymes in the bovine mammary gland at different functional stages. J Steroid Biochem Mol Biol 1996 Nov;59(3–4):339–47.

125 Zwirner M, Fawzy MM, Bopp FC, Klemm-Wolfgram E, Handschuh D, Voelter W, et al. Radioimmunoassay of 5 alpha-pregnane-3,20-dione. A metabolite of placental progesterone. Arch Gynecol 1983;233(4):229–40.

126 Rauschmann MA, Heine MC, Thomann KD. [The German Orthopedics Society 1918–1932. Developments and trends]. Orthopade 2001 Oct;30(10):685–95.

127 Waters JA, Kondo Y, Witkop B. Photochemistry of steroids. J Pharm Sci 1972 Mar;61(3):321–34.

128 Atkinson SK, Marlatt VL, Kimpe LE, Lean DR, Trudeau VL, Blais JM. Environmental factors affecting ultraviolet photodegradation rates and estrogenicity of estrone and ethinylestradiol in natural waters. Arch Environ Contam Toxicol 2011 Jan;60(1):1–7.

129 Linden KG, Rosenfeldt EJ, Kullman SW. UV/H2O2 degradation of endocrine-disrupting chemicals in water evaluated via toxicity assays. Water Sci Technol 2007;55(12):313–9.

130 Vulliet E, Falletta M, Marote P, Lomberget T, Paisse JO, Grenier-Loustalot MF. Light induced degradation of testosterone in waters. Sci Total Environ 2010 Aug 1;408(17):3554–9.

131 Katzenellenbogen JA, Ruh TS, Carlson KE, Iwamoto HS, Gorski J. Ultraviolet photosensitivity of the estrogen binding protein from rat uterus. Wavelength and ligand dependence. Photocovalent attachment of estrogens to proteins. Biochemistry 1975 Jun 3;14(11):2310–6.

132 Lee EJ, Lim HK, Shin MK, Suh DH, Lee SJ, Kim NI. An open-label, split-face trial evaluating efficacy and safty of photopneumatic therapy for the treatment of acne. Ann Dermatol 2012 Aug;24(3):280–6.

133 Shamban AT, Enokibori M, Narurkar V, Wilson D. Photopneumatic technology for the treatment of acne vulgaris. J Drugs Dermatol 2008 Feb;7(2):139–45.

134 Danby FW. Commentary: unroofing for hidradenitis suppurativa, why and how. J Am Acad Dermatol 2010 Sep;63(3):481–3.

135 van der Zee HH, Prens EP, Boer J. Deroofing: a tissue-saving surgical technique for the treatment of mild to moderate hidradenitis suppurativa lesions. J Am Acad Dermatol 2010 Sep;63(3):475–80.

136 Hazen PG, Hazen BP. Hidradenitis suppurativa: successful treatment using carbon dioxide laser excision and marsupialization. Dermatol Surg 2010 Feb;36(2):208–13.

137 Wortsman X, Jemec GB. Real-time compound imaging ultrasound of hidradenitis suppurativa. Dermatol Surg 2007 Nov;33(11):1340–2.

138 Mullins JF, McCash WB, Boudreau RF. Treatment of chronic hidradenitis suppurativa: surgical modification. Postgrad Med 1959 Dec;26:805–8.

139 Barron J. The surgical treatment of perianal hidradenitis suppurativa. Dis Colon Rectum 1970 Nov;13(6):441–3.

140 Rambhatla PV, Lim HW, Hamzavi I. A systematic review of treatments for hidradenitis suppurativa. Arch Dermatol 2012 Apr;148(4):439–46.

141 Kishi K, Nakajima H, Imanishi N, Nakajima T. Extended split superior gluteus maximus musculocutaneous flap and reconstruction after resection of perianal and lower gluteal hidradenitis suppurativa. J Plast Reconstr Aesthet Surg 2009 Aug;62(8):1081–6.

142 Chen E, Friedman HI. Management of regional hidradenitis suppurativa with vacuum-assisted closure and split thickness skin grafts. Ann Plast Surg 2011 Oct;67(4):397–401.

143 Na JI, Suh DH. Red light phototherapy alone is effective for acne vulgaris: randomized, single-blinded clinical trial. Dermatol Surg 2007 Oct;33(10):1228–33.

144 Kwon HH, Lee JB, Yoon JY, Park SY, Ryu HH, Park BM, *et al.* The clinical and histological effect of home-use, combination blue-red LED phototherapy for mild-to-moderate acne vulgaris in Korean patients: a double-blind, randomized controlled trial. Br J Dermatol 2013 May;168(5):1088–94.

145 Pinto C, Schafer F, Orellana JJ, Gonzalez S, Hasson A. Efficacy of red light alone and methyl-aminolaevulinate-photodynamic therapy for the treatment of mild and moderate facial acne. Indian J Dermatol Venereol Leprol 2013 Jan;79(1):77–82.

146 Akaraphanth R, Kanjanawanitchkul W, Gritiyarangsan P. Efficacy of ALA-PDT vs blue light in the treatment of acne. Photodermatol Photoimmunol Photomed 2007 Oct;23(5):186–90.

147 Strauss JS, Kligman AM. Effect of x-rays on sebaceous glands of the human face: radiation therapy of acne. J Invest Dermatol 1959 Dec;33:347–56.

148 Black HS, Tsurumaru Y, Lo WB. Rapid photolysis of cholesterol. Res Commun Chem Pathol Pharmacol 1975 Jan;10(1):177–80.

149 Holick MF, Clark MB. The photobiogenesis and metabolism of vitamin D. Fed Proc 1978 Oct;37(12):2567–74.

150 Slominski AT [personal communication]. Communication to F.W. Danby 2013 April 17.

151 Chang KC, Wang Y, Oh IG, Jenkins S, Freedman LP, Thompson CC, *et al.* Estrogen receptor beta is a novel therapeutic target for photoaging. Mol Pharmacol 2010 May;77(5):744–50.

152 Ekiz O, Balta I, Sen BB, Dikilitas MC, Ozuguz P, Rifaioglu EN. Vitamin D status in patients with rosacea. Cutan Ocul Toxicol 2014 Mar;33(1):60–2.

153 Mayser P, Pape B. Decreased susceptibility of *Malassezia furfur* to UV light by synthesis of tryptophane derivatives. Antonie Van Leeuwenhoek 1998 May;73(4):315–9.

154 Kalayciyan A, Oguz O, Bahar H, Torun MM, Aydemir EH. In vitro bactericidal effect of low-dose ultraviolet B in patients with acne. J Eur Acad Dermatol Venereol 2002 Nov;16(6):642–3.

155 Faergemann J, Larko O. The effect of UV-light on human skin microorganisms. Acta Derm Venereol 1987;67(1):69–72.

156 Boldeman C, Beitner H, Jansson B, Nilsson B, Ullen H. Sunbed use in relation to phenotype, erythema, sunscreen use and skin diseases. A questionnaire survey among Swedish adolescents. Br J Dermatol 1996 Nov;135(5):712–6.

157 Schwarz T. Photoimmunosuppression. Photodermatol Photoimmunol Photomed 2002 Jun;18(3):141–5.

158 Schwarz T. 25 years of UV-induced immunosuppression mediated by T cells-from disregarded T suppressor cells to highly respected regulatory T cells. Photochem Photobiol 2008 Jan;84(1):10–18.

159 Ho SG, Chan HH. The Asian dermatologic patient: review of common pigmentary disorders and cutaneous diseases. Am J Clin Dermatol 2009;10(3):153–68.

160 Kim RH, Armstrong AW. Current state of acne treatment: highlighting lasers, photodynamic therapy, and chemical peels. Dermatol Online J 2011;17(3):2.

CHAPTER 9

Acne in pregnancy

Babies are precious, so the management of acne before an intended pregnancy and during pregnancy is limited in several ways. Obviously, the first concern is the protection of the unborn child. This means that there is much greater need for care in the selection of therapy than usual.

The subjects that most mothers-to-be worry about are the drugs and other chemicals in the environment. Some of the threats posed by medications are real, they are proven, and they are based on science, as is the case with isotretinoin (better known as Accutane, Roaccutane, and about 10 other generic names around the world). Other reported risks are suspected but unproven, or based on less than perfect science, such as the suggestion that topical salicylic acid be avoided (discussed further in this chapter). And then there is the broad field of untested drugs and "supplements."

Because of the threat of litigation in the event of a less than perfect baby being born, universal caution is advised and risk avoidance has become the general self-protective rule for all cautious advisors and prescribers. The legal situation is made even more unsatisfactory for both physicians and patients by the lack of available safety data. This is, of course, because it is obviously impossible to conduct appropriately blinded medication trials in the "population at risk." You will never hear "We have this new drug, Mrs. Jones, and we'd like to have you try it during your pregnancy to see what will happen." That means that information on virtually all drugs is incomplete, and any use of any drug prior to conception and during pregnancy is considered on the basis of risk versus benefit. Every case is different.

Despite this problem, safe and rational management of acne prior to and during pregnancy is available. That means first of all that one should step back and take a cautious look from a distance. First, we need to consider whether the problem being treated is preventable. If so, then prevention should be the prime consideration, a subject covered in Section 8.1. Then we need to look at the active therapies available, and we need to know what is likely to happen *without* the medication that is being considered. Then the question of active therapy should be considered by carefully *searching first for the safest approach possible*. This means avoiding *any* topical or systemic medications that might cast a shadow across the unborn child's future.

9.1 Epidemiology

The incidence of acne in pregnancy is really not relevant in a population that suffers an 85–90% lifetime risk of this disorder. Epidemiology studies populations, not single pregnancies. Furthermore, epidemiology is of no use in predicting or explaining the appearance of significant acne in a single pregnancy. The practical approach says simply, "A problem will either happen, or it will not—it is 50:50." The difficulty is that acne may arrive totally unexpectedly and may be totally unrelated to the mother's prior clear-skinned, nonpregnant state. The only thing that is predictable is that acne's appearance in pregnancy is unpredictable. Preexisting acne can disappear with the same unpredictability.

Acne: Causes and Practical Management, First Edition. F. William Danby.
© 2015 John Wiley & Sons, Ltd. Published 2015 by John Wiley & Sons, Ltd.

9.2 Pathogenesis

To define the strategy for managing acne in pregnancy, one first needs an understanding of three facets of the disease:

1 The primary pathological processes that lead to the microcomedo that plugs the pore
2 The inflammatory reactions downstream from the primary disease process
3 The various treatments (including prevention) that are generally recognized as safe (and are as effective as possible).

The first two points are covered in previous chapters (Chapter 3 and Section 8.1), and this chapter will deal with prevention and therapy of acne before, during, and after pregnancy.

For many years, acne in pregnancy had been thought to be caused by the pregnancy itself. It was known that there were increases in the amount of normal male hormones (androgens and some relatives that can turn into androgens) made by the ovaries and by the adrenal (stress) glands. We thought these normal hormones were supplemented by more adrenal androgens that were caused by the stresses of pregnancy.

Indeed, this was considered an exaggerated form of the changes that Lucky demonstrated in showing the relationship of acne flares to the hormones produced during the luteal phase of the menstrual cycle [1] The luteal phase is the time after midcycle, so it is just after ovulation and before the period arrives, when the ovary produces more progesterone than at any other time, getting the uterus ready for a baby. If there is no baby, the progesterone level drops, the lining of the uterus is shed as period flow, and the "period acne" clears.

But, if there IS a pregnancy, the spot on the ovary that produced the egg goes on to form a yellow bump on the ovary called the *corpus luteum* (Latin for *yellow body*). In the initial stages of pregnancy, this collection of cells produces substantial amounts of progesterone (30 mg per day) and 5α-pregnanedione [2, 3]. Both these chemicals can turn into androgen, especially dihydrotestosterone (DHT), right in the folliculopilosebaceous unit (FPSU) itself. And DHT is the major cause of acne.

This ovarian influence normally fades beginning at six weeks of gestation, and the mother's placenta takes over as a prime source of progesterone, producing up to 300 mg per day of progesterone until delivery, and twice that or more in twins or multiple pregnancies [4]. The placenta also produces several other steroids, many of which are androgen precursors. This hormone output, which is supposed to go to the baby, is normally kept on the baby's side of the placenta, but some does reach the mother's circulation, mainly to maintain the link between the uterus and the placenta in good shape, and this may cause acne in some pregnancies. More research on placental hormones needs to be done, particularly in view of the fact that early studies were done on term (nine-month or post-delivery) placentas. These are basically aging placentas whose hormonal metabolic activities are slowing down. Ultimately they are failing or have failed as a fetal support system, and it is this failure that brings on labor contractions. But obtaining fresh healthy first-term and midterm placentas to study is understandably almost impossible.

The other possible source of hormones that turn into DHT in a small percentage of pregnancies may be from persistent corpus luteum progesterone production, beyond that described here. In other primates (like monkeys), this can be caused by the corpus luteum being exposed to an early rise in pregnancy-induced chorionic gonadotropin from the placenta [5]. The problem here is that what we *don't* know about the hormones produced by the human placenta would likely fill several books. This is understandable given the difficulties involved in studying such tissue.

The stress of pregnancy itself can be expected to produce both adrenal androgens (more DHT precursors) [6, 7] and more corticotropin-releasing hormone (CRH) [8]. Both of these tend to promote acne. CRH turns on the steroid hormones from the adrenals through its messenger, ACTH, but it also seems to have a direct effect on the FPSU as well. The CRH story is new, so you will need to look at Section 1.41 (and Figure 1.40) for further details.

In addition to starting the comedo/blackhead poreplugging process, the androgens attaching to the androgen receptors on the FPSU also stimulate an overproduction of sebum at the same time. There are steps in between that make for a very complicated set of reactions all in a row, all leading to the plugged pore. Remember that the acne process is ultimately regulated by the androgen (male) receptor. The problem in managing acne in pregnancy is that there is no medicine considered safe during pregnancy that we can use to actively block this receptor. It would be great to keep the receptor closed to prevent it from catching any androgens, but this is not practical. The only easily available, safe, and reasonably effective approach is to reduce the level of androgen receptor activity by reducing the levels of both insulin and IGF-1. That will allow the androgen receptor to return to its normal adult repressed (unreceptive and resting "closed") state, allowing the androgen-driven system to cool down, and the resulting acne to fade.

In summary, there is no available, acceptable, safe, and specific medication that can be used during pregnancy to block the effect of these important but acne-causing hormones, and of course investigation and development of such molecular intervention are next to impossible because of the risks to the study population (mom and baby).

9.3 Team up with Mother Nature

Fortunately, there is a simple, physiological, totally time-tested, and indeed healthy approach available. All that is needed is total dairy avoidance, preferably combined with a diet with serious restriction of high-glycemic-load (HGL: sugary and glucose-producing) foods. It is a big step for those of us raised on a Western diet, but simple science suggests that moving to such a diet is the most logical of all possible steps in the right direction. If you cannot do without some sort of fluid "milk," then it is time to try dairy substitutes. Look around for those made with soy, almonds, rice, coconut, or hemp, but take care to select only those that are "unsweetened" to lower the glycemic load. Save the chocolate and the French vanilla for occasional special treats only.

Then there is another simple "no-brainer." **Stop smoking.** Smoking as a possible cause of acne has been recognized anecdotally for years, but there is some new science to think about. Smoking is now linked with comedonal post-adolescent acne (so-called *adult acne*) as well as acne inversa/hidradenitis suppurativa (AI/HS) [9, 10]. In addition to discontinuing smoking for its deleterious cardiac and pulmonary effects on the mother, it should be eliminated in all patients with acne, and particularly in pregnancy, because of fetal concerns. The same is true in AI/HS.

9.4 Targeting therapy

There are three traditional targets of acne therapy. These are the physical plugs that require prevention and comedolytics, the organisms and debris in the duct that need various drugs for their control and elimination, and the inflammation that requires cooling. All three targets must be addressed in organizing a logical attack on acne. The solutions to the problem are limited by the "delicate condition" of pregnancy.

9.4.1 Clinical manifestations

There is really no difference in the presentation of acne between pregnant and nonpregnant women. Acne may suddenly appear in its most aggressive form for the first time in previously clear skin, or previously active acne may simply vanish in the glow of a new pregnancy. Similarly, it may disappear after delivery or it may recur in the postpartum period. Curiously, it may occur in some pregnancies but not others, despite identical parents. Every case, like every woman, is unique.

9.4.2 Pathology

There are no pathologic findings that are specific to acne in pregnancy that differentiate it from the acnes (vulgaris, rosacea, or inversa) of nonpregnancy.

9.4.3 Diagnostic evaluation

All true acne at any time is driven by hormones. The additional complexity of pregnancy hormones requires a careful evaluation of all sources of acnegenic hormones, both steroids and polypeptides. An extensive historical review of dietary habits is essential. Expensive laboratory investigation should be reserved for those whose acne is unusual. By that I mean it is sudden in onset, is accompanied by signs of androgen excess, is highly inflammatory, fails to respond to the exclusion of exogenous acnegens (including those supplied or induced by dairy and HGL diets), or is otherwise inexplicable. Drug history is especially important, as the offending substance (such as anabolic steroids used by bodybuilders—even some women) may be illicit and may be carefully hidden away behind maternal guilt. Diplomatic probing for a history of bodybuilding, use of whey- and casein-containing protein powder, and use of other bodybuilding supplements can lead gently to the question of anabolic steroid use.

In searching for acnegens, both the physician and the pregnant patient must realize that the elevations in insulin and IGF-1 that lead to de-repression (opening) of the androgen receptor are triggered by fluid milk (whether skim or whole) [11] and by ingestion of the whey and casein found in protein supplements [12], in addition to all the more easily recognized dairy products and the sugars and their easily digested carbohydrates. The androgen receptors, sensitized by dietary polypeptide hormones, open up and wait for the steroid hormones from both the normal nonpregnant sources (ovaries, adrenals and the intracrine system) and the overflow from the daily production of 300 mg of progesterone plus related steroids from the placenta [4]. Detecting anabolic steroids added from the outside is more important here than in Olympic athletes.

9.4.4 Overview and general approach to treatment

In the vulnerable mother and unborn baby, *prevention* of the disorder should take logical priority, so the first order of business is to define the steps that can be directed at the primary lesion, the comedo. Tactics must be designed and implemented to prevent the formation of new plugs, stop the progression of plugs that have gotten underway, and empty out the established plugs.

The single, and the healthiest, change (for both mother and baby) available to all is to adopt a zero-dairy and low-glycemic-load (LGL) diet. Dairy products, refined sugar, and refined wheat-based products were simply not part of the human diet until relatively recently, and the amounts of these we presently consume are immense compared to what our grandparents grew up with. For example, in the United States, the volume of cheese consumed per person is five times now what it was 35 years ago. In Japan, the amount of dairy product consumed per person per year went up from 5.5 lbs. to an astounding 117.4 lbs. between 1950 and 1975 [13]. Our bodies were simply not designed to handle these changes.

Fortunately, there is an answer to all this, the so-called Paleolithic diet. There is no diet available that more closely conforms to the diet that our bodies were designed for than this diet. For instance, consider lactose intolerance. Although some of the human population experienced the mutation of a gene about 15,000 years ago that now permits lactose in our diets, most of the human race has simply not evolved to handle the lactose in milk. Dairy products also normally contain significant levels of reproductive hormones, numerous polypeptide hormones, and growth factors. Refined wheat products fill the shelves of our grocery and "convenience" stores. Sugars are presented to us in seductive, attractive, and even addictive modern foods. These come to us courtesy of modern farming, selective breeding, and food production and marketing techniques. The milkman, the bread man, and the snack, soda, and soft drink sales force did not visit the caveman and his pregnant mate, nor should they visit the modern pregnant woman.

The Aché tribe studied by Cordain considers the practice of drinking the milk of another species "abhorrent" [14]. It strikes me as very curious that *we* think that *they* are primitive. It is disconcerting at best to realize that we know more about the hormonal exposure of Olympic athletes, baseball players, Tour de France winners, Greek weightlifters, and racehorses in Pennsylvania than we do about the hormones in the dairy products we feed to our children, grandchildren, and expectant mothers.

Drinking milk and eating dairy-based products are, quite simply, not a challenge for which evolution has prepared us. No other species knowingly exposes its pregnant females, let alone their offspring in utero, to the hormones and growth factors in dairy products. To resort to instructive hyperbole, we all need to be acutely aware that cows do not drink milk after weaning or while pregnant, and they most certainly are not fed milk from pregnant humans. Likewise, adult humans generally recognize that they should respect the weaning process as far as their own mothers are concerned.

9.4.5 Milk and pregnancy

It is not generally recognized that pregnancy itself can be negatively impacted by milk. Even "getting pregnant" is more difficult for dairy consumers [15]. Its consumption during pregnancy is also associated with increased infant size at birth [16]. Whether plumper babies are healthier babies remains to be seen, but they do increase obstetrical risk. As the authors state, "Milk intake was associated … with an increased risk of 'large for gestational age' babies, and a rapid early growth rate may be a risk factor for obesity." Dairy intake during pregnancy has other negative effects on the offspring, including later obesity [17], increased risk factors for cancer of the breast [18–20], and reduced longevity [20]. Less well-known effects on pregnancy include the impact of dairy intake on twinning rates. Steinman reports, "Vegan women, who exclude dairy products from their diets, have a twinning rate which is one-fifth that of vegetarians and omnivores" [21].

Of note, there are absolutely no countervailing studies that support dairy consumption during pregnancy as a benefit; indeed, a PubMed search of "benefits … milk … ingestion … pregnancy" yields eight articles with nothing of significant value.

It has been pointed out that "absence of evidence is not evidence of absence." While this is true, the market forces that drive the dairy industry have never shied away from any opportunity to use science on their side of the debate. If there is a positive side to consuming dairy during pregnancy, in an otherwise healthy population consuming a normal diet, I have yet to encounter evidence of it.

It is long past time to stop the party line that insists that pregnant women drink three cups of milk a day to have a healthy baby [22]. Recognizing this, the Healthy Eating Pyramid from the Harvard School of Public Health advises that pregnant women "limit milk and dairy to one or two servings per day" [23]. Combining the Harvard Pyramid with the US Department of Agriculture's (USDA) recognition of soymilk as equivalent to cow-sourced dairy [22], I'm comfortable recommending one or two servings of soy daily during pregnancy, but water would be just fine, "or, if you like, tea or coffee with little or no sugar," as Harvard advises [23]. There appear to be no risks to mother or child in following this advice.

The USDA "encourages consumers to make dairy products a regular part of their meals." From a scientific point of view, the USDA's recommendations are unsupportable. No other animal drinks milk to nourish its unborn. If this were simple harmless nonsense, there could be no reasonable objection. Yet research has shown little benefit, and considerable potential for harm, of such high dairy intakes. While moderate consumption of milk or other dairy products—one to two servings a day—may be fine, and has some benefits for undernourished children, it is not essential for adults or children for a host of reasons. That's why the (Harvard) Healthy Eating Plate recommends "limiting milk and dairy products to one to two servings per day, and drinking water with meals instead" [23]. This is excellent advice for the mother-to-be. Humans have, after all,

being safely drinking water as a preferred source of hydration for millions of years.

In summary, a healthy LGL and dairy-free diet during pregnancy provides nothing but positive influences. The impact we seek as dermatologists is to reduce to an absolute minimum the hormonal drive to comedo formation and the downstream inflammatory epiphenomena that constitute acne. Even more important from a public health standpoint is the opportunity for all physicians and other caregivers and health advisors to teach a healthy diet that a healthy mother can pass along to her healthy offspring, now and in future pregnancies. An additional benefit exists: those physicians who, like the author, had almost no training in diet and nutrition in medical school and postgraduate training could perhaps use the opportunity to learn about the interactions involved. There is an immense amount of science here, and a great deal more for most of us to learn.

9.4.6 Active therapy
9.4.6.1 Avoidance of harm
Teratogens are chemicals that cause damage to the structure and function of the unborn. Avoidance of fetal damage caused by teratogens is a prime consideration in choosing acne therapy for a pregnant patient.

The US Food and Drug Administration (FDA) divides the teratogenic risk of topical and systemic anti-acne therapies into five categories. This categorization varies among countries internationally, with a classification agreement of only 26% among three systems reviewed [24]. In May 2008, the FDA proposed major revisions to prescription drug labeling. The proposed regulations eliminate the current pregnancy categories A, B, C, D, and X. The intent is to label drugs with a risk summary, clinical consideration to support patient care decisions and counseling, and a data section that includes more detailed information. As of August 2014, the Final Rule is still in the writing and clearance process [25].

Meanwhile, I predict either very large labels or very small print.

The present categories apply to acne therapies:
Category A: Studies show no risk in any trimester.
  No acne therapy is Category A. This is basically because no studies have been done, and that in turn is because testing for side effects in this population is "problematic."

Category B: Animal studies show abnormalities, but risk to the fetus is remote.

Erythromycin topically seems to be very low risk clinically as well as in toxicology studies.

Clindamycin topically, despite the B rating, is avoided by many dermatologists because of the low but nonzero risk of colitis from absorption through the skin.

Metronidazole topically appears to present little risk; its mechanism of action is unknown other than it is anti-inflammatory, but it appears more useful in acne rosacea than in acne vulgaris.

Azelaic acid has been tested in several animal species and holds FDA approval for acne rosacea but not for acne vulgaris. The manufacturer cautions, "Because animal reproduction studies are not always predictive of human response, this drug should be used only if clearly needed during pregnancy." Because it is of limited potency, it is of limited use, and there is a difference in efficacy that is vehicle dependent, introducing another variable.

Erythromycin and azithromycin orally are listed in category B, but cardiovascular malformations have recently been reported for oral erythromycin [26] and, for azithromycin, a small increase in cardiac death "among patients with a high baseline risk of cardiovascular disease" [27].

Category C: Studies have not been conducted on humans; risk to the fetus is possible.

Topical benzoyl peroxide and the retinoids, despite their identical C rating, are not considered by clinicians to have the same safety profile in practice. Dermatologists cite a half-century history of safe use of topical benzoyl peroxide versus rare (and therefore, I suspect, coincidental) reports of teratogenicity associated with topical tretinoin. The FDA's new rating system will be useful in this instance, and we can hope for an "executive summary."

Adapalene (Differin® and its generics) is often avoided in pregnancy for legal reasons, there being no data upon which to base a medical decision.

Dapsone gel (Aczone®) for use in pregnancy likewise has no data.

Oral spironolactone is avoided because of its capacity as an androgen blocker that could theoretically produce hypospadias or other genital feminization syndrome or endocrine epigenetic effects in male babies. No actual cases have been reported. The animal study results are discussed at Section 8.6.2.1.

Category D: There is demonstrated risk to the fetus, although benefit may outweigh any risks.

Tetracycline is a risk to dentition after the first trimester, to bones, and to the maternal liver, but is no longer easily available in the United States. Its analogs doxycycline, minocycline, and lymecycline are likewise avoided.

Trimethoprim, with or without sulfamethoxazole, is an option if a serious condition such as Gram-negative folliculitis warrants. It is a folate antagonist so concurrent folic acid supplementation is advised, especially in the first trimester.

Category X: Evidence of risk to the fetus is documented.

Oral isotretinoin (Accutane® in the past, now Amnesteem®, Claravis®, Sotret®, and others in the United States, and RoAccutane® and others worldwide)

Oral acitretin, isotretinoin's chemical brother, which is used for psoriasis, other "disorders of keratinization," and, increasingly, AI/HS

Topical tazarotene (Tazorac®) is a potent "retinoid," and is listed despite no evidence for tazarotene-induced fetal damage in the literature.

The FDA also lists numerous other teratogens, some of which may be encountered occasionally in pregnant acne patients. Higher risk items are printed in **bold**.

ACE inhibitors (benazepril, captopril, enalapril, fosinopril, lisinopril, moexipril, quinapril, ramipril, and trandolapril)

Aminopterin

Androgenic hormones

Busulfan

Chlorobiphenyls

Cigarette smoking

Cocaine

Coumarin anticoagulants

Cyclophosphamide

Diethylstilbestrol

Etretinate

Fluconazole (high doses)

Iodides

Isotretinoin (Accutane®)

Lithium

Mercury, organic

Methimazole

Methotrexate (methylaminopterin)

Methylene blue (via intra-amniotic injection)

Misoprostol

Penicillamine

Phenytoin

Tetracyclines

Thalidomide

Toluene (abuse)

Trimethadione

Valproic acid

And, as possible teratogens:

Binge drinking

Carbamazepine

Colchicine

Disulfiram

Ergotamine

Glucocorticoids

Lead

Primidone

Quinine (suicidal doses)

Streptomycin

Vitamin A (high doses)

Zidovudine (AZT)

Zinc deficiency

All of these should ideally be considered in counseling women prior to, or early in, their pregnancy.

9.4.6.2 Lesion-directed therapy

Because the primary lesion is the comedo, it is appropriate that it be the prime target for therapy when prevention has not been adequate. Comedolytics are indicated to "lyse" (dissolve) the comedones but the most effective comedolytics of all, the oral retinoids, are absolutely contraindicated because of undisputed teratogenicity.

The first topical retinoid (tretinoin) was reviewed by Canada's Motherisk program, which considered 94 women who used topical tretinoin products during their pregnancies. The authors stated, on the basis of very limited data, "Available evidence suggests that topical tretinoin does not increase teratogenic risk in humans" [28]. On the other hand, teratogenicity associated with use of (but not proven due to) topical tretinoin is reported [29, 30], so even the topical retinoids, and the non-vitamin-A-derived drugs classified as retinoids, because of the threat of litigation, are best not used at all in pregnancy nor in those attempting pregnancy.

9.4.6.3 Nonprescription topicals

Topical salicylic acid has come under suspicion on the Internet, probably undeservedly, because of its chemical relationship to Category D acetylsalicylic acid (Aspirin®).

While it is possible to raise the level of salicylates in blood to detectable levels, there are no reports of secondary fetal damage. Damage to the skin from the direct action of the salicylic acid would likely limit the amount applied.

Topical elemental sulfur seems harmless in the 1%, 2%, and up to 5% concentrations usually encountered.

Tea tree oil 5% appears to compare favorably with benzoyl peroxide 5% clinically [31]. It has antimicrobial effects against *Staphylococci, Streptococci, Propionibacterium acnes*, and *Malassezia* [32]. *Demodex* has recently been added to that list [33]. No appropriate studies in pregnancy are available, so it is unrated as to teratogenicity.

The alpha-hydroxy acids were shown to be teratogenic in high-dose studies performed in 1999 [34]. Subsequent recent work by the same laboratory 12 years later shows evidence in rats that suggests no significant risk to human consumers [35], but no similar studies have actually been done in humans. Glycolic acid, the most used of the alpha-hydroxy acids, is exceedingly variable in its clinical impact, depending upon concentration, vehicle, pH, and length of exposure time. It is also operator variable. Caution is advised; the safety of alpha-hydroxy acids in pregnancy has not been documented.

9.4.6.4 Antimicrobials

Erythromycin and azithromycin orally are Category B, and the latter is favored for its much better gastrointestinal tolerance. It can be pulsed (three days of 500 mg daily) to cover 10 days of therapy, and other regimens are in use. It carries a new warning concerning arrhythmias [27].

Sodium sulfacetamide 10% topically is Category C. It has an excellent safety record with the exception of rare contact dermatitis, and it is available in 10% lotion or cream combined with 5% precipitated sulfur. It is applied from 3 to 14 times weekly. This allows adjustment to avoid overdrying from the sulfur component. It can be used either locally over the entire involved area or as a "spot" treatment.

Trimethoprim–sulfamethoxazole orally is Category C/D, whereas trimethoprim alone is Category C and might be considered for monotherapy if the situation warranted. There are no controlled data in human pregnancy, so trimethoprim should only be given during pregnancy with folic acid supplementation and "when benefit outweighs risk." It would be useful to have clearer guidelines, but both benefit and risk are in the mind of the estimator and flexibility is essential to avoid "cookbook" prescribing, and to avoid being locked into published guidelines that can be weaponized by lawyers.

9.4.6.5 Combination topicals

Several expensive combination topicals have appeared and most are Category C. Those containing retinoids or clindamycin are best avoided in pregnancy, which leaves only the erythromycin–benzoyl peroxide combination as a defensible option. The product insert states, "There are no well-controlled trials in pregnant women with Benzamycin Topical Gel. It also is not known whether Benzamycin Topical Gel can cause fetal harm when administered to a pregnant woman or can affect reproductive capacity. Benzamycin Topical Gel should be given to a pregnant woman only if clearly needed." Nevertheless, "when benefit outweighs risk," many dermatologists are comfortable prescribing this combination in pregnancy.

9.4.6.6 Anti-inflammatories

Dapsone gel (Aczone) is category C and is useful in mild acne.

Ibuprofen has been used as an oral anti-inflammatory in acne but was statistically effective only in combination with oral tetracycline, now no longer economically available [36]. Although most nonsteroidal anti-inflammatory drugs (NSAIDs) are likely safe in pregnancy, they should be avoided in the last six to eight weeks of pregnancy to prevent prolonged gestation due to inhibition of prostaglandin synthesis, premature closure of the ductus arteriosus (part of the baby's developing heart), and maternal and fetal complications from antiplatelet activity [37].

Corticosteroids may be used carefully in the later stages of pregnancy. Systemic doses must be coordinated with the attending obstetrician because, although these drugs may enhance lung maturity with occasional use, repeated doses may risk slowing the normal rate of myelination in the brain. The foreign body reaction component of acute acne flares may be cooled with short systemic pulses, or alternate-day therapy, of corticosteroids, using oral prednisone or methylprednisolone. Instead of oral steroids, triamcinolone acetonide given intramuscularly as 1 mg/kg at intervals of at least a month in the third trimester will allow time for the restrictive dietary therapy to achieve results. Although

no clinical trials are reported, the drug is in common use in the nonpregnant, and the safety of this modality is unparalleled when it is used judiciously [38].

The major risk of using systemic steroids is the phenomenon generally known as *rebound*. The flare following discontinuation of the steroid may be either a return to the original condition (for which I prefer the term *recurrence*) or a flare that is significantly worse than the original (for which I reserve the term *rebound*). I believe but cannot prove that rebounds occur when steroids suppress the competence of the immune response to phagocytize and eliminate bacterial and yeast pathogens. This is the system that is attempting to locate and physically remove and so eliminate microorganisms. So what actually happens? The microbes multiply in the absence of the inflammatory clearance response, and are present in even greater numbers when the steroid wears off. This triggers the enhanced flare we see as the *rebound phenomenon*. This can, of course, be minimized by using concurrent antibiotics and anti-yeasts orally, but in pregnancy this concurrent antidote presents other problems to mother and child.

Deep nodules and acne pseudocysts sometimes require intralesional injections of very small volumes of saline-diluted triamcinolone acetonide. We use 1–3.3–5 mg/mL using a tuberculin syringe and a 30-gauge needle. These injections may be repeated at intervals of 3 or 4 weeks.

Careful assessment is needed to avoid these medications when Gram-negative bacterial folliculitis may be present.

9.4.6.7 Hormone blockers

Spironolactone in massive doses has been shown in pregnant rats to produce genital abnormalities in male offspring [39] but not in very high (400 mg) human dose equivalents [40]. More recent work suggests a longer, likely epigenetic effect at very high doses on both male and female offspring, certainly sufficient evidence to avoid its use during pregnancy [41]. Its inclusion here is not to suggest its use in pregnancy but to provide support for its safe but cautious use in women of childbearing age. While it must be stopped if a pregnancy occurs, the risk of untoward effects on a male fetus is remote. In women unprotected against pregnancy, consider using spironolactone for 10 consecutive days per month, starting on the first day of menses. All other hormonal blockers, including finasteride, dutasteride, and flutamide, must be avoided in women *at risk of pregnancy*, whether or not they *intend* pregnancy.

9.4.6.8 Procedural therapies

Lasers, visible light, and even ultraviolet light when used alone for management of acne in pregnancy are generally considered safe.

The anti-inflammatory and desquamative effects of sunlight, even in moderation, can be very beneficial, and pure red, blue, or ultraviolet light is generally recognized as safe in pregnancy. The obvious trade-off is the aging effect of sun exposure, so moderation is advised. Each must be considered on its own merits for use in pregnancy.

The chemicals used as peeling agents and as photosensitizers, however, being designed to penetrate or substantially modify the epidermis and its appendages, present an undefined risk to mother, child, and physician because they have not been proven harmless to the unborn. On general principles, in the absence of safety data and given medicolegal considerations, peels and photodynamic therapy are best avoided.

9.5 Discussion

"Know thy enemy," counseled Sun Tzu. We now know about disease mechanisms that have been mysteries for decades, we now know about organisms whose impact has been ignored for decades, and we now know how the enemy responds to medications that have been available for decades. We know the enemy better now than ever before.

That acne runs on hormones is not new—that the hormones that tip the balance toward acne are sourced from our daily diet is becoming apparent. Indeed, it now appears that milk is indeed "nature's perfect food"—perfect for the creation of acne. Dairy products increase levels of both IGF-1 [42] and insulin [43]. This combined IGF-1 and insulin stimulus (IIS) opens the androgen receptors in androgen-responsive cells. The androgenic reproductive steroid hormones in dairy foods thereby gain access to those androgen receptors and populate them with bovine androgens. These milk-sourced hormones, made naturally by the cows that produce the milk, activate those open receptors. The androgens produced by the mother's ovaries, adrenal glands, the intracrine system of the pilosebaceous units themselves,

and the potent placental progesteroids of pregnancy are thus given unprecedented access to the androgen receptors in these cells.

The other half of this dietary (IIS) stimulus package comes from the high glycemic load of Western-type diets, which raise and prolong the elevations of insulin, further opening the androgen receptors [44].

The synergism of a HGL diet with a high-dairy diet further compounds the synergism of IGF-1 and hyperinsulinemia, producing maximal androgen receptor access long after normal weaning should have occurred.

One of evolution's challenges is to develop protection against chemicals that are not normally produced by the human body and that are not expected to be absorbed into it. These foreign chemicals are called *xenobiotics*, and this definition also covers substances present in much higher concentrations than are usual. Both insulin and IGF-1, when produced in excess in response to dairy, fit the definition of xenobiotics. This is the situation in humans with acne, whether pregnant or not. We humans have simply not evolved to handle this challenge. The most efficient way to remove these influences is simply to adopt, as closely as is practically possible, a truly xenobiotic-free diet.

Such a diet, if instituted before, followed during, and continued long after pregnancy, would likely go a long way toward improving the general health of each and every one of us.

9.6 Summary and conclusion

The time has come for true strategic management of acne in pregnancy. We must work toward, as Kligman has written, "the ultimate goal in medical practice, namely prevention" [45].

The prime strategy in acne is to prevent the follicular canal from plugging. For this reason, anything that opens the androgen receptor must be avoided, neutralized, or blocked if possible, to prevent the unwanted pore-plugging effects of the dietary dairy hormones and growth factors as well as the increased impact of normal steroidal reproductive hormones and other hormones, like those in the birth control methods used prior to pregnancy.

Taking dietary steps for the *prevention of acne is still the best way* to reduce the risk to a healthy baby. This will help all concerned in avoiding or minimizing the need for more aggressive therapy that may threaten the fetus.

In the absence of prevention, careful selection of acne therapy is mandatory for the health of both mother and baby.

References

1 Lucky AW. Quantitative documentation of a premenstrual flare of facial acne in adult women. Arch Dermatol 2004 Apr;140(4):423–4.

2 Backstrom T, Andersson A, Baird DT, Selstam G. The human corpus luteum secretes 5 alpha-pregnane-3,20-dione. Acta Endocrinol (Copenh) 1986 Jan;111(1):116–21.

3 Zwirner M, Fawzy MM, Bopp FC, Klemm-Wolfgram E, Handschuh D, Voelter W, et al. Radioimmunoassay of 5 alpha-pregnane-3,20-dione. A metabolite of placental progesterone. Arch Gynecol 1983;233(4):229–40.

4 Melmed S, Polonsky KS, Larsen PR, Kronenberg HM. Williams textbook of endocrinology. 9th ed. Philadelphia: WB Saunders; 1998.

5 Ottobre JS, Stouffer RL. Persistent versus transient stimulation of the macaque corpus luteum during prolonged exposure to human chorionic gonadotropin: a function of age of the corpus luteum. Endocrinology 1984 Jun;114(6): 2175–82.

6 Chiu A, Chon SY, Kimball AB. The response of skin disease to stress: changes in the severity of acne vulgaris as affected by examination stress. Arch Dermatol 2003 Jul;139(7): 897–900.

7 Yosipovitch G, Tang M, Dawn AG, Chen M, Goh CL, Huak Y, et al. Study of psychological stress, sebum production and acne vulgaris in adolescents. Acta Derm Venereol 2007;87(2): 135–9.

8 Ganceviciene R, Graziene V, Fimmel S, Zouboulis CC. Involvement of the corticotropin-releasing hormone system in the pathogenesis of acne vulgaris. Br J Dermatol 2009 Feb;160(2):345–52.

9 Capitanio B, Sinagra JL, Bordignon V, Cordiali FP, Picardo M, Zouboulis CC. Underestimated clinical features of postadolescent acne. J Am Acad Dermatol 2010 Nov;63(5):782–8.

10 Hana A, Booken D, Henrich C, Gratchev A, Maas-Szabowski N, Goerdt S, et al. Functional significance of non-neuronal acetylcholine in skin epithelia. Life Sci 2007 May 30;80(24–25):2214–20.

11 DiLandro A., Cazzaniga S, Parazzini F, Ingordo V, Cusano F, Atzori L, et al. Family history, body mass index, selected dietary factors, menstrual history, and risk of moderate to severe acne in adolescents and young adults. J Am Acad Dermatol 2012 Dec;67(6):1129–35.

12 Silverberg NB. Whey protein precipitating moderate to severe acne flares in 5 teenaged athletes. Cutis 2012 Aug;90(2):70–2.

13 Kagawa Y. Impact of Westernization on the nutrition of Japanese: changes in physique, cancer, longevity and centenarians. Prev Med 1978 Jun;7(2):205–17.

14 Cordain L, Lindeberg S, Hurtado M, Hill K, Eaton SB, Brand-Miller J. Acne vulgaris: a disease of Western civilization. Arch Dermatol 2002 Dec;138(12):1584–90.

15 Chavarro JE, Rich-Edwards JW, Rosner BA, Willett WC. Diet and lifestyle in the prevention of ovulatory disorder infertility. Obstet Gynecol 2007 Nov;110(5):1050–8.

16 Olsen SF, Halldorsson TI, Willett WC, Knudsen VK, Gillman MW, Mikkelsen TB, et al. Milk consumption during pregnancy is associated with increased infant size at birth: prospective cohort study. Am J Clin Nutr 2007 Oct;86(4): 1104–10.

17 Melnik BC. The role of transcription factor FoxO1 in the pathogenesis of acne vulgaris and the mode of isotretinoin action. G Ital Dermatol Venereol 2010 Oct;145(5):559–72.

18 Ahlgren M, Wohlfahrt J, Olsen LW, Sorensen TI, Melbye M. Birth weight and risk of cancer. Cancer 2007 Jul 15; 110(2):412–9.

19 Michels KB, Trichopoulos D, Robins JM, Rosner BA, Manson JE, Hunter DJ, et al. Birthweight as a risk factor for breast cancer. Lancet 1996 Dec 7;348(9041):1542–6.

20 Samaras TT, Elrick H, Storms LH. Birthweight, rapid growth, cancer, and longevity: a review. J Natl Med Assoc 2003 Dec;95(12):1170–83.

21 Steinman G. Mechanisms of twinning: VII. Effect of diet and heredity on the human twinning rate. J Reprod Med 2006 May;51(5):405–10.

22 United States Department of Agriculture. Nutritional needs during pregnancy [Internet]. 2013 Feb 16. Available from: http://www.choosemyplate.gov/pregnancy-breastfeeding/pregnancy-nutritional-needs.html

23 Harvard School of Public Health. Healthy eating plate and healthy eating pyramid [Internet]. 2013 Feb 16. Available from: http://www.hsph.harvard.edu/nutritionsource/pyramid/

24 Addis A, Sharabi S, Bonati M. Risk classification systems for drug use during pregnancy: are they a reliable source of information? Drug Saf 2000 Sep;23(3):245–53.

25 US Food and Drug Administration. Pregnancy and lactation labeling. Washington, DC: US Food and Drug Administration; 2011 Feb 11 [cited 2011 Mar 29]. Available from: http://www.fda.gov/Drugs/DevelopmentApprovalProcess/DevelopmentResources/Labeling/ucm093307.htm

26 Kallen BA, Otterblad OP, Danielsson BR. Is erythromycin therapy teratogenic in humans? Reprod Toxicol 2005 Jul;20(2):209–14.

27 Ray WA, Murray KT, Hall K, Arbogast PG, Stein CM. Azithromycin and the risk of cardiovascular death. N Engl J Med 2012 May 17;366(20):1881–90.

28 Shapiro L, Pastuszak A, Curto G, Koren G. Is topical tretinoin safe during the first trimester? [Internet]. 1998 March

[cited 2011 Mar 29]. Available from: http://www.motherisk.org/women/updatesDetail.jsp?content_id=301

29 Colley SM, Walpole I, Fabian VA, Kakulas BA. Topical tretinoin and fetal malformations. Med J Aust 1998 May 4;168(9):467.

30 Navarre-Belhassen C, Blanchet P, Hillaire-Buys D, Sarda P, Blayac JP. Multiple congenital malformations associated with topical tretinoin. Ann Pharmacother 1998 Apr;32(4):505–6.

31 Bassett IB, Pannowitz DL, Barnetson RS. A comparative study of tea-tree oil versus benzoylperoxide in the treatment of acne. Med J Aust 1990 Oct 15;153(8):455–8.

32 Raman A, Weir U, Bloomfield SF. Antimicrobial effects of tea-tree oil and its major components on *Staphylococcus aureus, Staph. epidermidis* and *Propionibacterium acnes*. Lett Appl Microbiol 1995 Oct;21(4):242–5.

33 Koo H, Kim TH, Kim KW, Wee SW, Chun YS, Kim JC. Ocular surface discomfort and *Demodex*: effect of tea tree oil eyelid scrub in *Demodex blepharitis*. J Korean Med Sci 2012 Dec;27(12):1574–9.

34 Carney EW, Freshour NL, Dittenber DA, Dryzga MD. Ethylene glycol developmental toxicity: unraveling the roles of glycolic acid and metabolic acidosis. Toxicol Sci 1999 Jul;50(1):117–26.

35 Carney EW, Tornesi B, Liberacki AB, Markham DA, Weitz KK, Luders TM, *et al.* The impact of dose rate on ethylene glycol developmental toxicity and pharmacokinetics in pregnant CD rats. Toxicol Sci 2011 Jan;119(1):178–88.

36 Wong RC, Kang S, Heezen JL, Voorhees JJ, Ellis CN. Oral ibuprofen and tetracycline for the treatment of acne vulgaris. J Am Acad Dermatol 1984 Dec;11(6):1076–81.

37 Risser A, Donovan D, Heintzman J, Page T. NSAID prescribing precautions. Am Fam Physician 2009 Dec 15;80(12):1371–8.

38 Robins DN. Intramuscular triamcinolone: a safe, effective and underutilized dermatologic therapy. J Drugs Dermatol 2009 Jun;8(6):580–5.

39 Hecker A, Hasan SH, Neumann F. Disturbances in sexual differentiation of rat foetuses following spironolactone treatment. Acta Endocrinol (Copenh) 1980 Dec;95(4):540–5.

40 Rose LI, Regestein Q, Reckler JM. Lack of effect of spironolactone on male genital development. Invest Urol 1975 Sep;13(2):95–6.

41 Jaussan V, Lemarchand-Beraud T, Gomez F. Modifications of the gonadal function in the adult rat after fetal exposure to spironolactone. Biol Reprod 1985 Jun;32(5):1051–61.

42 Hoppe C, Molgaard C, Dalum C, Vaag A, Michaelsen KF. Differential effects of casein versus whey on fasting plasma levels of insulin, IGF-1 and IGF-1/IGFBP-3: results from a randomized 7-day supplementation study in prepubertal boys. Eur J Clin Nutr 2009 Sep;63(9):1076–83.

43 Hoyt G, Hickey MS, Cordain L. Dissociation of the glycaemic and insulinaemic responses to whole and skimmed milk. Br J Nutr 2005 Feb;93(2):175–7.

44 Smith RN, Mann NJ, Braue A, Makelainen H, Varigos GA. The effect of a high-protein, low glycemic-load diet versus a conventional, high glycemic-load diet on biochemical parameters associated with acne vulgaris: a randomized, investigator-masked, controlled trial. J Am Acad Dermatol 2007 Aug;57(2):247–56.

45 Kligman A. Letter of welcome. Second International Conference on the Sebaceous Gland, Acne & Related Disorders 2008 Sep 13.

CHAPTER 10
Putting it all together

Managing acne requires teamwork. There are two sides to the story, the patient side and the physician side. Physicians can provide education, instructions, guidance, specialized knowledge, empathy, encouragement, experience, and prescriptions from their side, but much of what needs to be done has to come from the patient side.

From the physician's point of view, it really is pretty simple to write the prescriptions for topicals or oral medications, even isotretinoin (with birth control pills for female patients as appropriate), and stand in a supportive role for four to six months. The patient will get better with no untoward incidents most of the time. The physician is there for emergencies, but the main challenge is explaining the reasons for the therapy being used and how to use it.

The problem is that unless the patient looks after his or her side of the story, the acne (no matter which type) will be right back again. The lifestyle choices made by patients dictate the activity of the acnes. In all the acnes, exogenous hormones are the most important thing to reduce or eliminate. This is best achieved by reduction in dairy content and adoption of a low-glycemic-load diet. I consider this approach essentially proven in acne vulgaris. The results are "pending" (the study is partly done but "on hold" due to lack of funds) in acne rosacea. Increasing clinical experience supports the need to respect the zero dairy and low glycemic load diet in acne inversa/hidradenitis suppurativa (AI/HS) as well. The long timeline of AI/HS makes this a difficult disorder to investigate, because doing so in a "blinded trial" is essentially impossible, and one cannot simply discontinue all dairy and wait a year or so for results. Just blowing out the match will not stop the fire.

So we need to look at choices. That means an overview of patient lifestyle choices first, then a practical overview and implementation of physicians' therapeutic choices.

10.1 Lifestyle choices and the acnes

Acne is a disorder of the folliculopilosebaceous units (FPSUs), driven by hormones, and those hormones are to a major extent mediated by lifestyle, whether they are produced within our bodies (endogenous) or are provided from the outside (exogenous). Whether from inside or outside, there are two main hormone types, steroids and short proteins called *polypeptides*. Detailed discussions of each are at Section 4.2.4.1. What follows is a brief reminder.

Endogenous hormones include:

Steroids
  Reproductive (sex) hormones from the ovaries and testes
  Adrenal hormones: secondary to stress
Polypeptides
  Insulin-like growth factor-1 (IGF-1): increased normally at puberty—stimulated by endogenous growth hormone (GH)
  Insulin: stimulated by dietary glucose
  Corticotrophin-releasing hormone (CRH): from stress

Acne: Causes and Practical Management, First Edition. F. William Danby.
© 2015 John Wiley & Sons, Ltd. Published 2015 by John Wiley & Sons, Ltd.

Exogenous hormones include:

Steroids

Oral contraceptives and other birth control methods

Dairy sources of acnegenic hormones

Anabolic steroid acnegens: illicit and legal

Polypeptides

IGF-1: stimulated by dairy (casein) ingestion

Insulin: stimulated by dairy (whey) and high glycemic load

Other growth factors: from dairy protein source

Although the arrival of normal puberty is not a lifestyle choice, its premature arrival is increasingly attributed to dietary influences. Although diet is mainly a parental choice in preteens, it is a lifestyle choice nonetheless. In addition, pregnancy is a lifestyle choice, as are stress, the use of oral contraceptives (or not), and the ingestion of the hormones in dairy products. Most require little explanation, but there are some new players on the field.

Acne secondary to stress has for decades been considered a response to adrenocorticotropic hormone (ACTH). (See Section 2.10.) Recent studies show that the FPSU sebocytes have a functional CRH receptor system, and this seems likely to be responsive to hypothalamic-sourced CRH [1].

Sugar and other carbohydrate metabolites are intimately involved with insulin, IGF-1, and GH. Acne is associated with the syndrome X complex, which includes insulin resistance, type II diabetes, polycystic ovaries, infertility, obesity, and hyperandrogenemia. Brand-Miller notes, "Increasing obesity and habitual consumption of high-glycemic-load diets worsens insulin resistance and increases the risk of type 2 diabetes in all populations" [2]. Older studies showed that acne improves with insulin-sensitizing drugs such as the biguanide metformin [3], and its use in treating hidradenitis suppurativa shows definite promise [4]. Investigation of the thiazolidinediones to reduce sebum output has been considered [5], but clinical effectiveness has not yet been demonstrated to outweigh the risk of side effects. Meanwhile, low-glycemic-load diets reduce testosterone and fasting glucose levels while increasing sex hormone–binding globulin (SHBG) and improving insulin resistance. Although the relationships are complex, the net effect is a strong dietary influence on acne.

Polyunsaturated fatty acids (PUFAs) in Westernized diets tend to include omega-6/omega-3 ratios higher than those in the Paleolithic diet. Dietary manipulation that yields increased omega-3 and lowered omega-6

intake tends to suppress inflammation [6]. Although there is no formal study to show that an increased intake of lean meats will attenuate acne, "consumption of fish was associated with a protective effect" [7].

Oral contraceptives are now available containing progestins that are not only non-androgenic but also androgen blockers. Drospirenone has fewer metabolic side effects than cyproterone acetate, so it is generally favored, but recent concerns about thrombo-embolic events (blood clots) associated with these two progestins have led to a shift toward norgestimate and norelgestromin. These are both less efficient molecules for treating acne but can be supplemented with spironolactone (see Section 10.2).

Milk and the many products derived from it are the source of numerous hormones, growth factors, and other chemicals. The list includes over 60 molecules. (See Section 8.3.1.) Why all the growth factors in milk? Milk is designed to make things grow [8].

Milk also contains several important precursors of 5α-dihydrotestosterone (DHT). In addition to progesterone, there are several 5α-reduced compounds including 5α-pregnanedione and 5α-androstanedione [9], each of which is only a few enzymatic steps away from the most powerful acnegen, DHT.

Even the simple ingestion of milk invites more acne. There is a fourfold disparity in area under the curve (AUC) comparisons between the rise in serum insulin levels induced by the ingestion of milk when compared to the AUC expected based on milk's carbohydrate (mainly lactose sugar) content [10]. This reactive hyperinsulinemia opens the androgen receptors and empowers the androgens that drive the increased production of intraductal keratinocytes. These are the cells whose failed terminal differentiation and failed separation from each other lies at the base of the formation of the comedo, and that takes us back to where the story begins.

To stop the acnes, it is necessary to start at the beginning. Only by stopping the beginning of the process can we prevent progress to the end of the process. Prevention means no dairy at all during the teen years—and it also usually means limited dairy after the teens. Failure of prevention reflects poor lifestyle choices and means years more acne.

This part of the story is up to the patient. Just "going to the doctor" doesn't do the job. Patients need to follow the rules in this partnership, otherwise, as I occasionally point out, the "my way/your way" rule applies.

If you do it my way and it doesn't work, it may
be my fault;
    I will try something else.
If you do it your way and it doesn't work, it is
likely your fault;
    You get to try another dermatologist.
After all, it's your acne. You need to look after it.

10.1.1 The "processed cheese queen"

I met Mo when she was 17 and she already had extensive nodular acne. Her family doctor had tried just about
everything he could think of. She had a lovely classic
1940s cover girl face, but it was covered with acne and
the process had been going on long enough that she
had extensive scarring. She was an early candidate
for isotretinoin (Accutane). As soon as I could get her on
birth control pills, she was started on full doses of the
oral retinoid. She didn't like the side effects much, and
birth control pills in those days tended to put on weight,
but she persevered. And she cleared.

Once she finished the course of Accutane, things
looked great. To avoid further birth control pill side
effects, she discontinued those as soon as she could.
About four months later, she was back in the office,
pretty much back where she started. She denied any
dairy intake but was stressed by a boyfriend and school.
So we got to work with the second course of isotretinoin. She went on the same birth control pill, the same
dose, got the same clearing response, again came off the
birth control pills, and I turned her loose again.

This time, the good results lasted for almost 8 months,
probably because we were working with a somewhat
miniaturized set of oil glands by now. And then she was
back again, almost as bad as before, very discouraged,
tearful, and angry. She didn't like the birth control pills,
she didn't like the weight she was putting on, and she
didn't like giving up her ice cream and cheese and milk.
I was getting the message that I was on her "dislike" list
as well. I certainly wasn't living up to her expectations.
So around we went again, birth control pills and
Accutane, and success once again.

The same thing happened again for her fourth course,
and at age 22 she showed up once again with nodular
facial acne, but now with acne on the upper back and
shoulders as well. She had hoped that she would "grow
out of it" in the intervening couple of years since I had
seen her, but it had just gotten worse. Nevertheless, she
knew that if she got back on the birth control pills and the
isotretinoin, she would be cleared in about 4 months. But

this time she had a question. "Doc, is 'X' a dairy product?" X is a processed cheese whose product brand name
I cannot mention here. "Yes, Mo, why do you ask?"

Well, it seems that Mo was a Product X addict. In
Canada at that time it was available in tall 32-ounce
glass jars with a screw-on top. Not only was she
consuming at that time a full jar of 32 ounces of
processed cheese every 2 weeks, but also she had
been doing so since I met her 5 years previously. I
thought that the brand name was a pretty good hint
that it contained cheese, but I guess that hint wasn't
broad enough for Mo.

Mo's fifth course of Accutane was, fortunately, her
last. It took about 2 years for her facial skin to mold. The
scars on her shoulders and upper back were fading when
I last saw her, and she never had any more active acne.

Lesson learned: Keep asking about the diet, forever.
Sometimes the source of the trouble is hidden, whether
intentionally or not.

Note: While processed foods in general have been criticized for years, the makers of Product X and similar
dairy-based products have come under fire for using
an illegal, or at least unapproved, additive called milk
protein concentrate, or MPC. In the case of processed
cheese, MPC is used primarily to eliminate some of
the inherent problems of cheese solids. When milk is
filtered through an ultrafine mesh, the result is a
concentrated form of milk protein that has the ability
to lock in more whey and water than traditional
cheese proteins. MPC has not been approved as a food
additive by the U.S. government, however, so its continued use in products such as Product X is somewhat
controversial.

10.2 Therapeutic choices and the acnes

To take an objective look at a subject, the view as seen
through the eyes of a mythical Martian has often been
considered. So if a Martian took a look at "the acnes"
and the therapeutic choices available for their care,
what would Martian medicine for the acnes look like?

10.2.1 Acne vulgaris

The first thing needed is to stop plugging the pores. Total
dairy avoidance for the entire population is a choice that
I wholeheartedly and unreservedly advocate for all.
This choice avoids not only acne but also numerous
other problems from dairy products, likely including the

contribution to national obesity. At the same time, consumption of high-glycemic-index foods and the high-glycemic-load diets they make up should be sharply reduced. In all women of childbearing age, consider the temporary (6–12 months) use of one of the less androgenic birth control pills, to be discontinued as soon as possible when the zero-dairy diet has had its effect. Spironolactone is a second choice or may be added to birth control pills or other methods for increased effect. That should stop new pores from getting plugged.

Next, the plugs in the pores need to be emptied. Whether in males or females, the most effective therapy is isotretinoin. It should be the obvious first choice, and I believe that it should ideally be used in all stages of acne, as soon as the disorder appears. It not only clears the follicular ducts but also shrinks the sebaceous glands and improves the quality of life for patients even before the acne spots are healed. This will not only clear the pores of their plugs but reduce the overpopulation by *Propionibacterium acnes* as well. This is now possible at low risk with the low-dose regimens now in use.

Because isotretinoin does not fully clear the *Malassezia* population, the yeasts should be reduced as close to zero as possible with the oral ketoconazole routine, and then oral ketoconazole may be needed for the long term at a maintenance dose of 200–400 mg once monthly, reinforced with a 1% selenium sulfide shampoo weekly. No formal clinical trials of this combination have been done, but it is remarkably successful in private practice.

The choices given here can usually do away with the need for (and the risks of) both oral antibiotics and topical antibiotics. The topical benzoyl peroxide products and the topical retinoids are retained as long-term preventives, to be used as maintenance after the initial isotretinoin clearance, in conjunction with diet and, if appropriate, hormone control for females.

10.2.2 Acne rosacea

Looking at the likelihood that sun damage is a major contributor to both the actinic telangiectasia and the follicular wall weakness that predispose to papulopustular acne rosacea, our Martian would suggest lifelong sun avoidance. Proper cover would include broad-brimmed hats and sunglasses and parasols, as well as full-spectrum nontoxic sunscreen coverage. This would be needed from the cradle (and the stroller) well into late middle age as a preventive and would necessitate the use of supplemental vitamin D in full dose for the lifetime of all fair-skinned as

well as darker skinned individuals. Our Martian would have access to the rosacea and dairy intake data and would conclude that there is an association, compatible with the findings in acne vulgaris, and recommend the same dietary restrictions noted for both acnes.

In the event that some of the population at risk missed out on these adequate preventive measures, a thorough cleanout of all the plugged pores using oral isotretinoin would be an objective Martian-based medicine first choice. This would eliminate most *P. acnes*, the *Demodex*, and most of the *Malassezia*, cooling the fires considerably.

If isotretinoin clearance could not be undertaken, topical metronidazole in whatever vehicle and in whatever concentration will look after most acne rosacea lesions and should be tried next. Eliminating *Bacillus oleronius* from the gut of the *Demodex* [11, 12], if indeed metronidazole will do this job, may prove to be the key here, but in the event of further inflammation, the other potential contributors will need to be eliminated. That will mean resorting to the doxycycline–minocycline options for *P. acnes*, topical crotamiton, or oral ivermectin (Stromectol®) for *Demodex*, and topical selenium sulfide and oral ketoconazole for the *Malassezia*. Judicious selection of these oral agents provides effective customized management of the inflammatory causes of acne rosacea.

10.2.3 Acne inversa/hidradenitis suppurativa

Our Martian, recognizing the familial pattern of AI/HS, would realize that the prevention of this disorder would need to start with genetic counseling, even though the links are crude and the specific genetic defects so far only partially defined. He would also take note of the impact of dietary influences and recommend a return to a more natural diet, free of dairy, and free of high-glycemic-index foods and high-glycemic-load meals. Total hormone control would be put in place with the appropriate birth control pills and spironolactone blockade in women, and the dutasteride blockade in men. Acitretin would be instituted whenever possible [13], as would metformin [4]. All patients would take both vitamin C 500 mg and zinc gluconate 30 mg three times a day mixed into meals [14, 15]. Aggressive anti-inflammatory measures using tumor necrosis factor-alpha (TNFα) inhibitors or other biologicals would be used to shut down all active inflammatory areas. Then, a full surgical unroofing [16, 17] of all nodules and sinus tracts, plus removal of dilated and multiple-headed "tombstone" comedones and small epidermoid cysts, would be undertaken. Ideally, this should occur at one sitting in a regional operating theatre specially equipped and staffed for this purpose. The team would be capable of full wide excisional surgery of Hurley III lesions, with the ability to construct flaps, apply fenestrated grafts, and provide appropriate aftercare.

10.3 Conclusion

The mind-set of medicine has developed a progressive, incremental, and reactive therapeutic approach to much of the disease burden we try to contain. I believe "the acnes" would benefit from aggressive and continuous prevention, early utilization of the modalities that we know can stop the progress of the disease, and an emphasis on long-term preventive maintenance.

These diseases, especially if one factors in the social costs, are very expensive. The linked disorders (from prostate cancer to national obesity) are a huge additional burden that could be considerably reduced through adherence to the dietary aspect of this care. I strongly believe that making such healthy choices should be an international priority and that these choices will not only provide better care at lower cost but also contribute to a far healthier world.

In 2008 I was one of 66 speakers at the Second International Conference on Sebaceous Gland, Acne, Rosacea and Related Disorders. The subtitle was "Basic and Clinical Research, Clinical Entities and Treatment." I was the only speaker to touch on prevention, but was very pleased that the late Professor Albert Kligman had sent a letter of greeting in which he expressed the hope that the attendees would learn to help our patients help themselves "to actually achieve the ultimate goal in medical practice, namely prevention" [18]. We are getting closer.

References

1 Ganceviciene R, Graziene V, Fimmel S, Zouboulis CC. Involvement of the corticotropin-releasing hormone system in the pathogenesis of acne vulgaris. Br J Dermatol 2009 Feb;160(2):345–52.

2 Brand-Miller JC, Griffin HJ, Colagiuri S. The carnivore connection hypothesis: revisited. J Obes 2012;2012:258624.

3 Pasquali R, Gambineri A. Insulin-sensitizing agents in polycystic ovary syndrome. Eur J Endocrinol 2006 Jun;154(6): 763–75.

4 Verdolini R, Clayton N, Smith A, Alwash N, Mannello B. Metformin for the treatment of hidradenitis suppurativa: a little help along the way. J Eur Acad Dermatol Venereol 2013 Sep;27(9):1101–8.

5 Schuster M, Zouboulis CC, Ochsendorf F, Muller J, Thaci D, Bernd A, et al. Peroxisome proliferator-activated receptor activators protect sebocytes from apoptosis: a new treatment modality for acne? Br J Dermatol 2011 Jan;164(1): 182–6.

6 Simopoulos AP. The importance of the omega-6/omega-3 fatty acid ratio in cardiovascular disease and other chronic diseases. Exp Biol Med (Maywood) 2008 Jun;233(6):674–88.

7 DiLandro A., Cazzaniga S, Parazzini F, Ingordo V, Cusano F, Atzori L, et al. Family history, body mass index, selected dietary factors, menstrual history, and risk of moderate to severe acne in adolescents and young adults. J Am Acad Dermatol 2012 Dec;67(6):1129–35.

8 Koldovsky O. Hormones in milk. Vitam Horm 1995; 50:77–149.

9 Darling JA, Laing AH, Harkness RA. A survey of the steroids in cows' milk. J Endocrinol 1974 Aug;62(2):291–7.

10 Hoyt G, Hickey MS, Cordain L. Dissociation of the glycaemic and insulinaemic responses to whole and skimmed milk. Br J Nutr 2005 Feb;93(2):175–7.

11 Lacey N, Delaney S, Kavanagh K, Powell FC. Mite-related bacterial antigens stimulate inflammatory cells in rosacea. Br J Dermatol 2007 Sep;157(3):474–81.

12 O'Reilly N, Menezes N, Kavanagh K. Positive correlation between serum immunoreactivity to Demodex-associated Bacillus proteins and erythematotelangiectatic rosacea. Br J Dermatol 2012 Nov;167(5):1032–6.

13 Boer J, Nazary M. Long-term results of acitretin therapy for hidradenitis suppurativa. Is acne inversa also a misnomer? Br J Dermatol 2011 Jan;164(1):170–5.

14 Brocard A, Knol AC, Khammari A, Dreno B. Hidradenitis suppurativa and zinc: a new therapeutic approach. A pilot study. Dermatology 2007;214(4):325–7.

15 Brocard A, Dreno B. Innate immunity: a crucial target for zinc in the treatment of inflammatory dermatosis. J Eur Acad Dermatol Venereol 2011 Oct;25(10):1146–52.

16 Danby FW. Commentary: unroofing for hidradenitis suppurativa, why and how. J Am Acad Dermatol 2010 Sep;63(3): 481–3.

17 van der Zee HH, Prens EP, Boer J. Deroofing: a tissue-saving surgical technique for the treatment of mild to moderate hidradenitis suppurativa lesions. J Am Acad Dermatol 2010 Sep;63(3):475–80.

18 Kligman A. Letter of welcome, Second International Conference on the Sebaceous Gland, Acne & Related Disorders. Rome; 2008.

CHAPTER 11

Appendices

11.1 Appendix A: the rosacea "classification and staging" controversy

The nomenclature of acne rosacea has presented problems for many years. In 2002 and in 2004, an Expert Committee looked at the question and published a document "on the classification and staging of rosacea" [1].

The document contained changes that I felt were ill-advised and tended to mislead the public, as outlined in the following letter, published in the Journal of the American Academy of Dermatology:

To the Editor: For the past year or so, dermatologists have been the ambivalent recipients of referrals and self-referrals of patients who either believe or have been told that they have rosacea. And some of them do—the papular and papulopustular disorder known as acne rosacea in times past.

But many do not. Instead they present with a history of intermittent flushing (triggers varying from emotional overload to estrogen depletion) or a background facial erythema (sometimes demonstrably genetic but more commonly actinic) of varying color depth, or telangiectasia of the sun-exposed areas that rosacea favours, or all three.

Some have already been treated with the metronidazole-containing products that represent the standard of care, making the diagnosis a little difficult if the characteristic papules and pustules have disappeared. The problem is that these patients are usually complaining that their rosacea "is still there." By this they mean the background erythema and telangiectasia that, alone or together, do not make a diagnosis of acne rosacea even though they are common companions of that disorder.

We dermatologists are presented with two problems, in addition to sorting out whether the patient actually has (or had) acne rosacea.

The first is education, actually re-education, defining the disorder for the patient and pointing out where he or she fits. This is a challenge, because an Expert Committee has recently suggested a change in the criteria for the diagnosis of rosacea (sic) and a new disorder, erythematotelangiectatic rosacea, has been included. Details were published in the June issue of the Journal. The criteria, also published online at http://www.rosacea.org/class/classystem.html, are such that anyone with persistent central facial erythema (with or without telangiectasia) fits this diagnosis, even though they suffer from nothing more than actinic (i.e., sun-induced) erythema, once known simply as "high colour" in the British literature.

I make no claim that these features are not part of rosacea, just that the diagnosis cannot hang on the vascular changes alone, because these features are quite capable of existing by themselves. I have begun to diagnose such patients as having "pseudorosacea." It seems a better fit than "inconstant vasodilatory and actinic telangiectatic non-rosacea."

The second problem is what to do about the patients' unreasonable expectations. Patients are sent (or come driven by advertising) to us in the expectation that we will be able to "fix" them. Well, of the six components of rosacea, two (the papules and the pustules) are easily managed in most (but not all) cases by topical metronidazole or sulfur/sulfacetamide products, with or without oral antibiotics. It is not unreasonable to expect a good outcome here, and of course there will be a diminution of some of the erythema as the inflammation associated with these components lessens. That leaves us with the need to explain that the two vascular components are manageable only with a vascular laser

Acne: Causes and Practical Management, First Edition. F. William Danby.
© 2015 John Wiley & Sons, Ltd. Published 2015 by John Wiley & Sons, Ltd.

(there are several) for the telangiectases or an intense pulsed light (IPL) unit for the background erythema, or both. While this presents dermatologists who own such equipment with a golden opportunity to market the procedure, one can understand that the somewhat suspicious medical public will wonder whether they are becoming victims of clever "bait and switch" marketing. The fifth component, the famous W. C. Fields rhinophyma, now referred to as "phymatous rosacea," will require surgical reduction in one of several ways, usually requiring another referral. Sixth and last, if the patient responds to careful questioning that an itchy or scratching or gritty feeling in the eyes is part of the problem, then a diagnosis of ocular rosacea and a referral to an ophthalmologist should be considered.

So how should the front-line primary care practitioner confront suspected rosacea? I would suggest that the presence of papules and pustules at a minimum is required for a diagnosis of acne rosacea and treatment should be with topicals supplemented as needed with oral cyclines and other anti-inflammatories. Failure to respond should trigger a referral to a dermatologist for consideration of at least seven differential diagnoses mentioned in neither the above reference nor the above Web site (post adolescent acne, contact dermatitis, drug reaction, seborrheic dermatitis, perioral dermatitis, polymorphous light eruption, and facial psoriasis). In the absence of the papules and pustules, where only flushing and telangiectasia exist, actinic erythema and/or actinic telangiectasia would be better referring diagnoses. The consultant dermatologist should be able to confirm the diagnosis, consider the several alternatives, and direct the patient to appropriate care, including sun avoidance techniques and truly broad-spectrum sunscreens.

One further thought: the concept of marketing actinic telangiectasia as a form of rosacea (or pre-rosacea) amenable to topical pre-emptive or preventive therapy seems to be part of this whole picture. Proof is lacking that the former is a predictor or precursor of the latter, making such therapeutic innovations premature at this time. A multicenter phase IV clinical study is underway nevertheless. Meanwhile the predictive diagnosis of prerosacea must remain impossible to make until adequate and tested diagnostic criteria are developed. For now it might be fair to accept the diagnosis, but only when made retrospectively.

In any case, it would be best if the patient were not led to believe that the topicals will "cure" the problem, or, in the alternative, that these same topicals have actually failed to do what was expected. Unfulfilled unreasonable expectations tend to breed dissatisfied patients.

The Chair of the Expert Committee informs me by letter that he welcomes reports on the usefulness and limitations of these criteria. I write in the hope that this contribution will help with both patient care and patient-physician communication. [2]

The response from the Expert Committee is as follows:

To the Editor: The National Rosacea Society Expert Committee on the Classification and Staging of Rosacea read with interest the letter of Dr F. William Danby to this journal with comments relating to the standard classification of rosacea. As noted in its publication, and in the more recent publication of a standard grading system, this is a provisional system that is expected to require modification as the pathogenesis and subtypes of rosacea become clearer, and as its relevance and applicability are tested by researchers and clinicians The committee, therefore, welcomes reports on the usefulness and limitations of these criteria.

We believe that the letter by Danby contains a number of observations that are reasonable and accurate about the problems of treating patients with rosacea today; for example, that current therapies for rosacea offer limited success, especially in treating the erythema of rosacea, and this often poses a problem in managing patient expectations. However, we are concerned that some mistaken assumptions and implications about the classification system could easily be interpreted as critical and might cloud the intended benefits of the new system to researchers, physicians, and their patients.

It may first be useful to clarify what the standard classification system is not. First, it should be recognized that these standard diagnostic criteria have nothing to do with the promotion of treatment. In fact, they meticulously avoid treatment recommendations, either specific or general.

Secondly, the standard classification system does not represent a sudden, revolutionary, or arbitrary change in the definition of rosacea. Rather, it reflects the predominant informal classifications of rosacea that evolved during recent years in individual publications as the disorder became increasingly recognized and understood. These usually consisted of categories or stages of rosacea that included vascular, inflammatory (acne rosacea in an earlier era), phymatous, and ocular. Unlike earlier systems devised by one or two individuals, however, the new system was developed by a consensus committee and review panel of 17 experts worldwide, and is based on current scientific knowledge alone to be free of assumptions on pathogenesis and progression.

The genesis of the standard classification system was recognition that standard criteria are essential to perform research, analyze results, and compare data from different sources. Beyond this, the new system can serve as a diagnostic reference in clinical practice, and standard terminology is fundamental for clear communication among a broad range of researchers, practicing physicians, health administrators, patients, and the general public. The ultimate goal is to set the stage for a better understanding of rosacea by fostering communication and ultimately facilitating the development of a research-based classification system.

Regarding the comment of Danby on subtype 1, we agree that there may be clinical overlap between erythematotelangiectatic rosacea and actinically damaged skin, and some patients with rosacea have a background of actinically induced changes. However, the correct diagnosis may be identified by obtaining a patient history to differentiate between rosacea and isolated photodamage. For example, any patient whose occupation or lifestyle has involved extensive sun exposure may experience photodamage, whereas patients with a history of flushing alone are more likely to have rosacea. In addition, in the case of rosacea, erythema and telangiectasia tend to present with a central facial distribution rather than at the peripheries. These points will be emphasized in future publications. Meanwhile, the nature of the relationship between sun exposure and rosacea is becoming increasingly defined by ongoing research supported by the National Rosacea Society.

Concerning the comments by Danby about the unpredictability of progression, the published standard classification system points out that evolution from one subtype to another may or may not occur. Regardless of subtype, however, each individual characteristic may progress from mild to moderate to severe.

Regarding the comments of Danby on patient expectations and communications, we believe that the usual role of the physician includes addressing both of these issues on a case-by-case basis as part of patient care. Because rosacea varies substantially from one patient to another, treatment and potential outcomes must be explained on the basis of which components of the disorder are involved, as he points out. Rather than making this more difficult, however, we believe the standard criteria and terminology of the new classification system should make it easier for physicians to clearly communicate those important distinctions to their patients. Rosacea is a typology with many potential presentations, and there is no single treatment that is effective against them all.

We believe rosacea is a condition that warrants concern and compassion from the medical community. Fortunately, as with other significant disorders, patient care should continue to improve as a result of the ongoing efforts of both medical researchers and practicing physicians. [3]

11.2 Appendix B: the dairy versus carbohydrate controversy

Following the publication of the "Western Diet" paper by Cordain [4] in 2002, several papers appeared that looked into the relationship between acne and diet [5–10]. The group that produced the best-designed prospective studies eventually published several papers on various aspects of their studies [11–14]. The work that has received the most attention from the media is that published in the *Journal of the American Academy of Dermatology* [12]. The diets in those studies were designed with a balanced caloric intake and carefully calculated percentages of high- and low-glycemic-load protein, fats, and carbohydrates. At the time of their design, there was no recent literature to suggest the possibility that dairy intake might be a confounder. The authors kindly provided details of the diets used, and a review of the contents shows significant differences in composition of the diets beyond their intentionally different glycemic loads.

1 The high-glycemic-load (HGL) group, in addition to having appropriately targeted nondairy modifications such as white bread, potato chips, and corn- or rice-based cereal and cereal bars, also had an *additional* 45 g of low-fat cheese and 100 g of low-fat ice cream *daily* beyond the dairy content of the low-glycemic-load (LGL) group.

2 Although the HGL milk component was "skinny" (the Australian equivalent of "skim") rather than "low-fat" cow milk, a higher volume of 200 g daily was provided to HGL subjects versus 160 g in the LGL group, for an additional 280 g of skim milk weekly. In addition to the 25% increase in volume, note that skim milk (two glasses daily) was the type of milk most closely associated with acne in the first Harvard University study, with a prevalence ratio of 1.44 [5]. Subsequent studies in Italy and Malaysia with comparable skim milk volumes produced odds ratios of 2.20 [15] and 3.988 [16], respectively.

3 We are now aware that "cereal bars," unless specifically non-dairy-based, contain whey, casein, and caseinates, and they may be labeled as containing milk isolates, milk solids, and so on. It is known that increased insulin-like growth factor 1 (IGF-1) and insulin levels are induced by dietary casein (IGF-1) and whey (insulin) ingestion [17].

4 Of special note, the members in the HGL group in one study were also treated daily to a "piece" (size and weight not reported) of an Australian delicacy called a Lamington, a chocolate-frosted white flour cake; the cake is made with 113 g of butter and 150 g sugar plus 120 mL milk, and the "frosting" recipe calls for 454 g icing sugar, 42 g butter, and 120 mL milk [18]. Rough calculations based on very conservative percentages of butterfat content in cheese, ice cream, and the Lamington servings show that the content of dairy hormone in the Smith–Mann HGL diet was from 50% to over 300% higher than that in the LGL diet.

Smith and Mann's conclusion is indisputable, that the demonstrated improvement in acne was a result of the study participants consuming the diet labeled as "low glycemic load," but it is now apparent that the control (HGL) diet was significantly higher in dairy products than the LGL diet, meaning that the LGL diet was significantly lower in dairy products by comparison. *Indeed, this carefully done work is equally supportive of the views that the diet that improved the acne was lower in dairy components and that the improvement was due to the LGL diet.*

Based upon Cordain's work, Smith and Mann were looking for a carbohydrate connection. The Adebamowo group at Harvard University, based upon my clinical suspicions and the unpublished work [19] of Dr Jerome Fisher, was looking for a dairy connection. It seems now apparent that the Smith–Mann data support both theories.

Recently, revelations at the molecular level have been elucidated that tie these contributing acnegens together, as Melnik has extensively discussed [20–23]. Furthermore, all of these threads trace back to what Cordain has called the Western diet, a dietary amalgam of both high-dairy and HGL foods.

Two further studies of glycemic load as the primary driver of acne have since appeared. In the first study, Reynolds *et al.* addressed the question in 58 adolescent Australian males. Facial acne improved on both diets. The results on the low glycemic index (GI) diet (GI = 51)

were better than those on the high GI diet (GI = 61), but the difference between the results did not reach significance [24].

In the second, Kwon *et al.*, in a carefully designed Korean study, showed that a closely supervised LGL diet decreased the overall acne severity and the lesion counts of both inflammatory and non-inflammatory lesions at 10 weeks by significant amounts ($p < 0.05$). This was accompanied by statistically significant reductions in the histologic size of sebaceous glands, in the expression of sterol regulatory element-binding protein 1 (SREBP-1), and in the interleukin 8 (IL-8) levels [25].

On the dairy side of the argument, another published paper has added to the data favoring the dairy–acne link. Silverberg described five adolescent males whose acne was associated with protein supplements containing whey protein [26].

One might speculate that the original Adebamowo studies of acne and dairy consumption [5–7] were less definitive than the Italian study, being based on a population in the United States that has a heavy dairy background while the Italian study, with a dietary emphasis leaning more toward olive oil, may have been less confounded by background dairy. The same explanation might be offered in the Reynolds and Kwon studies, the difference between the heavier dairy tradition in Australia and the lighter load in Korea, allowing a statistical separation in Korea that was not achieved in Australia. The Malaysian study, in which the amounts of dairy would appear to be almost below threshold level by American standards, also emphasize the dairy impact on the background of a lighter Malaysian dairy tradition.

Knitting these dietary influences together, Melnik's recent work recognizes a nutrient-sensitive kinase *mammalian target of rapamycin complex 1* (mTORC1) as the central signaling node in cellular metabolism for stimulation of both growth and cell proliferation. Milk is a species-specific endocrine signaling system that activates this pathway, and that activation is enhanced by high GI foods in HGL diets [27, 28]. Milk thus acts not only to activate androgen-sensitive organs such as the FPSU, the breasts, and the prostate, but also to stimulate growth in general through mTORC1.

In summary, it would now appear that the synergistic actions of insulin, IGF-1, steroid and polypeptide hormones, and other growth factors, both present in and induced by dairy products and HGL diets, work together to produce the lesions of the acnes.

Curiously, this synergism is paralleled by the efforts of several investigators and their teams: Fisher, Cordain, Adebamowo, Smith and Mann, DiLandro Kwon, Ismail, Silverberg, and Melnik. They comprise a living example of scientific synergism; working separately, they have defined, to my satisfaction at least, the pathogenesis of acne vulgaris. I suspect that, with further work, all acnes including acne rosacea and acne inversa (formerly hidradenitis suppurativa) may be found to be driven by the same forces.

This brings us closer now than ever before to recognizing the molecular cause of acne. It also points us in the direction of modifying the dietary causes of acne, fulfilling Kligman's admonition "to actually achieve the ultimate goal in medical practice, namely prevention" [29].

References

1 Wilkin J, Dahl M, Detmar M, Drake L, Liang MH, Odom R, et al. Standard grading system for rosacea: report of the National Rosacea Society Expert Committee on the classification and staging of rosacea. J Am Acad Dermatol 2004 Jun;50(6):907–12.

2 Danby FW. Rosacea, acne rosacea, and actinic telangiectasia. J Am Acad Dermatol 2005 Mar;52(3 Pt 1):539–40.

3 Odom R. Rosacea, acne rosacea, and actinic telangiectasia: in reply. J Am Acad Dermatol 2005 Dec;53(6):1103–4.

4 Cordain L, Lindeberg S, Hurtado M, Hill K, Eaton SB, Brand-Miller J. Acne vulgaris: a disease of Western civilization. Arch Dermatol 2002 Dec;138(12):1584–90.

5 Adebamowo CA, Spiegelman D, Danby FW, Frazier AL, Willett WC, Holmes MD. High school dietary dairy intake and teenage acne. J Am Acad Dermatol 2005 Feb;52(2):207–14.

6 Adebamowo CA, Spiegelman D, Berkey CS, Danby FW, Rockett HH, Colditz GA, et al. Milk consumption and acne in adolescent girls. Dermatol Online J 2006;12(4):1.

7 Adebamowo CA, Spiegelman D, Berkey CS, Danby FW, Rockett HH, Colditz GA, et al. Milk consumption and acne in teenaged boys. J Am Acad Dermatol 2008 May;58(5):787–93.

8 Cordain L. Implications for the role of diet in acne. Semin Cutan Med Surg 2005 Jun;24(2):84–91.

9 Cordain L, Eaton SB, Sebastian A, Mann N, Lindeberg S, Watkins BA, et al. Origins and evolution of the Western diet: health implications for the 21st century. Am J Clin Nutr 2005 Feb;81(2):341–54.

10 Magin P, Pond D, Smith W, Watson A. A systematic review of the evidence for "myths and misconceptions" in acne management: diet, face-washing and sunlight. Fam Pract 2005 Feb;22(1):62–70.

11 Smith R, Mann N, Makelainen H, Roper J, Braue A, Varigos G. A pilot study to determine the short-term effects of a low glycemic load diet on hormonal markers of acne: a nonrandomized, parallel, controlled feeding trial. Mol Nutr Food Res 2008 Jun;52(6):718–26.

12 Smith RN, Mann NJ, Braue A, Makelainen H, Varigos GA. The effect of a high-protein, low glycemic-load diet versus a conventional, high glycemic-load diet on biochemical parameters associated with acne vulgaris: a randomized, investigator-masked, controlled trial. J Am Acad Dermatol 2007 Aug;57(2):247–56.

13 Smith RN, Mann NJ, Braue A, Makelainen H, Varigos GA. A low-glycemic-load diet improves symptoms in acne vulgaris patients: a randomized controlled trial. Am J Clin Nutr 2007 Jul;86(1):107–15.

14 Smith RN, Braue A, Varigos GA, Mann NJ. The effect of a low glycemic load diet on acne vulgaris and the fatty acid composition of skin surface triglycerides. J Dermatol Sci 2008 Apr;50(1):41–52.

15 DiLandro A, Cazzaniga S, Parazzini F, Ingordo V, Cusano F, Atzori L, et al. Family history, body mass index, selected dietary factors, menstrual history, and risk of moderate to severe acne in adolescents and young adults. J Am Acad Dermatol 2012 Dec;67(6):1129–35.

16 Ismail NH, Manaf ZA, Azizan NZ. High glycemic load diet, milk and ice cream consumption are related to acne vulgaris in Malaysian young adults: a case control study. BMC Dermatol 2012;12:13–8.

17 Hoppe C, Molgaard C, Dalum C, Vaag A, Michaelsen KF. Differential effects of casein versus whey on fasting plasma levels of insulin, IGF-1 and IGF-1/IGFBP-3: results from a randomized 7-day supplementation study in prepubertal boys. Eur J Clin Nutr 2009 Sep;63(9):1076–83.

18 Jaworski S. The joy of baking: Lamingtons recipe [Internet]. 2010 [cited 2010 Oct 22]. Available from: http://www.joyofbaking.com/Lamingtons.html#ixzz125gkhBKv

19 Fisher JK. Acne vulgaris; a study of one thousand cases [Internet]. JK Fisher; 2006 [cited 2014 Aug 24]. Available from: http://www.acnemilk.com/fisher_s_original_paper

20 Melnik BC. Milk—the promoter of chronic Western diseases. Med Hypotheses 2009 Jun;72(6):631–9.

21 Melnik BC, Schmitz G. Role of insulin, insulin-like growth factor-1, hyperglycaemic food and milk consumption in the pathogenesis of acne vulgaris. Exp Dermatol 2009 Oct;18(10):833–41.

22 Melnik BC. Is nuclear deficiency of FoxO1 due to increased growth factor/PI3K/Akt-signalling in acne vulgaris reversed by isotretinoin treatment? Br J Dermatol 2010 Jun;162(6):1398–400.

23 Melnik BC. The role of transcription factor FoxO1 in the pathogenesis of acne vulgaris and the mode of isotretinoin action. G Ital Dermatol Venereol 2010 Oct;145(5): 559–71.

24 Reynolds RC, Lee S, Choi JY, Atkinson FS, Stockmann KS, Petocz P, *et al.* Effect of the glycemic index of carbohydrates on acne vulgaris. Nutrients 2010 Oct;2(10):1060–72.

25 Kwon HH, Yoon JY, Hong JS, Jung JY, Park MS, Suh DH. Clinical and histological effect of a low glycaemic load diet in treatment of acne vulgaris in Korean patients: a randomized, controlled trial. Acta Derm Venereol 2012 May;92(3):241–6.

26 Silverberg NB. Whey protein precipitating moderate to severe acne flares in 5 teenaged athletes. Cutis 2012 Aug;90(2):70–2.

27 Melnik BC. Diet in acne: further evidence for the role of nutrient signalling in acne pathogenesis. Acta Derm Venereol 2012 May;92(3):228–31.

28 Melnik BC, Zouboulis CC. Potential role of FoxO1 and mTORC1 in the pathogenesis of Western diet-induced acne. Exp Dermatol 2013 May;22(5):311–5.

29 Kligman A. Letter of welcome, Second International Conference on the Sebaceous Gland, Acne & Related Disorders. Rome; 2008.

CHAPTER 12
The handouts

It is the rare doctor who can teach all that is needed in the short time allotted. The patient who can remember all the details necessary to carry out the instructions is even rarer. Handouts are essential in managing all skin disorders. Proper handouts, kept relevant and up-to-date, reflect the standard of care provided in physicians' offices.

These are ours. They are available at www.acnemilk.com and are updated as new information becomes available.

Acne: Causes and Practical Management, First Edition. F. William Danby.
© 2015 John Wiley & Sons, Ltd. Published 2015 by John Wiley & Sons, Ltd.

12.1 Acne

Acne is caused by a blockage of the duct leading to the skin surface from the oil glands. This blockage occurs because of sex hormones (mainly the male ones—chemicals called *androgens*). These hormones are present in both men and women. They regulate the activity of the oil glands and the lining cells of the ducts in the pores on the face and upper back and chest. They are particularly good at turning on and plugging up these ducts in persons with a family tendency to develop acne.

The duct clogs with too many lining cells, and this results in a plug of material that is either open to the surface as a blackhead (called a *comedo*) or closed and visible under the surface (called a *whitehead*). Within this blocked material are trapped hairs and skin cells and bacteria and yeast. The bacteria and yeast increase in number, the wall leaks, and eventually the body's reaction to these materials is a pustule (pimple). If the whole pore shatters, there is an explosion of pore wall material, bacteria, yeasts, white blood cells, and other foreign material under the skin, and a deep red acne papule is created. A blackhead takes three to four months to be formed from the initial plugging of a pore; pustules or papules take about 6 months.

Because acne is due to sex hormones and growth hormones as well, it onsets at puberty, in girls from 9 to 11 years and boys from 11 to 13. Eighty percent of teens "grow out" of acne by 18–22 years. About 10% of women and 3% of men go on to have adult acne. Acne occurring to a marked degree in women over 22 or 24 years of age is often due to a persisting minor hormone imbalance, ovarian or adrenal, and it is sometimes necessary to investigate the hormone system. Most acne settles in the late teens or early 20s as these hormones stabilize, but long-term stress is also a factor and other hormonal influences can make acne worse. Nicotine is a contributor. Birth control pills (BCPs) with a tendency to a male hormone–type balance (such as Ovral and Lo-Ovral) should be switched to a BCP that helps block male hormones. Ocella/Yasmin is the best for this; Gianvi/Yaz is good for smaller women; and there are some other alternatives.

Oil-based cosmetics can make acne worse.

Dairy products (containing numerous hormones from the pregnant cows that produce the milk) play a role.

Milk, cream, butter, cottage cheese, cheese, pizza, yogurt, ice cream, protein powder shakes, and milkshakes are all best totally avoided. Skim milk is even worse than 2% or whole milk. Recent work strongly suggests that a low-glycemic-load diet (low sugar, and low levels of simple carbohydrates) will also help clear acne faster.

It is really important that harmful habits are discontinued—these are little habits such as absent-mindedly picking, touching, rubbing, or pinching your face. These trigger flares of preexisting acne. Pressure causes the contents of the pores to leak into the tissue surrounding the pore, and this starts the hot inflammatory lesions known as cysts or "blind pimples." Picking worsens acne and leaves scars—often the scar from the picking is worse than that produced by the acne itself.

Therapy is aimed at five things:

1 *Opening and emptying plugged pores.* Special applications such as Differin®, Retin-A®, or Tazorac® are used to do this. Blackhead removal by the doctor may be necessary. Oral isotretinoin (originally Accutane® or Roaccutane®) does this job best.

2 *Preventing new plugged pores.* This is most important but takes the longest time. Sometimes years of care using Differin®, Retin-A®, or Tazorac® are required.

3 *Killing bacteria and yeast that cause pus formation, and calming inflammation.* Benzoyl peroxide wash or cream or lotion, and antibiotic pills (doxycycline or minocycline) or lotions (erythromycin or clindamycin). Low dose oral ketoconazole is excellent for clearing the yeast.

4 *Reducing acne production and sebaceous gland activity in women using hormone-blocking medications.* Birth control pills (BCPs), preferably Yasmin®/Ocella®/Zarah®/Syeda® or Yaz®/Gianvi®, are best, and spironolactone (Aldactone®) may also be used.

5 *Shutting down oil and sebaceous gland production, and emptying plugged pores in severe, scarring, or resistant acne using oral isotretinoin* (one of the generics—Amnesteem®, Sotret® or Claravis®).

PLEASE NOTE: Picking or squeezing is generally forbidden. "Acne surgery" is best done by your dermatologist unless you have had special instructions.

THIS TREATMENT TAKES <u>TIME</u>. IT IS <u>NOT</u> A FAST CURE. It takes three to four months to slow oil gland production.

You will need to work at this daily for <u>months to clear</u> and <u>years to stay clear</u>.

The things that cause acne do not disappear quickly and so the treatment is prolonged.

With good advice, good medicines, and your regular care, you should do well.

TREATMENT

Wash with Dove® Beauty Bar for Sensitive Skin (Fragrance Free), Cetaphil® Cleanser for Normal and Oily Skin, Ivory®, Oil of Olay®, or Neutrogena®. Just use soapy hands. Then rinse, repeat, and rinse again until "squeaky clean." Be thorough, but **do not scrub**. Avoid face cloths. Be sure to rinse well, especially around the ears and hairline. Twice or three times a day is usual.

Alcohol swabs may be used after exercise to remove oil and sweat, but a soap-and-water shower would be better.

Creams, gels, lotions, and washes—You will be using one or more of the following:

1 *Retinoids*: Differin® or Retin-A® or Tazorac® (cream, gel, or solution) for blackheads. Start using every second night and slowly increase to nightly or even twice-daily use. If you are too irritated, skip an application or two. These materials work by bringing the plugs in the pores up to the surface. This should make your acne appear worse for a while but, once the "garbage" has been put out, things gradually settle down. Apply with fingers only, not cotton balls. Rinse fingers well after use. Apply to the entire involved area, not just to pimples, because long-term use of these retinoids, after isotretinoin for example, is needed to prevent further plugging.

Tazorac® must never be used in women who may become pregnant.

2 Benzoyl peroxide (BP) cream, lotion, gel, or wash (for pimples): start using PanOxyl® 10 Wash or Clearasil® or another 2%, 4%, 5%, or 10% lotion (cheap and over the counter [OTC]) to wash every second evening for about two minutes and, if there is no irritation, increase slowly to every evening and then to twice a day if necessary. Use it in the shower and rinse well to avoid bleaching bath mats and towels, or you can use a BP cream or gel or lotion in the same area, after the bath or shower, and leave it on. It will bleach sheets and pillowcases. If you are too irritated, skip an application or two, or reduce the strength or the time of the exposure. Apply to the entire involved area. Stinging on application is normal for many of these products. They work by drying up the pimples, killing germs, peeling off dead skin, and reducing oil production.

One of the Proactiv® products is a mild 2% benzoyl peroxide version, but Acne Free® is even cheaper.

PersaGel 10® and ZapZyt are other OTC BP products. Both are cheap and effective for overnight application to "hotspot" pimples. The expensive prescription varieties seem to be no better.

Warning
All benzoyl peroxide products bleach clothes and hair and towels and bedclothes.

Benzamycin®, BenzaClin®, EpiDuo®, Duac®, and Plexion® lotion: Apply every day, morning or night, or both. These help kill the acne bacteria. Most do not kill the *Malassezia* yeast.

If you are using two or more products, you may choose which is for morning, for evening, and for night.

Some degree of irritation is expected.

If you are uncomfortable, slow the therapy a bit—but DO NOT STOP.

If you are worried, call the office.

Pills and capsules (antibiotics): Doxycycline is used most often and, like minocycline (Minocin), it **can** (and **should**) be taken with food. Tetracycline very expensive and cannot be mixed with food, milk, or antacids—they neutralize it, so take pills one hour before or two hours after eating, with water (one full glass) only.

For easily upset stomachs, Doryx® (and its generic) is best but it is expensive.

Side effects are rare with all of these, but diarrhea longer than three days or a vaginal discharge or itch may be due to yeast and must be reported. Phone the office. Malassezia is worse with all antibiotics.

Sunburn may occur with less sun exposure than usual, especially with doxycycline, so be careful (skiers and vacationers take note). If doxycycline is taken with the evening meal, this risk is reduced almost to zero, but be sure to take it at midmeal with a large glass of water.

Pregnancy means "stop the pills". Completely. No questions. Do not take any 'cycline with isotretinoin (Accutane® or generic).

If another doctor orders penicillin for you, stop the 'cycline.

Ketoconazole: 200 mg tablets–two tabs are taken in a single dose weekly for *Malassezia* yeast infection.

Sunlight: If you are using any 'cycline and/or retinoids (see above), the treated areas may be more easily sunburned than before. It is very important to use a sunscreen when taking either tetracycline or doxycycline—minocycline is less photosensitizing but has other side effects.

The best chemical sunscreens are Anthélios L 60® or Vichy® Capital Soleil. The best nonchemical full-spectrum sun blocks are Vanicream® 35 and 50+ or the CoTZ group.

Never "bake" in the sun. High skin temperatures make acne worse. Stay cool.

Cosmetics and moisturizers: Lipstick, eye shadow, mascara, and powder blush are permitted. Safe cosmetics include any Almay® product and any product that bears the word "non-comedogenic." You can apply your moisturizer and/or makeup and/or sunscreen on top of Differin® or Tazorac®. Use Almay®, Vanicream®, Cetaphil®, or any "non-comedogenic" product.

Medicines: Report all medications to your doctor, even aspirin and vitamins and supplements and health foods and naturopathic therapies.

More information:

http://www.acnehelp.org.uk (for Dr. Danby's papers)

http://www.acnemilk.com (for animation, historical information and nondairy dietary instructions)

http://www.glycemicindex.com (for dietary advice)

http://www.thepaleodiet.com

12.2 The "zero-dairy" diet

Why avoid milk products?

Milk and milk products cause acne because milk contains hormones that "turn on" oil glands. The cows that give the milk are pregnant and milking most of their lives. These hormones are not injected into the cows—they are natural hormones that cows make during every "menstrual" cycle—but during pregnancy these hormones are produced at high levels and so are found in all cow milk, pregnant and nonpregnant.

What about hormone-free milk?

There is no such thing as "hormone-free" milk. The confusion was caused by a company in the United States that sold a hormone (BST or rBGH) for injection into cows to make them produce more milk. Some milk producers (both organic and not) have made the point that they do not use this injection, by advertising that the milk is "hormone-free." It obviously does not contain the injected hormone, but all the natural cow hormones are still in the milk. We do not know yet what the injected hormones do to the levels of natural cow hormones in milk.

Is lactose-free milk or "organic" milk ok?

No. Lactose intolerance has nothing to do with acne, and "organic" simply means that the pesticides and insecticides the cows are allowed to be exposed to in their food are less toxic than usual. The "organic" cows are healthier and have higher levels of natural hormones, and so they are likely *worse* for acne.

What are the options?

There are two ways to handle dairy restriction:

The first (and simplest) way is to just stop consuming all milk, cream, cheese, ice cream, butter, sour cream, cream cheese, cottage cheese, cheeseburgers, pizza, yogurt, and protein powders or bars or shakes containing casein or whey—anything that contains a significant amount of milk or milk solids. It is best to avoid "anything that comes from the south end of the cow."

Goat milk and goat cheese are not alternatives, because they are not hormone-free, either.

The second way is to find dairy-like substitutes for whatever you are missing. Soy-based products are the most convenient and include substitutes for milk, creamer, chocolate milk, yogurt, ice cream, cheeses of various types, and even butter. Almond, coconut, rice, pea, mixed vegetable protein, and hemp products also can be useful.

You don't **need** to eat soy or other substitutes, just stay away from cow dairy.

How do the cow hormones make Acne?

Oil gland pores are plugged by the overproduction of the cells that line the pore—basically a "traffic jam" happens in the pore. This overproduction is caused by hormones, and there are three sources. The first is ovaries or testicles, the second is from stress, and the third is dairy products. These three "stack up" on each other, and when the amount of hormone present is enough to plug up the pore, acne is started.

Some lucky people just do not have the gene for acne, but just about everybody has a different level of hormone where this happens (this is the *acne threshold*). Many young women pass this threshold just before their period every month, others stay above the threshold for years because of milk and milk products, and others cross the threshold with stress (first-year college is the most common stressor in late teens). By removing dairy from your diet, you will usually be able to get down below your personal threshold, making your acne much less with time. This threshold is also influenced by your family history, so if one or both of your parents had acne, your threshold will be lower, making acne risk higher.

How long do I need to do this?

The "zero-milk" diet has three phases.

First is the **total restriction** phase. That means NO DAIRY AT ALL. That is what "zero" means. It is essential to minimize the production of new plugs in the pores, and this lasts at least six months. With proper therapy, you are expected to clear during this time.

Second is the **maintenance** phase, and it lasts through all the teen years into the early 20s. During this phase, **zero** dairy intake is best, but some patients can have a little bit.

Third is the **cautious reintroduction** phase, usually possible in the early 20s. But, depending on individual thresholds, some acne patients can never return to dairy.

What else can I do for my hormones?

For males, there is no generally accepted anti-hormone therapy.

Unfortunately, there is almost nothing to be done about stress hormones in males or females.

Young women have the option of controlling their ovarian hormones with BCPs. We prefer to call these *hormone control* or *acne control pills*, but they are all the same as BCPs, really, and are given for medical reasons. The products we prefer are not only the least "male" of all "birth control" pills, but the best, *drospirenone*, also blocks the acne-making hormones coming from other sources (like the stress glands). Most young women with previous acne have almost no acne after six to 12 months on this "pill," especially if they stop all dairy.

What about my calcium intake?

Remember first of all that there are hundreds of thousands of growing teens in this country, and millions in the world, who are either genetically lactose intolerant or allergic to milk. They do not drink milk but grow up just fine. It also helps to realize that cows have big strong bones and healthy teeth, produce milk during most of their lives, and also produce a calf every year—with its own bones—yet they drink no milk and take no calcium supplements in nature (although when they are being "factory milked," they get supplements). It is also a fact that it is very difficult to design a low-calcium diet for those few medical conditions that require it.

It is far more important for maintenance of bone health to make sure you have regular bone-stressing exercise, a healthy diet containing adequate sources of calcium, a normal amount of estrogen in your body if you are female, and an adequate intake of vitamin D. **We recommend Vitamin D3 only, 2000 IU daily, taken with food, as both safe and wise. We consider 2000 IU daily a minimum. Others consider it maximum.**

What else does dairy hormone do?

There are studies that suggest that consuming dairy products may be associated with breast cancer, ovarian cancer, and prostate cancer. Further studies are necessary, but if you have a family history of any of these kinds of cancer, you should consider avoiding dairy intake. Dairy also reduces women's fertility, favors the conception of twins, is associated with greater weight gain during pregnancy, leads to larger unborn babies, and increases the risk of difficult deliveries and Caesarian sections.

Enjoy your new face! ☺

Take a look at:

http://www.acnehelp.org.uk/dairy.htm#Dairy2 http://dermatology.cdlib.org/124/original/acne/danby.html
http://www.acnemilk.com
http://www.godairyfree.org
http://www.thepaleodiet.com
http://www.glycemicindex.com

12.3 The risks and benefits of isotretinoin

Introduction and History

With Thanks to Dr. James Baumgaertner

Isotretinoin (originally marketed as Accutane®) is a powerful oral acne medication that has been on the market in the United States since 1982. It is a synthetic retinoid and it is closely related to vitamin A. Isotretinoin is a natural part of the metabolic cycle of vitamin A in our bodies—we all have a low level of isotretinoin in our blood, but obviously not enough to keep acne away. Isotretinoin is dramatically effective for all types of acne, including severe scarring cystic acne and even (in very low doses) hidradenitis suppurativa. There is simply no better treatment for resistant acne.

Drs Danby and Margesson have both been practicing dermatology for over 38 years, and isotretinoin is the only medicine that we would categorize as a real miracle drug. Before isotretinoin became available in 1982, dermatologists had no consistently effective treatment for the most severe forms of acne. Despite the use of dangerous cortisone pills, sulfa medicines, chemical peels, ultraviolet light, X-ray therapy, surgery, and high doses of various antibiotics, severe acne would frequently continue unabated. Patients suffered for years with painful nodules that would scar their faces and severely damage their fragile psyches.

Isotretinoin changed all that. Over the last 32 years, millions of people all over the world (and 700,000 per year in the United States) have successfully and safely used isotretinoin to clear their resistant acne. Perhaps more importantly, isotretinoin has converted thousands of reclusive, depressed young adults with ravaged faces into clear-faced, smiling, outgoing, and self-confident individuals. Isotretinoin is not just a face saver; it is also a real lifesaver.

Side effect concerns

Although isotretinoin is a truly miraculous drug, it does have some well-known and potentially serious side effects. Virtually all medications, including Aspirin, penicillin, Tylenol, and even vitamin pills, have potential side effects. For comparison, there are 70,000 emergency room admissions (and 100 deaths) each year in the United States from Tylenol.

Isotretinoin has come under increased scrutiny over the past few years by the public, the media, and the US Food and Drug Administration (FDA) because of charges that it may have induced serious depression in some patients. Tragically, a number of patients (about 40), while on courses of isotretinoin, committed suicide. Of course, many individuals over the last two decades who were not on isotretinoin also became depressed and some of these (about 100,000 between the ages of 18 and 24) even committed suicide. What was scientifically unclear until June 2005 is whether or not there might be a real increased risk of depression and mental status changes in people on isotretinoin compared to similar people not on isotretinoin. In a study published in the *Archives of Dermatology*, the authors concluded, "The use of isotretinoin in the treatment of moderate-severe acne in adolescents did not increase symptoms of depression. On the contrary, treatment of acne either with conservative therapy or with isotretinoin was associated with a decrease in depressive symptoms." This has been our personal experience and that of thousands of other dermatologists.

In a previous study published in the *Archives of Dermatology* (Jick SS, *et al.* Accutane use and risk of depression, psychotic symptoms, suicide, and attempted suicide. Arch Dermatol 2000 Oct;136:1231–6), 7535 acne patients treated with isotretinoin were compared to 14,376 acne patients treated with oral antibiotics. "There was no evidence that use of isotretinoin is associated with an increased risk for newly diagnosed depression, other psychiatric disorders, or suicidal behaviour."

Nevertheless, despite this large study, we personally think it is still possible that isotretinoin could be a factor in the development of depression in a very small subset of patients. There are certainly documented cases of patients who have developed depression while on a 20-week course of isotretinoin. Some of these patients noted improvement in their depression when the isotretinoin was stopped, and some later noted worsening of their depression when isotretinoin was reintroduced. This certainly suggests to us a possible cause-and-effect relationship in this small subset of isotretinoin-treated patients. This is called an *idiosyncratic response*. It is unpredictable and is very rare. There are also reports of depression developing three or more months after coming off of isotretinoin. We know that isotretinoin is completely out of the body approximately two weeks after stopping the drug, and so these reports suggest to us a coincidental relationship rather than a cause-and-effect relationship. We fear that individuals who happen to develop depression many months or even years after taking isotretinoin may now try to blame isotretinoin for their condition.

Does isotretinoin cause depression? It is unlikely; however, what is certain is that depression can and does occur in some young people and it can, unfortunately, lead to some very serious, and sometimes fatal, consequences. Therefore, it is vitally important that all persons, and particularly those who are prescribed isotretinoin, should be carefully observed by family, physicians and friends for signs or symptoms of altered mental status, particularly depression. If such changes are noted, isotretinoin should be stopped immediately and appropriate therapy should be initiated at the earliest opportunity.

Isotretinoin medication guide: "Be Smart" booklets and the iPLEDGE rules

Because of the FDA's increasing concern over these potential psychiatric side effects, an isotretinoin "Medication Guide" was produced and distributed by the manufacturer in January 2001. The FDA and the original drug manufacturer (Roche Laboratories) directed that all patients who were to receive isotretinoin must be given this guide. The FDA also mandated that pharmacists provide this information sheet every time an isotretinoin prescription was filled or refilled. Subsequently, this was replaced when the iPLEDGE program was introduced. The FDA, the drug manufacturers, and all dermatologists want to be sure that every patient who is placed on isotretinoin understands all of the drug's potential side effects.

Our concerns

We have read the new isotretinoin iPLEDGE material issued by the manufacturers and we feel it covers the main risks quite thoroughly. We are, however, concerned that it is written in a slanted way that raises excessive fears about other risks that are either extremely rare or simply not related to isotretinoin. We are also worried that patients, or their families, who read the iPLEDGE material may conclude that isotretinoin is a terribly dangerous drug. This is simply not the case. Because of these unrealistic fears, parents may refuse to allow the drug to be used for their children when it is really needed. We fear that some of our younger patients will be forced to endure years of painful acne with resultant facial and psychological scarring because of unwarranted fears over potential and rare isotretinoin side effects. In essence, we have seen FDA-induced fear lead to denial of a very valuable drug.

Our perspective

Having personally prescribed isotretinoin over 7000 times since 1982, we can assure you that isotretinoin is actually a very safe medication when properly used. Proper use means that the physician prescribes it correctly and the patient follows all of the directions and keeps all of the appointments. In our practice, if we feel the risk of isotretinoin in an individual patient exceeds the potential benefit, we will not prescribe it. If a simpler, safer, and/or less expensive medication will control the acne, we will use that therapy and not prescribe isotretinoin. If a patient is unable or unwilling to follow the isotretinoin directions and keep the necessary appointments, we will not prescribe it, or we will refuse to continue therapy. For most patients who have treatment-resistant acne, and who understand the risks and who agree to follow the rules, we will be very happy to prescribe this excellent medication.

For your information, we would like you to know that we have prescribed isotretinoin for one of our own daughters. You should also know that we have no financial interest in prescribing isotretinoin; as a matter of fact, we would make more money with much less liability risk if we simply kept prescribing less effective acne treatments for years on end rather than clearing (and usually curing) the stubborn acne with a single 16—20-week course of isotretinoin. Our goal as dermatologists is to clear, and if possible to cure, skin diseases as quickly, safely, and efficiently as possible. We do not want you to be denied the use of an excellent medication because of unrealistic and exaggerated fears.

Just one other thing—isotretinoin will almost certainly clear your acne, but you still need to do all the other hormone management discussed at your visits to prevent recurrences, including birth control pills, the "zero-dairy" or "Paleolithic" diet, avoidance of stress if possible, and spironolactone and Differin® if ordered.

So what are the real risks of isotretinoin?

Isotretinoin is a powerful medicine and it does have side effects. It would be nice if we had medicines that were highly effective, inexpensive, and without any side effects for all of our diseases. Unfortunately, that just isn't the case. Isotretinoin is highly effective, is moderately expensive, and has some potentially severe side effects. So what are the real side effect risks?

Pregnancy and teratogenesis

For fertile female patients, the most serious and the most feared side effect has to do with isotretinoin's teratogenic potential. That means simply that isotretinoin can definitely cause serious birth defects. The birth defects usually develop in the first few weeks after conception. This can occur before the woman even recognizes that she is pregnant. Therefore, every fertile woman anticipating isotretinoin usage must take measures to absolutely ensure that she will not be pregnant for one month prior to the start of isotretinoin therapy; and that she will not conceive while on the treatment or for one month after the treatment. At least two forms of contraception must be used simultaneously. Isotretinoin is out of the body just a few weeks after stopping the medication, and so it will not affect future pregnancies.

For all fertile female patients, there will be mandatory discussions about pregnancy, contraception, and the need for periodic pregnancy testing. Please do not be embarrassed. Even with seemingly effective contraception, pregnancies can rarely happen. Therefore, any sexually active female must decide in advance what she would do in the event that she did become pregnant while on isotretinoin. A deformed and/or handicapped baby is a tragedy that must be avoided. Such an event can ruin lives and severely disrupt families. More complete discussion of isotretinoin's potential for birth defects will be provided in the handouts. Absolute abstinence is an acceptable form of contraception … but it must be absolute. Sudden love affairs are a constant risk, and the risk of nonconsensual (forced) sex is always present.

Mental status changes and depression

Another potentially serious side effect has to do with mental status changes and, in particular, depression. In well over 30 years of prescribing isotretinoin, we can recall only one patient who developed serious depression while on isotretinoin. This may have been due to the birth control pill (an early high-estrogen type) in her case, or it may have been coincidental because acne and depression are both quite common in the teenage years. In our experience, and the experience of our colleagues, the development of serious depression while on isotretinoin is certainly a very rare event. We have, however, treated many patients (perhaps 100 or more) who were depressed prior to starting isotretinoin. Some were under psychiatric care and on antidepressants. We do not recall any aggravation of the symptoms of depression in any of these closely watched patients while on isotretinoin. We do recall that many of these patients had a dramatic clearing of their depression as their acne cleared. We believe most dermatologists would agree that isotretinoin is much more likely to improve depression than to induce depression in our patient population. Nevertheless, it is vitally important that patients and their friends or family inform their physician of any changes in mood, activities, appetite, concentration, sleep habits, or suicidal thoughts, as these could be signs of depression. This is good advice at any time, not just for patients on isotretinoin.

Lipid abnormalities

Isotretinoin and other vitamin A analogs (related synthetic retinoids) can occasionally induce elevations of circulating levels of certain fats, including triglycerides and, less commonly, cholesterol. This is rarely a problem in young people, but it is not uncommon in older patients. For this reason, the lipid levels may need to be monitored to ensure that there are not any significant elevations. If the lipid levels become markedly elevated, there is a remote chance that a serious inflammation of the pancreas (acute pancreatitis) could occur that would induce abdominal pain. We are aware of one fatal case of pancreatitis that occurred in a teenage male in another state and there is a known association of pancreatitis with alcohol, so alcohol is best avoided. In our own practice, we have had a few patients experience moderate elevations of their triglyceride levels. Rarely, some of these patients required lipid-lowering drugs (*statins*) while on the isotretinoin. A far healthier approach is to shift to a zero-dairy, low-glycemic-index, and low-carbohydrate diet, which usually solves the problem. One of our patients (not on isotretinoin) brought her triglyceride level from over 4100 to 297 by simply going on the Paleolithic diet for 2 weeks.

Pseudotumor cerebri

A swelling of the brain called *pseudotumor cerebri* has been rarely reported with isotretinoin. High-dose (hundreds of thousands of units) vitamin A ingestion and the use of other drugs, including tetracycline, can also rarely cause this problem. If this occurs, patients first experience headache symptoms and if the headaches persist and become severe, patients can also develop blurred vision, nausea, and vomiting. This is a very rare side effect but it can occur. Therefore, patients are cautioned to contact their physician if a headache develops and particularly if it is persistent and severe. We do not recall ever having any cases of isotretinoin-induced pseudotumor cerebri in our practice, and it is very unlikely to occur with the low doses we now use.

Visual problems

Altered night vision has been reported with isotretinoin. It may be related to inadequate body stores of natural vitamin A. We do recommend that our patients eat plenty of colorful vegetables and take a multivitamin. The manufacturers of isotretinoin warn not to take extra vitamin A pills, but there is no scientific evidence to back up their concern and we do not find any problems with the small amount of vitamin A present in a multivitamin. We feel it is protective and often recommend "filling up" vitamin A receptors by taking 10,000–12,000 IU of vitamin A daily for 7–10 days before starting isotretinoin. If visual problems do develop, the isotretinoin should be stopped. Isotretinoin can also cause slight drying of the eyes by interfering with the lipid (oily) part of the tear film, and this may make it more difficult to wear contact lenses. Usually this is not a problem with wearers of soft contact lenses.

Dry lips and other skin problems

Dry skin and chapped lips will occur in virtually every patient on isotretinoin. The lips require regular hydration with water followed by lubrication with petrolatum or lip balms. If the lips become too dry, the isotretinoin can be stopped for a week to allow the lips to recover. The lining of the nose may also get dry, and this may lead to minor nosebleeds. Hydration with plain water and a thin film of petrolatum up the nose will minimize these common problems. Occasionally there can be some increased hair shedding while on isotretinoin. We have also noted occasional patients whose hair becomes curlier while on isotretinoin. Nails may become thinner, and ingrown toenails may be more likely to develop. All these changes generally reverse when isotretinoin is decreased or discontinued. We have seen one case of hives attributed to the preservative or dye in the original version of isotretinoin capsule; that is very rare. Occasionally, isotretinoin can make nodular acne lesions a bit more inflamed during the first few weeks of therapy. The dose is then reduced. Isotretinoin can also make the skin more sensitive to trauma. Because of this increased fragility, patients should not undergo electrolysis removal of hair, waxing of hair, or chemical peeling while on isotretinoin and must avoid dermabrasion or laser facial treatments for a year after coming off the isotretinoin.

Musculoskeletal problems

With higher doses of isotretinoin, there may be a potential for muscle inflammation. This is probably on the basis of dehydration. This may be particularly common if the patient is on high doses of isotretinoin and engaged in vigorous sports, such as long-distance running. Proper hydration, electrolyte replacement, and isotretinoin dose adjustment should minimize the likelihood of this developing. Consider avoiding strenuous and hard contact sports during isotretinoin therapy. Abnormalities of bone have not been a significant problem with isotretinoin in acne.

Miscellaneous side effects

We are not aware of any problems with hearing or the induction of deafness. It must be extremely rare if it occurs at all. Inflammation of the liver is also extremely rare with isotretinoin, although it occasionally did occur with another related synthetic retinoid no longer available. Too much alcohol can inflame the liver and raise triglyceride and enzyme levels, and so it is a good idea to decrease or eliminate alcohol use while on isotretinoin, especially just before blood tests.

Summary

This discussion is an attempt to put into proper perspective the real risks and the real benefits of isotretinoin. Isotretinoin is actually a very safe drug, but it does have some potentially severe side effects that must be watched for. Therefore, it is imperative that the patient and the family understand the potential side effects and keep in close contact with the prescribing physician. Please remember that dermatologists have the knowledge and the experience to use this effective medication, and they would not prescribe it if it were felt that the risks outweigh the benefits. Trust your dermatologist, follow his or her instructions, keep educated, and never hesitate to ask questions.

12.4 The Paleo diet

With Thanks to Dr. Ben Balzer, Family Physician
There are thousands of people who are all slim, stronger, and faster than us. They all have straight teeth and perfect eyesight. Arthritis, acne, diabetes, hypertension, heart disease, stroke, depression, schizophrenia, and cancer are absolute rarities for them. These people are the last 84 tribes of hunter-gatherers in the world. They share a secret that is over 2 million years old—their diet—a diet that has changed little from that of the first humans 2 million years ago, and their predecessors up to 7 million years ago. Theirs is the diet that humans evolved on, the diet that is coded for in our genes. It has some major differences from the diet of the "civilized world."

Their diet is usually referred to as the *Paleolithic diet*, referring to the Paleolithic or Stone Age era. It is also referred to as the *Stone Age diet, caveman diet*, or *hunter-gatherer diet*. More romantic souls like to think of it as the diet that was eaten in the "Garden of Eden," and they are correct in thinking so.

The basic principles of the Paleolithic diet are simple. It consists of a fully integrated, comprehensive, and holistic dietary theory combining the best features of all other dietary theories, eliminating the worst features, and simplifying it all.

All major dietary components are covered—vitamins, fats, proteins, carbohydrates, antioxidants, phytosterols, and so on. It is the only diet that is coded for in our genes—it contains only those foods that were "on the table" during our long evolution, and ignores those that were not.

Basics of the paleolithic diet

For millions of years, humans and their relatives have eaten meat, fish, fowl, and the leaves, roots, and fruits of many plants. One big obstacle to getting more calories from the environment is the fact that many plants are inedible in their raw state.

Around 10,000 years ago, an enormous breakthrough occurred. It changed the course of history, and our diet, forever. This breakthrough was the discovery that cooking these foods made them edible—the heat released nutrients and made them more easily digested and absorbed. Grains like wheat, corn, barley, rice, sorghum, millet, and oats entered the diet. Grain use led to secondary products such as flour, bread, noodles, and pasta entering the menu of New Stone Age (Neolithic) humans, and Paleolithic diet experts refer to them as *Neolithic foods*.

The cooking of grains, beans, and potatoes had an enormous effect on our food intake:
- doubling the number of calories that we could obtain from the plant foods in our environment
- permitting storage for long periods
- enabling easy transport
- allowing ready farming of the species.

Despite these advantages, our stomachs and intestines and our sugar-handling system never really evolved and adapted to grains, beans, and potatoes, and so we are still not fully "in tune" with them.

Then followed the harnessing of dairy products, which allow humans to obtain far more calories from the animal over its lifetime than if it were simply slaughtered for meat. Dairy products are interesting as they combine a variety of components—some of which our genes were ready for and some not. While cow milk is ideal for calves, there are several very important differences between it and human milk. For example, the brain of a calf is only a tiny fraction of its body weight, whereas humans have very big brains. Not surprisingly, cow milk is low in critical nutrients for brain development, particularly omega-3 fats.

Since the Neolithic era, many other substances have entered the diet—particularly salt, sugar, and more recently a huge variety of chemicals including caffeine, then all sorts of other additives, colorings, preservatives, pesticides, anti-oxidants, and so on. We have not evolved at all to handle these.

Grains, beans, and potatoes (gbp)

These are all rich sources of carbohydrate, and once cooked this is often rapidly digestible—and basically that means they are easily and quickly broken down into simple sugars and then rapidly absorbed into the bloodstream. The word *hyperglycemia* is made of the ancient words for a common sugar (*glucose*) and the active part of blood (*heme*); fast absorption of sugar into the blood produces a high (*hyper*) sugar (*glyc*) level in the blood (*[h]emia*)—hyperglycemia. A food that produces a sugar spike like that has a *high glycemic index*. Eating a lot of that food produces a *high glycemic load*. They are poor sources of vitamins (particularly vitamins A, B-group, folic acid, and C), minerals, and antioxidants.

Essentials of the Paleolithic diet
Eat the following:

Meat, chicken, and fish, including organ meats (liver and kidneys) (if you can—some can't)

Eggs

Fruit

Vegetables, especially root vegetables including carrots, turnips, parsnips, rutabagas, and Swedes (Swedish turnips), but not including potatoes or sweet potatoes

Nuts, such as walnuts, Brazil nuts, macadamias, and almonds. Do not eat peanuts (a bean) or cashews (a family of their own).

Berries: strawberries, blueberries, raspberries, and so on.

Eat none of the following

Grains—including bread, pasta, and noodles

Beans—including string beans, kidney beans, lentils, peanuts, snow-peas, and peas

Potatoes

Dairy products

Sugar

It will take some time for your body to adjust to the changes after all these years.

There will be a huge surge in your vitamin intake and a huge decrease in your toxin intake.

Start with breakfast for few days. This is the easiest place to start as most people eat it at home, and it tends to be the least Paleolithic meal of the standard three daily meals. Then move on to lunch or dinner for a few days and then to all three meals. If you work or go to school, you will often find it easier to take your lunch. School menus are often high glycemic load—just what you are trying to avoid. For weight loss you will eventually need to reduce your overall carbohydrate intake.

But if you are doing this for acne or hidradenitis suppurativa, zero dairy is the most important part. That means all milk, cream, ice cream, cheese, yogurt, plus casein and whey-containing protein has to go.

See: www.thepaleodiet.org
www.godairyfree.org
www.glycemicindex.com
www.acnemilk.com

The table below is from Harvard's School of Nutrition. We recommend you **avoid GI over 55**.

Glycemic index and glycemic load for 100 foods.

FOOD	Glycemic index (glucose = 100)	Serving size (grams)	Glycemic load per serving
BAKERY PRODUCTS AND BREADS			
Wheat tortilla	30	50	8
Coarse barley bread, 75–80% kernels, average	34	30	7
Vanilla cake made from packet mix with vanilla frosting (Betty Crocker)	42	111	24
Apple, made with sugar	44	60	13
Sponge cake, plain	46	63	17
Apple, made without sugar	48	60	9
Banana cake, made with sugar	47	60	14
100% Whole Grain™ bread (Natural Ovens)	51	30	7
Corn tortilla	52	50	12
Banana cake, made without sugar	55	60	12
Pumpernickel bread	56	30	7
50% cracked wheat kernel bread	58	30	12
Hamburger bun	61	30	9
Pita bread, white	68	30	10
White wheat flour bread	71	30	10
Whole wheat bread, average	71	30	9
Bagel, white, frozen	72	70	25
Kaiser roll	73	30	12
Wonder™ bread, average	73	30	10
Waffles, Aunt Jemima (Quaker Oats)	76	35	10
Baguette, white, plain	95	30	15

(Continued)

(Continued)

FOOD	Glycemic index (glucose = 100)	Serving size (grams)	Glycemic load per serving
BEVERAGES			
Tomato juice, canned	38	250 mL	4
Apple juice, unsweetened, average	44	250 mL	30
Orange juice, unsweetened	50	250 mL	12
Coca Cola®, average	63	250 mL	16
Fanta®, orange soft drink	68	250 mL	23
Cranberry juice cocktail (Ocean Spray®)	68	250 mL	24
Gatorade	78	250 mL	12
Lucozade®, original (sparkling glucose drink)	95 +/− 10	250 mL	40
BREAKFAST CEREALS AND RELATED PRODUCTS			
Pearled barley, average	28	150	12
Whole wheat kernels, average	30	50	11
Converted, white rice (Uncle Ben's®)	38	150	14
Bulgur, average	48	150	12
Brown rice, average	50	150	16
Quinoa	53	150	13
All-Bran™, average	55	30	12
Oatmeal, average	55	250	13
Sweet corn on the cob, average	60	150	20
Raisin Bran™ (Kellogg's)	61	30	12
Couscous, average	65	150	9
Cream of Wheat™ (Nabisco)	66	250	17
Muesli, average	66	30	16
Quick cooking white basmati	67	150	28
Special K™ (Kellogg's)	69	30	14
Cream of Wheat™, Instant (Nabisco)	74	250	22
Grapenuts™, average	75	30	16
Coco Pops™, average	77	30	20
Puffed wheat, average	80	30	17
Instant oatmeal, average	83	250	30
White rice, average	89	150	43
Cornflakes™, average	93	30	23
GRAINS			
COOKIES AND CRACKERS			
Shortbread	64	25	10
Rye crisps, average	64	25	11
Graham crackers	74	25	14
Soda crackers	74	25	12
Vanilla wafers	77	25	14
Rice cakes, average	82	25	17
DAIRY PRODUCTS AND ALTERNATIVES			
Milk, skim	32	250 mL	4
Reduced-fat yogurt with fruit, average	33	200	11
Ice cream, premium	38	50	3
Milk, full fat	41	250 mL	5
Ice cream, regular	57	50	6

FOOD	Glycemic index (glucose = 100)	Serving size (grams)	Glycemic load per serving
FRUITS			
Grapefruit	25	120	3
Prunes, pitted	29	60	10
Pear, average	38	120	4
Apple, average	39	120	6
Orange, average	40	120	4
Peach, canned in light syrup	40	120	5
Dates, dried	42	60	18
Peach, average	42	120	5
Pear, canned in pear juice	43	120	5
Grapes, average	59	120	11
Banana, ripe	62	120	16
Raisins	64	60	28
Watermelon	72	120	4
BEANS AND NUTS			
Peanuts, average	7	50	0
Chickpeas, average	10	150	3
Soy beans, average	15	150	1
Cashews, salted	27	50	3
Kidney beans, average	29	150	7
Lentils, average	29	150	5
Black beans	30	150	7
Navy beans, average	31	150	9
Blackeye peas, average	33	150	10
Chickpeas, canned in brine	38	150	9
Baked beans, average	40	150	6
PASTA and NOODLES			
Fettucini, average	32	180	15
Spaghetti, wholemeal, boiled, average	42	180	17
Spaghetti, white, boiled, average	46	180	22
Macaroni, average	47	180	23
Spaghetti, white, boiled 20 min, average	58	180	26
Macaroni and Cheese (Kraft)	64	180	32
SNACK FOODS			
M & M's®, peanut	33	30	6
Corn chips, plain, salted, average	42	50	11
Potato chips, average	51	50	12
Snickers Bar®	51	60	18
Microwave popcorn, plain, average	55	20	6
Pretzels, oven-baked	83	30	16
Fruit Roll-Ups®	99	30	24
VEGETABLES			
Carrots, average	35	80	2
Green peas, average	51	80	4
Parsnips	52	80	4
Yam, average	54	150	20
Sweet potato, average	70	150	22

(Continued)

(Continued)

FOOD	Glycemic index (glucose = 100)	Serving size (grams)	Glycemic load per serving
Boiled white potato, average	82	150	21
Instant mashed potato, average	87	150	17
Baked russet potato, average	111	150	33
MISCELLANEOUS			
Hummus (chickpea salad dip)	6	30	0
Pizza, Super Supreme (Pizza Hut)	36	100	9
Chicken nuggets, frozen, reheated in microwave oven 5 min	46	100	7
Honey, average	61	25	12
Pizza, plain baked dough, served with parmesan cheese and tomato sauce	80	100	22

Source: Harvard Health Publications. Glycemic index and glycemic load for 100 foods [Internet]. Cambridge, MA: Harvard Medical School; n.d. Available from: http://www.health.harvard.edu/newsweek/Glycemic_index_and_glycemic_load_for_100_foods.htm
Note: The complete list of the glycemic index and glycemic load for more than 1000 foods can be found in the article "International tables of glycemic index and glycemic load values: 2008" by Fiona S. Atkinson, Kaye Foster-Powell, and Jennie C. Brand-Miller in the December 2008 issue of *Diabetes Care*, Vol. 31, number 12, p. 2281–3.

12.5 Acne inversa / Hidradenitis suppurativa (AI/HS)

Often mistaken for "boils" that keep coming back, hidradenitis suppurativa (HS) is a disease that starts with sore red lumps under the arms; under breasts; in the groin, buttock, and perianal areas; or under bra straps or beltlines. These spots appear suddenly, rapidly increase in size (with increasing pain), and then rupture, usually sideways under the surface of the skin, or they sometimes drain to the surface. Besides the painful cysts, blackheads and scars can form, and sinuses (tunnels under the skin) can drain smelly pus. It is more common in women than in men. This condition is also called *acne inversa* because it is caused by the same mechanism and hormones that cause common acne.

This is a chronic, recurrent skin disease. It affects the hair and oil gland follicles of the body, but especially the follicles that are in the hot, moist, sweaty, oil gland–bearing areas.

The basic problem is that people with HS have "weak pores" that rupture easily.

This is often hereditary, so ask other family members about similar problems or "boils."

What is the cause?

This condition develops due to blockage of the short tubular ducts that lead up to the skin pores. The pores are the tiny openings to the skin surface from the oil glands and hair follicles below. The same foods (dairy and high glycemic index—sugary—foods) that put on weight also plug the pores. When the duct wall (shaped like a short tube to the surface) makes too many "lining cells," they fill the tube with extra cells. A plug builds up in those blocked areas and starts expanding the duct. This causes it to leak its contents, and the oil duct and hair follicle eventually explode sideways underneath the skin. The body develops a strong irritant and allergic reaction to this foreign material under the skin, causing inflammation and irritation. The reaction is like the one you get from a buried splinter or ingrown hair. Large, red, hot, painful swellings develop. They eventually break down and drain pus, even though this is not an infection.

What are the factors that make this worse?

In addition to the family history, hormones cause this condition. It commonly starts around puberty. It often gets worse each month with the menstrual cycle. Stress can be a trigger. Friction in areas of involvement is often a problem. The walls of the pores or "follicles" in the sweaty areas of the body are "weak" and they rupture easily. Anything that rubs the areas (tight clothing, menstrual pads, etc.) can cause the plugged and swollen ducts to break down more easily. Try to avoid any friction or irritation. Squeezing these "boils" or "cysts" will always make things worse. Sweating can trigger a flare. No plucking, pinching, picking, or "needling"—they will stir the problem up further.

Is this an uncommon condition?

This is not rare. It affects up to 1 in 300 persons. Some say up to 1 in 25 if you include mild cases.

What does it look like?

First there are red, swollen bumps that develop into what look like "boils." These heal after weeks with pitted or pouting scars. The "boils" can be solitary, scattered in an area, or grouped together. Single and grouped blackheads may be seen. Some patients have 1–2 areas involved, while others will have many areas extensively involved. The grouped lesions may form a large swollen area that is connected by small tunnels under the skin, called *sinuses*. If you press on some areas of involvement, you can probably find pus coming out of openings nearby.

What does not cause hidradenitis suppurativa?

It is not due to infection or washing habits. It is **not** because one is overweight (millions of overweight people never get this), although it may make the condition worse because of increased friction or rubbing from clothes, especially bra straps and edges of underwear.

Antiperspirants have not been shown to cause it. Smoking does seem to make things worse and it likely is an actual cause in some patients, but half our patients never smoked.

How is it diagnosed?

The diagnosis is made by recognizing the typical skin changes in the typical locations. The pattern of recurrent "boils" in these particular areas, especially when they do not respond to standard antibiotics, is a good clue. There is no "test" for the disease.

Normal boils are caused by bacteria and respond quite well to antibiotics.

Normal boils usually do not come back in the same areas after treatment.

Normal boils come to a head and drain vertically to the surface, then heal with a scar and do not make horizontal tunnels under the skin.

Why is this problem overlooked or missed?

By its nature and location, this is a hidden disease. There is not much research money for this condition, so there is very little research being done. Most medical students get little to no education on this subject, so many doctors simply are not aware of the diagnosis. Patients often suffer in silence due to embarrassment or previous misdiagnosis and treatment difficulties. This is not an easy condition to manage, so failures with old types of treatment were frequent and patients (and some physicians too) often gave up.

How is hidradenitis suppurativa treated?

Treatment depends on severity and lesion type. Treatment may just involve medications that are used on the skin or taken orally. Long-term (but very low-dose) isotretinoin (formerly Accutane®) or acitretin (Soriatane®) can help prevent new plugging. Surgery of various kinds is useful in all stages.

To decide the best treatment for you it is helpful to know how severe your problem is, and this is done with a staging system using criteria set out by Dr. H.J. Hurley of Philadelphia.

Hurley's Stage I: there are some abscesses ("boils"), one or several, but they do not have the small tunnels under the skin (sinuses) and scarring is fairly minor.

Hurley's Stage II: there are recurrent abscesses ("boils") with small sinuses under the skin and scarring. There may be one or several of these complexes scattered in different areas, or small groups of them.

Hurley's Stage III: there are large areas involved with multiple interconnected tunnels (sinus tracts) and draining lesions with a lot of scarring.

General treatment

1 It is important to reduce any friction in the areas where you have recurrent spots. Change to loose cotton clothing such as loose boxer shorts (yes, ladies, too), and avoid underwear with seams that bind and rub in areas that give you new lesions. Wear clothing that is loose and cool so that you are not overheated and sweating in those areas. Take a change of underwear to work in a Ziploc® bag.

2 Avoid local injury to the area. Wash all clothing, towels, pajamas, sheets, and so on in a laundry detergent free of enzymes. Use ONLY "ALL®" Brand Free/Clear in the white jug, the only one easily found. Use no fabric softeners or dryer sheets.

3 Waxing? Don't even ask! Shaving is also pretty risky—but you may get away with it if you soften the hairs with a soak in water (tub or shower for 5 minutes), lubricate well and often with Dove® unscented cleansing bar lather, use a fresh blade each time, and shave only in the direction of hair growth.

4 Laser for bikini line hair removal? In experienced hands (very hard to find), this can reduce the size and coarseness of the hairs and has also been claimed to reduce the active HS itself. There are no controlled studies. If you wish to try this, get a small test area (about 10–20 hairs) done to see what happens. Do not allow the operator to pluck the hairs. Take pictures before and after.

5 Ingrown hairs? DO NOT PLUCK them out. The new hair may not be able to find its way to the surface, and then you will have a worse problem when it grows back under the skin. Use alcohol to clean the skin, then a sterile safety pin to nick the skin over the hair and "flick" it out onto the skin surface. Cut it short—¼ inch would be good—cover it with petroleum jelly, and leave it alone to heal. That way, a new follicle will grow and the hair can reach the surface.

6 Try hard to reduce obesity and get down to ideal weight. The best diet is the Paleolithic diet (www.thepaleodiet.com). It is a zero-dairy and low-glycemic-load diet. The most important part is TOTAL avoidance of ALL dairy products, and a slow steady loss to ideal weight. Yes, ALL dairy products, 100% More details below.

7 Metformin tablets improve HS. Start 500 mg/day and increase to tolerance.

8 There is reason to believe (but no proof yet) that vitamin C supplements may help strengthen the weak pores. Take 500 mg of vitamin C twice daily with your zinc supplement at mealtime, with your food. See below.

9 Antiseptic washes can be helpful. These do not cure anything but can help in areas of odor and drainage. Use a triclosan-containing cleanser like Dial® antiseptic daily. Otherwise use a mild soapless cleanser such as Dove® for Sensitive Skin—Fragrance Free or Cetaphil® Cleanser for Sensitive Skin.

10 Stopping all nicotine from any source is essential. Nicotine stimulates plugging of the pores. Also, toxins in smoke appear to interfere with proper healing, and smokers generally have low vitamin C levels. We have never successfully cleared a smoker of this disease. Don't try to be the first.

11 It is very important to block male hormones in both women and men.

   a This can be done using birth control pills (BCPs) such as Yasmin (or generics Ocella or Zarah) or Yaz (or its generic—Gianvi). They contain drospirenone, the best hormone blocker in BCPs. Depending on family history, a BCP containing norgestimate may be used instead, but it is a distant second for the control and blockade of male hormones.

   b We can add an extra hormone blocker called *spironolactone* to the drospirenone or the norgestimate BCP, or use spironolactone alone.

   c There are other male hormone blockers called *finasteride* and *dutasteride,* but they are less used than the BCP blockers. (Pregnancy must be strictly avoided with the use of such hormone blockers.)

   d Dutasteride has also made a big difference in some male patients.

12 To decrease inflammation, antibiotics are recommended. They can be given:

   a Topically—1% clindamycin lotion applied morning and night.

   b By mouth—antibiotics have traditionally been used for short periods of time or sometimes for weeks or months. Minocycline, doxycycline, clindamycin, amoxicillin/clavulanic acid, Bactrim, or combinations like clindamycin and rifampin are anti-inflammatory but are NOT capable of curing the disease because this disease is NOT due to infection.

13 To improve healing, and as an extra anti-inflammatory, add oral zinc to strengthen your innate immune system. Take one Solaray zinc 50 mg copper 2 mg amino acid chelate with breakfast and one with supper (order SLR284 from www.swansonvitamin.com).

14 For an odd painful spot, an injection of cortisone called *triamcinolone acetonide* (Kenalog®-10) right into the bump may be used. It usually quickly takes down the redness, swelling, and pain over 2–3 days. But if it comes back, go to 17 below.

15 Oral cortisone (prednisone or methylprednisolone) may be given for short periods or intermittently to temporarily cool inflammation. It may spread bacterial infection and can encourage yeast infections.

16 For Hurley Stage II—systemic anti-inflammatory antibiotics are used as in Stage I, for weeks or months. Clindamycin may be combined with rifampin. Intralesional triamcinolone may be used. Dapsone can be very useful.

17 Surgical treatment is important. Some early hotspots can be removed with simple punch biopsy drainage. If there are spots that keep coming back and breaking down, then you must assume that there is a proliferative (actively growing) mass trapped under the skin or that a cyst or a tunnel (referred to as a *sinus*) has formed. These are a tremendous source of inflammation, aggravation, odor, and pus. They will never heal spontaneously and must be surgically unroofed. This is done after gentle local anesthesia by cutting off the top the area with scissors, cleaning out all the problem material, then allowing it to heal in from below. No sutures are used. The unroofed area will heal in 2–3 weeks, usually eliminating pain within 2–4 days.

18 For the most severe Hurley Stage III, the treatment usually requires the help of a knowledgeable surgical team to remove the entire involved area. Usually this is in hospital and the patient is "put to sleep." Before surgery is carried out, the patient will need to be on anti-inflammatories, which may involve antibiotics or possibly systemic cortisone (prednisone) or other special medications, including the TNFα inhibitors and other "biologics." Remicade® is the best of the lot but must be given intravenously. Other "biologics" are being tried.

19 Ongoing work suggests that a strict zero-dairy diet will lead to or maintain clearing in many or most patients. The diet needs to be really well controlled. Nothing at all from cow or goat sources can be used. In addition to no milk, cream, cheese, butter, yoghurt, cream cheese, cottage cheese, ice cream, and derivatives like cheeseburgers and lasagna, this means checking protein powders and protein drinks to be sure there is no casein, whey, milk protein isolate, or milk solids. Egg, soy, hemp, pea, almond, and other vegetable and nut-sourced drinks and foods are acceptable, but should be the

unsweetened variety only. No French vanilla, and no sweetened chocolate.

20 Adding a low-glycemic-load diet as well as stopping dairy will help even more to stop the new lesions from forming. We encourage the use of metformin in all HS patients in the highest dose tolerated. See the special diet at www.thepaleodiet.org.

What will happen to me?

Some patients clear with early care and avoidance of all the precipitants the dairy and highly refined flour- and sugar-containing foods, male-type hormones, smoking, and the stresses that appear to trigger the problem. They can be kept in Stage I or actually cleared. Patients in Stage II can be brought back to Stage I with aggressive care, and some are cleared. And even some in Stage III can be brought back to Stage II and Stage I, and kept cool and quiet, but with scars left behind.

The diets and drugs (including metformin, zinc and copper, vitamin C, and hormone blockade) may need to be used for many years. Evidence points to heredity causing the weak follicular wall, and that is not something we can fix.

Clearance of Stage II and III lesions usually cannot be done with drugs and diet alone, but prevention of **new** lesions (for years) requires the dietary restriction here too.

Surgical treatment of the areas is often necessary but is usually nowhere near as difficult, nor as extensive, as most patients (and their physicians) imagine. The earlier this is done, the better. There are illustrated papers on unroofing and deroofing in the *Journal of the American Academy of Dermatology* (available at www.hs-foundation.com)

Remember that this takes time.

Your lesions take time to develop and time to disappear. You need to know that you have lots of little "time bombs"—nobody knows how many—under your skin. With the full routine outlined, you should develop no new ones, but it will take months.

Meanwhile, while stopping new ones, you need to use the time to get rid of the old ones by getting your doctor to unroof, punch biopsy, or excise active areas.

The only other way the nodules and pustules can be eliminated is to have them come to the surface on their own. This is messy, painful, disheartening, and depressing but the disorder will stop over weeks or months as the "time bombs" are all eliminated.

This disease can be cured, but it takes a lot of work, a cooperative and patient patient, and a knowledgeable, understanding doctor. Do it all, 100%—and keep doing it.

For more information:
www.hs-foundation.org
www.godairyfree
www.acnemilk.com
www.glycemicindex.com
www.thepaleodiet.com
www.uptodate.com

12.6 Yasmin/Ocella/Zarah or Yaz/Gianvi extended cycle for acne therapy

Acne is caused by hormones so, in treating acne, hormone control is essential. That means reducing the amount of "maleness" (acne and hair on the face are - sorry - "male" characteristics), so we need to do three things.

1 Use more female hormones.

2 Try to use **no** male-type hormones.

3 Block other male-type hormones (like the ones in milk).

We use Yasmin/Ocella/Zarah or Yaz/Gianvi when we can for this. They contain the usual type of female estrogen (ethinyl estradiol) and a unique progestin called *drospirenone*. Drospirenone's maleness rating is zero. It has the added advantage of being able to block some of the other male hormones, like the ones from your adrenal (stress) glands and from your ovaries, and those from your milk and other dairy food. ALL other progestins in other birth control preparations are male-like (androgenic) to various degrees. We tend to use Yaz/Gianvi in smaller women (less than $50\,kg = 110$ lbs.) because it has a lower female estrogen (ethinyl estradiol) content.

To increase the anti-acne effect of these drugs, it is possible to give them in an extended-cycle program, so instead of taking only 63 (3 times 21) active pills every three months, the extended cycle means taking it for 84 days in a row, then taking a seven-day break, giving a 91-day cycle. So then there are only four periods a year, one every 91 days.

For smaller women using the Yaz/Gianvi choice, we order 96 active pills (the "actives" from four packages of 24) taken daily, then seven days of the white blank placebo pills, so there is a period every 103 days.

The following is from *American Medical News*, July 10, 2006.

Note: We do NOT recommend the Lybrel, Loestrin, Seasonale or Seasonique products discussed below. They are useful for period control but may *worsen* acne.

New Birth Control Pills Give More Control over Menstruation

"Formulations allow women to have four periods a year or none at all, or shorten them to just a few days." By Victoria Stagg Elliott, AMNews staff. July 10, 2006.

A handful of new birth control pills either approved within the past couple of years or due soon to reach the marketplace is challenging the notion that women need to have a monthly cycle.

"There's nothing that says a woman has to have a period once a month or have it for six days," said LeRoy Sprang, MD, clinical professor of obstetrics and gynecology at Northwestern University Feinberg School of Medicine in Chicago.

The Food and Drug Administration is currently considering whether Lybrel, a hormonal birth control pill that would be taken every day without a breakthrough bleed, should be approved. Seasonale, which allows for only four periods a year, was approved in September 2003. Seasonique, with a second-generation version that replaces the placebo pills taken every three months with those that provide a low-dose estrogen, was approved in May. Yaz and Loestrin 24 FE were both approved earlier this year and provide 24 days of hormones rather than the traditional 21. The result is a shorter period than occurs with the standard formulations.

Not a New Function

Experts attribute the shift away from the pill's traditional 21/7 regimen -- long viewed as the gold standard -- on several converging factors. The pill has been around for decades, meaning that women are more likely to trust it to work without the need for the monthly reassurance that breakthrough bleeding provides.

"It was made to appear natural and be reassuring that you're not pregnant," said Leslie Miller, MD, associate professor of obstetrics and gynecology at the University of Washington in Seattle. "Forty-five years later, we don't need that."

Medications not just to cure disease but also to improve people's quality of life and, if possible, provide other benefits such as convenience, are an increasing focus.

"Women are more active and more involved in the world," said Nancy Church, MD, an ob-gyn at the Wellness Connection in Chicago. "There's no reason not to assist them."

Physicians also say the trend is an official acknowledgement that many women have been manipulating menstruation all along. Some have chosen to alter their pill doses to eliminate or shorten their period for convenience. Others were recommended by their physicians to take the pill continuously to deal with migraines or painful menstruation.

A 2003 survey by the Association of Reproductive Health Professionals found that nearly three-quarters of physicians who participated have prescribed menstrual suppression. Another 2003 poll, this one by the American College of Obstetricians and Gynecologists, found that about half their female members have used the pill to avoid their periods.

"It's not a totally new idea," Dr. Miller said. "Doctors' friends and families always knew that they could skip their periods."

But despite the fact that using the birth control pill to alter menstruation has been common on an off-label basis, many physicians welcome the new approved options because they might make women more at ease with altering their cycle.

"This makes it much more acceptable to the general community," Dr. Sprang said. "Women knew they could do it, but they were not always comfortable doing it."

Many physicians also say that the additional options lead to more interesting discussions with their patients.

"It does take a little bit more time, because there are more options to discuss, but it gives me a little bit more opportunity to find out about my patients as people," said Stephen A. Wilson, MD, MPH, assistant director of the family medicine residency program at the University of Pittsburgh Medical Center's St. Margaret Hospital.

"We have some different types of conversations that we may not have had otherwise."

Doctors note, though, that menstrual suppression is not for everyone. Even the most ardent supporters say that if a woman is doing well with her current birth control formulation, there's no need to bring up the newer options.

"I don't think that everyone should have no periods," Dr. Miller said. "If she's happy, I'm not going to waste my breath."

Physicians also say that some women still need to experience monthly reassurance that they are not pregnant. Others may view something abnormal in giving up their periods completely. They may prefer to stick with traditional regimens or switch to the versions of the pill that allow for shorter periods.

"Patients know no pill is 100%. Each person has that fear factor," said Tyrone Malloy, MD, an obstetrician-gynecologist in Decatur, Ga. He was one of the investigators for the trials of Loestrin 24 FE. "People also feel that it's natural to see something every month."

Index

Note: Page references in *italics* refer to Figures; those in **bold** refer to Tables

Acne: Causes and Practical Management, First Edition. F. William Danby.
© 2015 John Wiley & Sons, Ltd. Published 2015 by John Wiley & Sons, Ltd.